STUDY GUIDE FOR

Pharmacology and the Nursing Process

Sixth Edition

Linda Lane Lilley, PhD, RN
Shelly Rainforth Collins, PharmD
Scott Harrington, PharmD
Julie S. Snyder, MSN, RN-BC

Study Guide prepared by

Julie S. Snyder, MSN, RN-BC
Adjunct Faculty
School of Nursing
Old Dominion University
Norfolk, Virginia

Study Skills by

Diane Savoca
Coordinator of Student Transition
St. Louis Community College at Florissant Valley
St. Louis, Missouri

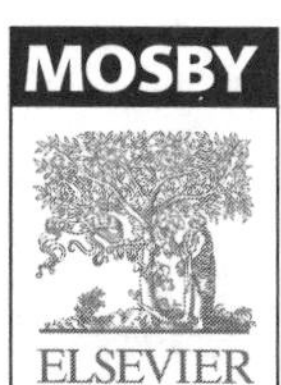

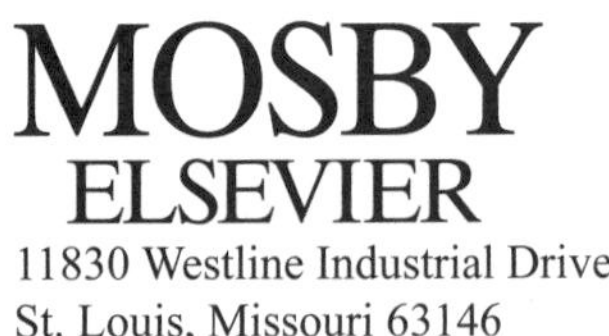

11830 Westline Industrial Drive
St. Louis, Missouri 63146

STUDY GUIDE FOR PHARMACOLOGY
AND THE NURSING PROCESS, SIXTH EDITION ISBN: 978-0-323-06660-0

International Standard Book Number 978-0-323-06660-0

Senior Editor: Lee Henderson
Associate Developmental Editor: Jacqueline Twomey
Publishing Services Manager: Jeffrey Patterson
Senior Project Manager: Clay Broeker
Publishing Services: Lisa Hernandez

Printed in the United States of America

Last digit is the print number: 9 8 7 6 5 4 3 2 1

Contents

	Student Study Tips	1
Chapter 1	The Nursing Process and Drug Therapy	21
Chapter 2	Pharmacologic Principles	23
Chapter 3	Life Span Considerations	25
Chapter 4	Cultural, Legal, and Ethical Considerations	27
Chapter 5	Gene Therapy and Pharmacogenetics	29
Chapter 6	Medication Errors: Preventing and Responding	31
Chapter 7	Patient Education and Drug Therapy	33
Chapter 8	Over-the-Counter Drugs and Herbal and Dietary Supplements	35
Chapter 9	Substance Abuse	39
Chapter 10	Photo Atlas of Drug Administration	41
Chapter 11	Analgesic Drugs	45
Chapter 12	General and Local Anesthetics	49
Chapter 13	Central Nervous System Depressants and Muscle Relaxants	53
Chapter 14	Central Nervous System Stimulants and Related Drugs	55
Chapter 15	Antiepileptic Drugs	57
Chapter 16	Antiparkinsonian Drugs	61
Chapter 17	Psychotherapeutic Drugs	63
Chapter 18	Adrenergic Drugs	65
Chapter 19	Adrenergic-Blocking Drugs	67
Chapter 20	Cholinergic Drugs	69
Chapter 21	Cholinergic-Blocking Drugs	71
Chapter 22	Heart Failure Drugs	73
Chapter 23	Antidysrhythmic Drugs	75
Chapter 24	Antianginal Drugs	77
Chapter 25	Antihypertensive Drugs	79
Chapter 26	Diuretic Drugs	83
Chapter 27	Fluids and Electrolytes	85
Chapter 28	Coagulation Modifier Drugs	87
Chapter 29	Antilipemic Drugs	89
Chapter 30	Pituitary Drugs	91
Chapter 31	Thyroid and Antithyroid Drugs	93
Chapter 32	Antidiabetic Drugs	97
Chapter 33	Adrenal Drugs	99
Chapter 34	Women's Health Drugs	101
Chapter 35	Men's Health Drugs	103
Chapter 36	Antihistamines, Decongestants, Antitussives, and Expectorants	105
Chapter 37	Bronchodilators and Other Respiratory Drugs	107
Chapter 38	Antibiotics Part 1	109

Chapter 39 Antibiotics Part 2 113
Chapter 40 Antiviral Drugs 115
Chapter 41 Antitubercular Drugs 117
Chapter 42 Antifungal Drugs 119
Chapter 43 Antimalarial, Antiprotozoal, and Anthelmintic Drugs 121
Chapter 44 Antiinflammatory and Antigout Drugs 123
Chapter 45 Immunosuppressant Drugs 125
Chapter 46 Immunizing Drugs and Biochemical Terrorism 127
Chapter 47 Antineoplastic Drugs Part 1: Cancer Overview and Cell Cycle–Specific Drugs 129
Chapter 48 Antineoplastic Drugs Part 2: Cell Cycle–Nonspecific and Miscellaneous Drugs 133
Chapter 49 Biologic Response–Modifying and Antirheumatoid Drugs 135
Chapter 50 Acid-Controlling Drugs 137
Chapter 51 Bowel Disorder Drugs 139
Chapter 52 Antiemetic and Antinausea Drugs 143
Chapter 53 Vitamins and Minerals 145
Chapter 54 Nutritional Supplements 147
Chapter 55 Anemia Drugs 151
Chapter 56 Dermatologic Drugs 153
Chapter 57 Ophthalmic Drugs 155
Chapter 58 Otic Drugs 157
Overview of Dosage Calculations 159
Answers 181

Student Study Tips

CHOOSE TO MANAGE YOUR TIME

Time and money have much in common. They can be spent, saved, invested, given away, stolen, and wasted. The big difference between these two commodities is that you can earn more money. Your time is limited. Learn to mange your time now and the quality of your life will increase because you will have more time to do what you enjoy.

You may not enjoy studying. What you want is to be a nurse, and studying is one choice that will get you what you want. Being a nurse will bring you the satisfaction that you need. I, for one, am very thankful that you have made this decision. The world needs dedicated skilled nurses. To meet this need, you must make the decision to manage your time effectively.

Establish Goals and Create Action Plans

One key to time management is having clear goals and an action plan to accomplish these goals. This is more than saying, "I want to be a nurse" or "I want to ace my pharmacology midterm." It is a decision to spend time now to get clarity and direction so that you will have more time later to relax. The following guidelines can help you get what you want.

Guidelines for Setting Goals

There are some basic guidelines to follow when setting goals:

- **Be realistic**. The goal must be something that you can reasonably expect to accomplish. A goal of scoring 100% on each and every unit test is not realistic, but a goal of scoring 85% or better is.
- **Be specific.** Goals must set out exactly what needs to be done. Do not simply state, "I will study for the exam." Specify how many hours, what days, and what times you will study. The more specific the goal statement, the easier it is to establish a plan, complete that plan, and thus achieve the goal set.
- **Establish a time limit.** Specify a time limit for completing each step in the plan and an overall deadline for accomplishing the goal.
- **Make the goal and actions measurable.** State the goal and each step in the plan for achieving it in a way that will enable you to measure your progress toward completion.

The following is an example of how this goal and action process works: You have a chapter test a week from today. The test will cover approximately 45 pages of text material, and there are 40 specific pharmacologic terms you must know. In addition, you have been given about 20 pages of supplementary handouts in class. What will you do in the next 7 days to prepare for this test?

Goal Statement:
I will study to make a good grade on this exam.
This is a poor goal statement because it is not specific, sets no time limits, and offers no real way to measure progress. The intent is good, but the implementation of such a vague goal is usually poor.

Revision 1:
I will spend 2 hours a day studying for the next chapter test in order to get at least an 80% score.
This is a better goal statement. If one assumes that 2 hours per day is realistic, then the goal is more specific, the grade goal is measurable, and there is a time limit of sorts. This goal statement might be good enough, but it could still be improved.

Final Version:
I will spend 2 hours per day, from 2:30 to 4:30 PM, for the next 7 days studying for the chapter test in order to score at least 80%.
This is what is needed. This version states how much time, when, how many days, and for what purpose. Setting clear goals helps you get started and serves as a motivator to keep you working.

Guidelines for Action Statements

A goal, no matter how well stated, is not enough. There must be action statements to help you make day-to-day progress toward meeting the goal. The guidelines that apply to defining your goal also apply to establishing the action statements—they should be realistic, specific, measurable, and time-limited. They spell out what is going to be done day to day. Here are three examples of good action statements for the sample goal:

- I will master six pharmacology terms each day.
- I will spend from 2:30 to 3:00 PM each day reviewing class handouts.
- I will review 10 pages of text material from 3:00 to 4:00 PM each day.

These examples should give you a good idea of how to go about developing a clear goal and a set of actions to carry out to achieve that goal.

Organize Tasks and Create Schedules

It takes time to make time. It is your choice. Either you set your schedule or others will do it for you. It is 2:30 PM. The phone rings and friends want you to go out or your boss wants you to work overtime or your sister wants you to watch the kids. When you have an action plan and a schedule, your choices are clear. This is the time you scheduled to review class handouts. Can you reschedule this review or do you want to keep this promise you have made to yourself to accomplish your goal? No matter what you decide, you have maintained control over your time.

Your goals and action plans are the foundation for your time management. The next key is to organize tasks and create schedules.

Guidelines for Organizing Tasks

1. Divide tasks into three categories:
    a. Jobs that **have to be done,** such as going to class, going to work, eating, and getting adequate rest. These jobs are the easiest to accomplish because the consequences of not doing them are serious. If you do not go to class, failure is almost a sure thing. If you do not go to work, soon there will be no paycheck. The consequences of not eating or sleeping are obvious.
    b. Jobs that **should be done,** such as studying, paying bills, cleaning the house, and all of those other necessary but unpleasant tasks that are part of life. The "should-be-done" jobs are the most difficult to accomplish because they are the jobs that are all too easy to put off doing. These are also the jobs for which time management skills are most essential.
    c. Things that you **want to do.** These include all of the fun things that provide pleasure and escape from the routines of class, study, and work. Most of us are very successful at finding time to do what we want to do, even when there is a sizable backlog of "should-be-done" chores waiting. This choice can lead to procrastination and stress. The important things are maintaining balance and staying focused on your goals.
2. Prioritize items in your **"have-to-be-done" category** based on your physical and mental health needs. Examine the consequences of not doing these activities. If you can live without doing an activity, then it is not a need.
3. Prioritize your **"should-be-done" category** based on your physical and mental health needs. Examine the consequences of not doing these activities. Can you accomplish your established goals without doing a given activity? If so, then it is not a need.
4. Prioritize your **"want-to-do" category.** Some recreational time is absolutely essential in any effective time management system. "Want-to-do" activities can often be used as incentives for completing what should be done.
5. Use incentives to accomplish what you should do. For each person the rewards will be different. Spend a little time determining what will work for you. It might be watching your favorite reality show, prime time drama, or comedy show; going to the movie theater to see a new release; reading a book for pleasure; or just spending some time with family or friends.

Guidelines for Creating Workable Schedules

You will need three types of schedule: **master, weekly,** and **daily.**

Start by developing a **master schedule** table on your computer that has seven columns and 15 to 17 rows. The columns are the days in the week and the rows are the hours in the day. The left-hand column will represent Sunday and the far right will be Saturday. Start at the top of each column with the time you usually get up in the morning and end each column with the time you usually go to bed. A typical master schedule might begin at 6 AM and end at 11 PM.

Once the blank schedule sheet is prepared, the next step is to fill in those hours that correspond to the activities you have to do. These are the hours others control, and the activities are those that occur at the same hour, on the same day or days, and for several weeks or longer. For example, the semester's schedule of classes is the first set of activities to enter into the master schedule. Other activities such as work, travel, worship services, and any other regular activities also belong in the master schedule.

The master schedule should contain only those recurring activities that cannot be done at any other time. Activities such as doing the laundry, watching television, and shopping should not be included, because the time when you do them is more flexible. The idea behind compiling the master schedule is to establish those times

	SUN	MON	TUES	WED	THUR	FRI	SAT
7:00		GET UP		GET UP		GET UP	
8:00		TRAVEL		TRAVEL		TRAVEL	
9:00	GET UP	CLASS		CLASS		CLASS	
10:00	CHURCH	CLASS	TRAVEL	CLASS	TRAVEL	CLASS	
11:00	CHURCH		PRACTICUM		PRACTICUM		
12:00		CLASS	PRACTICUM	CLASS	PRACTICUM		
1:00			PRACTICUM		PRACTICUM		
2:00		PERSONAL	PRACTICUM		PRACTICUM		
3:00		PERSONAL					
4:00		AEROBICS		AEROBICS		AEROBICS	
5:00							
6:00		DINNER	DINNER	DINNER	DINNER	DINNER	
7:00							FUN
8:00							FUN
9:00							FUN
10:00							FUN
11:00	BEDTIME	BEDTIME	BEDTIME	BEDTIME	BEDTIME	BEDTIME	FUN

Figure 1-1. The master schedule. This is an essential first step in managing time effectively.

of the day that are "spent" and therefore cannot be used for any other activities. The empty blocks that remain represent the time you have to do everything else. Figure 1-1 shows a sample master schedule.

Creating a master schedule takes no more than half an hour, and it will generally serve you for an entire semester. The only reason to compile a new master schedule is that a significant schedule change has occurred. You may get a new work assignment or your nursing practicum site may change and require an additional 15 or 20 minutes of travel time. Then a new master schedule should be drawn up to accommodate the increase in time that is now necessary. Once the master schedule is completed, make four or five copies of it. These copies will be used to prepare the detailed weekly schedule.

Next, move on to developing your weekly schedule. The master schedule helps you identify the time you have available to complete the "should-be-done" and "want-to-do" task lists. The weekly schedule is more complex. It is intended to help you plan for study, recreation, family time, and all those other activities that you want to fit into a typical week. To prepare the detailed weekly schedule, take one of the copies you made of the master schedule and begin to fill in activities in the open blocks of time. The first blocks of time you should assign are the most important ones for any student—study time. This is what time management is all about—scheduling the needed hours for study (Figure 1-2).

When filling in study hours, consider these important factors:

- **Amount of planned study time.** There is an old rule pertaining to study time, and even though it is an old rule, it is still a very good guideline. The rule is to plan 2 hours of study time for each 1 hour spent in class. For example, a three-credit-hour course meets 3 hours per week, so you need to plan 6 hours of study time per week for this course. Remember, this is a general rule. Some courses will not actually require as much time as you allot, whereas others will require more. The reason for beginning a semester with this approach is simple. It is easy to find things to do with time you do not need for study, but once a semester is under way it can be very difficult to find additional study time. If you do not plan enough study time at the beginning, you will soon find yourself in a constant battle to keep up. The result is frustration, anxiety, and a sense of impending doom—feelings you do not need when you want to perform at your very best.
- **Personal prime time.** Do you wake up early, ready to charge forward, but find it difficult to be productive after 10 PM? Do you do your best work in the afternoon and early evening and prefer to sleep until 10 AM? Are you a night owl? Answers to these questions will reveal your prime time, those times of the day when your ability to concentrate is at its best and you can accomplish the most. These are the times you want to use for study. It is not always possible, because of class and work schedules, to schedule all study time in your prime hours, but it is essential that those hours be used for study as much as possible. It

	SUN	MON	TUES	WED	THUR	FRI	SAT
7:00		GET UP		GET UP		GET UP	
8:00		TRAVEL		TRAVEL		TRAVEL	
9:00	GET UP	CLASS	*STUDY*	CLASS	*STUDY*	CLASS	
10:00	CHURCH	CLASS	TRAVEL	CLASS	TRAVEL	CLASS	*STUDY*
11:00	CHURCH	*LUNCH*	PRACTICUM	*LUNCH*	PRACTICUM	*LUNCH*	*STUDY*
12:00		CLASS	PRACTICUM	CLASS	PRACTICUM		*PERSONAL*
1:00		*STUDY*	PRACTICUM	*STUDY*	PRACTICUM	*STUDY*	*PERSONAL*
2:00	*FREE*	*STUDY*	PRACTICUM	*STUDY*	PRACTICUM	*STUDY*	*PERSONAL*
3:00			*TRAVEL*		*TRAVEL*		
4:00		AEROBICS		AEROBICS		AEROBICS	
5:00							
6:00		DINNER	DINNER	DINNER	DINNER	DINNER	
7:00	*STUDY*	*STUDY*	*STUDY*	*STUDY*	*STUDY*	*STUDY*	FUN
8:00	*STUDY*		*STUDY*		*STUDY*		FUN
9:00	*STUDY*	*REVIEW*	*REVIEW*	*REVIEW*	*REVIEW*		FUN
10:00							FUN
11:00	BEDTIME	BEDTIME	BEDTIME	BEDTIME	BEDTIME	BEDTIME	FUN

Figure 1-2. The detailed weekly schedule. Study times should be filled in first.

would be foolish to plan to study your toughest material between 9 and 11 PM when you know that is a time when just reading the daily paper is a challenge.

- **Study hours for specific courses and general study hours.** The reason for scheduling both general and specific study times is that the study demands of different courses vary from day to day and week to week. For instance, you will need some hours of study every week to master new material, terms, and concepts in pharmacology, but the study time demands will increase in the days just before exams, midterms, and project due dates. The hours set aside for specific courses are for accomplishing the day-to-day study demands; the unassigned study hours are for meeting the changing demands posed by these special circumstances. These unassigned study hours also let you meet unexpected demands. No matter how carefully you plan your time, something will happen to prevent you from using the time block you had set aside for learning.

Be patient and evaluate what works for you. It usually takes two or three attempts over a period of 3 weeks to arrive at a detailed schedule that works well for you. There is a tendency on the first attempt to try to schedule some important activity for every waking hour. Ultimately such a schedule will make you feel as though there is no time for fun. Determine what is not working for you and make appropriate adjustments. Each week your schedule will come closer to being realistic and effective. The need to evaluate and revise is the reason for making several copies of the master schedule. Or you may want to use an electronic calendar. It saves time in the revision process, and saving time is, after all, what time management is all about.

Your last scheduling activity is to create **daily schedules and lists.** No matter how carefully and thoughtfully you prepare the detailed weekly schedule, it cannot include all the tasks you will face. You will have small tasks, infrequent tasks, and unexpected tasks that will need to be added to your schedule. Each day as you think of things you want or need to do the next day, write them down. Carry a small notebook that will fit into a pocket or purse. Many cell phones have a list and/or calendar feature. Once a day, review the list and set priorities for the next day.

Consider the following when setting priorities:

- **There are only 24 hours in each day.** Be realistic about what you are able to accomplish. Do not plan to review three chapters of text material on a day when you know there will not be enough time to cover more than half of one chapter.
- **Not everything is important.** Rank your tasks as A, B, or C, with A being the most important and C being the least important. Then go about completing your As. Procrastinating about your B and C lists is not a sin. For example, going to the dry cleaners is critical if the outfit you must wear tomorrow is there, but if you do not absolutely have to have that outfit tomorrow, then the trip to the cleaners is a low priority and can be postponed to another day. Then it will be on your A list.

- **Rewriting to-do lists can steal your time.** You may want to make one weekly list and mark the tasks as A, B, or C. Put only A tasks on your daily to-do list. If you have extra time you can look at your weekly list. Or you can keep your tasks on note cards and then each day stack them in priority order.
- **Planning your route can save you time.** Look at the small tasks listed, such as picking up milk and dog food, dropping off dry cleaning, and going to the bank. Not only plan to do those errands but also think about the order in which they should be done. Planning your route so that it completes a circle from home to the cleaners to the grocery store to home will be much more time-efficient than going from home to the grocery store, back home, then to the cleaners, and finally back home again.
- **As you complete a job on the daily list, cross it off.** Crossing it off tells you that you are making progress and motivates you to move to the next item on the list. If not every item is crossed off, remember that tomorrow is another day. Celebrate what you did get done and create a plan for tomorrow that will help you accomplish your goals.
- **Remember your goals and planned action steps.** When unexpected daily tasks push them onto the B list, be sure to revise your plan to get back onto your time line. Put planning on your A list.
- **Waiting time can be a gift.** Small blocks of time are often lost or wasted because it does not seem as though anything significant could be accomplished during them. If you learn to use these small blocks effectively, you can free up larger blocks for more time-consuming or fun tasks. If a class ends 10 minutes early or if you are waiting for your ride, use the time for study. Take advantage of such "found" time to review five vocabulary terms, rework a set of class notes, or preview the next five pages of assigned reading. Using the odd minutes in the day to your advantage can really help you achieve your goals as a student.

Your time is a valuable resource for you to manage or to waste. The choice is yours. Stop for a few minutes and think over the previous strategies on how to manage your time: establishing goals and creating action plans, organizing tasks, and creating schedules. Which of these strategies will you choose to apply?

CHOOSE TO USE YOUR RESOURCES

This Study Guide is one of the resources that will help you be successful in this course. When you choose to apply these study tips, they will help you to be successful in all of your course work. Three other resources are your textbook, your instructor, and your classmates.

Your Textbook

The authors of your textbook have taken great care in organizing the information provided in a manner that will assist your learning. Each part starts with study skills tips that build on the tips that are presented in the Study Guide. At the beginning of each chapter, you will find specific objectives describing what you are expected to know and be able to do as a result of studying each chapter. Each chapter also contains learning activities and a glossary of terms. Take 10 minutes right now to perform a survey of your textbook so that you know what to expect over the term of this course. Look for chapter titles and Points to Remember. Later in this Study Guide you will find tips for mastering your textbook.

Your Instructor

Some students look at their instructor in awe. She or he is so smart and has so much experience. This is true, but he or she is also a teacher who cares about pharmacology and your learning. Your instructor wants to hear your questions because this demonstrates that you are interested in learning and you are actively engaged with the material in your textbook and lectures. The instructor is an expert on the content and the type of tests that will be given in the class. Ask questions about what will be covered on a test and the type of questions you can expect. Office hours are designed to make your instructor available to you. Choose to get your money's worth and use them!

Your Classmates

We all have different learning styles, strengths, and perspectives on the course material. Participating in a study group can be a valuable addition to your nursing school experience. These groups can be a fun way to learn. Teaching others helps us to learn and aids in organizing the course material. A study group is made up of students who are in the same class and who want to learn by discussing the course material. There are guidelines for organizing successful study groups.

1. Carefully **select members** for your group.
    - Choose students who have **abilities and motivation** similar to your own. Socializing and gossiping can eat up valuable study time. Noncommitted and underprepared classmates can be a drain.
    - Look for students who have a **common time to meet.**
    - Select classmates who have **different learning styles** from yours. They might understand the reading material or lecture material better than you. They may be able to draw a diagram that will help your learning.

- Find students who have good communication skills—people who know how to listen, ask good questions, and explain concepts.

2. Clarify the **group's purpose and expectations.**
   - Where and when will you meet?
   - How often will you meet? How long will the meetings be?
   - How much individual preparation between meetings is expected?
   - Can family members, children, or other students come to the meetings?
3. **Exchange names, phone numbers, addresses, and e-mail addresses.** Have a plan in case of emergencies.
4. **Plan an agenda** for each meeting.
   - Put the date and goal for the session on the top.
   - List the activities that will help you accomplish the goal.
   - At the end of the study session, list the results of your efforts and set the date and time for your next session.
   - Make assignments for the next session.

There are also some useful strategies to follow:

1. Exchange lecture notes and discuss content for clarity and completeness.
2. Divide up difficult reading material and develop a lesson to teach the information to each other.
3. Quiz each other by turning objectives at the beginning of each chapter into questions.
4. Use the Critical Thinking and Application and Case Study sections in this Study Guide as a basis for discussions.
5. Create and take your own practice tests. Discuss the results.
6. Develop flash cards that review key vocabulary terms.

This list could go on and on. Work with your group to design the strategy that works for you. Each study group you work with will be different.

Often in career programs like those in nursing, medical, and law schools, the course study group will turn into a learning group. **Learning groups may meet over several semesters even when the members are not taking the same classes.** Learning groups help you to prepare for licensing examinations, laboratory work, clinics, or practicum experiences. They focus on understanding and application in the field.

CHOOSE TO DEVELOP YOUR VOCABULARY

Participating in study groups and learning groups is an asset when you are working to develop a new vocabulary. Every specialty or discipline has its own language that must be learned for full mastery to occur. When you learn vocabulary with a group, you can hear others using the terms and they start to become real to you. Courses such as this one on pharmacology contain extremely complex material, and terminology is a major component of that complexity. As you learn to integrate this vocabulary into your discussions of the discipline, it will seem less like a foreign language. In technologic, scientific, and medical areas, mastering the vocabulary can make the difference between being successful and struggling constantly to understand the ideas and concepts being presented. It is therefore helpful to adopt some strategies that can make the process of vocabulary development easier and more effective. Working with a study group is one strategy, but there are several more.

Use Dictionaries

You must have a good current desk reference dictionary. *Current* means the most recent edition of whatever dictionary you choose. A dictionary published 10 or 15 years ago may contain most of what you need, but unless there have been periodic revisions, as shown on the copyright page, it is almost certain to lack some information, and this may cause you problems. A desk reference dictionary is a hard-bound dictionary and not a condensed or paperback version. Paperbacks are convenient to carry around, but to get the dictionary to this convenient size, some words have been omitted and some definitions have been shortened. This is not what you want. You need the most complete and current edition you can find and afford.

You may or may not need a medical dictionary. You will probably have access to one or more at your college or departmental library. The best way to decide whether you need to invest in such a specialized dictionary is to ask your instructor for his or her advice.

Reference the Text Glossary

As soon as you look at any of the chapters in this text, you will discover the glossary. A glossary is nothing more than a text-specific dictionary. It contains the terms and definitions the authors consider essential for a full understanding of the material. The glossary will not necessarily contain every term that is unfamiliar to you. (This is why you need a good dictionary.) You can begin the process of mastering vocabulary by paying particular attention to the glossary and key terms.

Create Flash Cards

Obtain a supply of note cards. Pick the size that best accommodates your handwriting style and size. If 5" × 7" cards do not fit into your notebook, pocketbook, or book bag and this discourages you from carrying them around with you, then use 3" × 5" cards. Remember, the flash cards these become are one of the best things you can study on the run.

Use What You Know

When you encounter an unfamiliar word, do not automatically assume that you have no idea what it means. Use the knowledge you have already acquired in other nursing courses and throughout your life.

For instance, *psychotherapeutic* appears in the chapter title for Chapter 17. Your first reaction may be that you do not know what this term means. By using what you know, however, you may be able to make an educated guess as to the meaning of the word without consulting either the text glossary or a dictionary.

This is how you make that educated guess. Consider that the first part of the word is *psycho.* By this point in your career as a student, you know that *psycho* refers to the mind. This is a good start. Now consider the next part of the word. The meaning of *therapeutic* may or may not be evident to you, but it should remind you of a simpler word, *therapy*, which is the treatment used to cure or alleviate an illness or condition. Put *mind and treatment* together, and it would seem that *psychotherapeutic* must refer to the treatment of mental problems.

Note that this is an educated guess. It may not be a perfect definition, but it will give you a basis for acquiring a fuller understanding when the term is defined in the glossary or introduced and defined in the text of the chapter. A sentence in Chapter 17 confirms that this educated guess is very close to the actual meaning: "The treatment of mental disorders is called *psychotherapeutics*." Using this approach to analyzing the meaning of a word not only confirms that you have a basic understanding of the word but also cultivates a mental link between what you know and the more specific definition provided in the text. Words and their meanings learned in this way are usually easier to grasp and easier to retain. Unfortunately, this technique will not work with some of the terms used in pharmacology because they are so specialized and specific to the field. This calls for the use of other techniques.

Hypercholesterolemia, a condition in which greater-than-normal amounts of cholesterol..

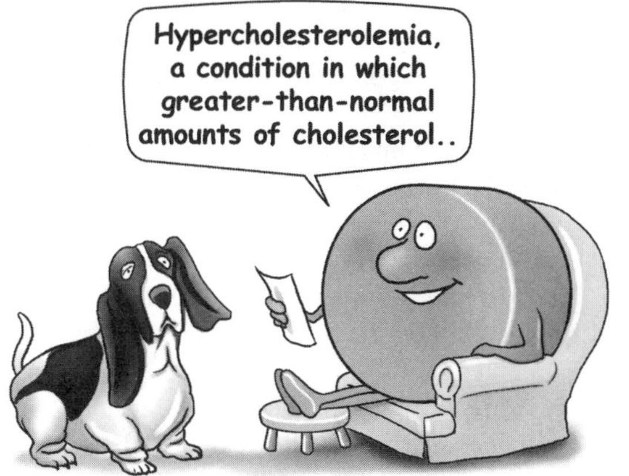

Learn the Standard Abbreviations

Make sure as you read that you pay attention to the "shorthand" used. For example, in Chapter 13, the abbreviation *CNS* is used repeatedly. The first time it is presented, the author identifies it as standing for *central nervous system* by putting the abbreviation in parentheses after the term. Thereafter, the abbreviation is used in lieu of the long term. The same thing is done for *REM* in this chapter. It is essential that you learn these abbreviations and recall each, not as a set of meaningless letters but as a key term that must be mastered.

Establish Relationships

REM is an abbreviation for *rapid eye movements*, and this term refers to a particular stage of sleep. Chapter 13 deals with CNS depressants. Relating REM to the focus of this chapter will help you remember that CNS depressants are used to influence sleep. The idea is to establish a clear relationship between the terms used and the ideas presented. Words should not be learned in isolation from the material; otherwise, you may know a lot of words and their meanings but not be able to relate them to ideas and content. *On tests, you are not likely to be asked just to repeat memorized definitions.* Instead, you will be asked to integrate these meanings into your answers to questions about nursing practices and applications.

Another important way of relating words to meanings is to link the meanings of closely related terms. The words *hypnotic* and *sedative* are good examples of this. In looking at the meanings in the glossary, you will find that each refers to a certain class of drugs. Both classes of drugs influence the CNS, but the drugs in each have a somewhat different effect. It is useful to start with the understanding that both affect the CNS but then to appreciate how the terms relate to each other. Sedatives inhibit the CNS but do not cause sleep; hypnotics at low dosages have the same effect, but at higher dosages they may induce sleep. In this learning method, you learn meanings by looking at the general similarities and then at the specific differences between terms. In doing this, you have learned both words and should never have any problems relating the words to their meanings.

CHOOSE TO TAKE EFFECTIVE LECTURE NOTES

Why Take Notes?

The primary reason for taking notes is to help your memory. It is impossible to remember everything that is said during a 1- to 2-hour lecture. The very act of writing something down helps strengthen learning and memory. In addition, note-taking helps to focus attention on the lecture. It is very easy to take mental vacations during a lecture; note-taking helps keep you involved.

Note-Taking Problems

1. **Selectivity** is the biggest challenge. How do you know what is really important?
2. **Unfamiliar vocabulary** causes confusion. This is particularly true in a course heavy in technical, medical, and pharmaceutical terminology such as this one.
3. Hard-to-read or even **illegible handwriting** is frustrating.
4. It is **difficult to listen and write at the same time.** It splits one's focus and often gets in the way of understanding.

Note-Taking Solutions

1. Realize that note-takers are made, not born. You can learn to be more effective as both a note-taker and note-user, but **this requires some practice** and a willingness to adopt new techniques.
2. **Use the vocabulary development** strategies previously discussed so that you will have a better understanding of the lecture material.
3. **Note-taking is a five-stage process** that is spread out over the days and weeks between lectures and the time when you are reviewing your notes in preparation for a test.

Stage 1: Be Prepared

Note-taking begins before the lecture. Read assigned material before class. This provides you with the background needed to listen intelligently to the lecture and to be selective when taking notes. You will have less unfamiliar vocabulary. The lecture will bring the textbook content to life for you.

Go to class a few minutes early and review your notes from the previous lecture. This will help warm up your brain so it will be ready to receive new information.

Stage 2: Active Listening

Taking quality class notes requires active listening. This is one of the most challenging aspects of being a good note-taker. It requires an awareness of both the lecturer's language and his or her nonverbal style. You have to pay attention not only to what is said, the verbal aspect, but also to the visual, nonverbal, aspect of the presentation.

Active listening requires selectivity. If you spend the lecture time trying to write down every word, you will not be able to listen to and therefore grasp the ideas. Focus on the most important ideas, terms, and facts to be recorded for later review. Writing less and listening more is a good rule to follow for note-taking.

Learn to listen for key words and phrases. These vary with the subject content and with the individual lecturer, so there is no way to provide a single, definitive list of them. However, there are some verbal signals (words) that will give you clues that the lecturer is about to give important information:

- Sequence words—*first, second, next, then, last, finally*
- Contrast words—*but, however, on the other hand*
- Importance words—*significant, key, main, main point, most important*

The use of words and phrases such as these is the lecturer's way of signaling the relative importance and progression of certain facts and ideas. As important as these words are, however, it is also necessary to be aware of the volume, tone, and pace of delivery. Some instructors will slow down or repeat ideas that are important. Other instructors may speak louder and point into the air to emphasize a point. Get to know your instructor's style and you will be able to anticipate what will be on the test. Of course, if the instructor says, "One of the most important drugs in the treatment of …," then you should immediately know that what follows is an important point for your notes. The instructor has even told you it is important. As you practice active listening and observing in the lecture environment, you will find that your ability to discern the important ideas will improve.

Stages 1 and 2 are preparation for the real work that goes on in the last three stages.

Stage 3: In-Class Note-Taking

The split-page note format requires a change in the way you set up your note paper. In this method, each sheet is divided into two parts by drawing a line down the full length of the page to create a left-hand column that is 2 1/2 to 3 inches in width and a right-hand column that is 5 1/2 to 6 inches in width. The right-hand column should be used for taking class notes. (The function of the left-hand column will be explained in the description of Stages 4 and 5.)

There is no magic formula for note-taking. Simply take the best notes you can. Remember, notes are personal. Do not judge your notes against those of other classmates. Some will take a lot of notes, and others with a different background and expectations will take far fewer notes. The key point is to do what works for you. When what you are doing stops working, then try another strategy.

Here are some tips for taking effective lecture notes that may make the process easier and more effective for you:

- **Write in your own words** most of the time. Writing ideas in your own style will make them easier to learn and remember.
- **Leave space** between main points. When you sense that the lecturer has moved to a new idea, leave a couple of lines blank on your note paper. That way,

if the lecturer returns to this point later, you will have room to add further notes. Even if there is no need for additional notes, the blank lines will help you see the organization of the ideas and the relationship between them. This space can also be used to add information that is from the textbook.

- Indicate **direct cues** from the lecturer, such as "This will be on the test," "This is a difficult concept," or even "Know this." Put a star or a check in your notes so you will remember to study this information when preparing for the test.
- Be especially aware of the **visual presentation.** This consists of information written on the chalkboard or presented using an overhead projector, slide projector, PowerPoint display, or other electronic display. Many lecturers outline key points on the chalkboard as a means of staying focused on the points they want to cover. Use this information to help you stay equally focused. Electronic displays are often chosen because the ideas can best be understood when they are presented visually.
- The **repetition** of certain points is the single most useful tip that they are really important. When an idea, term, or fact is important, the lecturer will almost certainly repeat it. For instance, the lecturer will introduce a new term, define it, give a couple of examples to clarify the definition, and finally redefine the term. This repetition is a signal that it is very important for you to learn the information.
- Be alert for **questions directed to the class.** These questions are another way the speaker stresses important information and are also a way for him or her to find out how well the students have understood what has been said. Such questions are thus also cues that certain information is important.
- Be **actively involved** in what is going on in class. This means being willing to respond to a question directed to the class. It also means asking questions when things are not clear. Do not feel that because no-one else is asking questions, you are the only person who does not understand something. It is highly probable that there are others who are just as confused. Your objective in class is to understand the lecture and record key ideas in your notes so that you can study effectively. Questions are not dumb if they relate to the material being presented.

Stage 4: Out-of-Class Reworking

The notes you take in class are only one part of the effective study of lecture material. Out-of-class reworking of these notes is critical, and this is where the left-hand column of your note paper comes into use. Ideally, this reworking should be done immediately after the class ends, but this is not always possible. It must be done within 24 hours, however, to get full benefit from this strategy. Reworking class notes will not take more than 10 to 15 minutes to complete, but it will save you hours of study time later on.

The following is the recommended method for reworking your class notes:

- **Read over the class notes.** Look for major topics, key ideas, terms, and the organization pattern. At this point you are not trying to remember everything you got from the lecture. You are looking for places where your notes are incomplete or confusing. If you read your notes soon after the lecture, you will be able to clarify points or add missing material because most of what was said will still be fresh in your mind. If you wait until the next day (or worse, the next week), what is now only confusing will by then be a complete mystery. Taking the time to read your notes over soon after you take them will save much time and frustration later on.
- **Write topic heads for lecture segments** in the empty left-hand column of your notes. As you read your notes, identify the major topics that were discussed. For example, look at Chapter 12 in the text. The chapter title tells you that it is about general and local anesthetics, but the information does not stop there. Further topics are discussed and divided into subgroups. Headings are necessary to break down very complex material into understandable blocks. You should be doing the same thing with your notes. Limit your labels to three to five words. You are not trying to rewrite class notes but to make the organization of the ideas crystal clear. Sometimes the notes on the chalkboard or PowerPoint slide will provide the labels for you. Sometimes the labels will be included in a lesson outline furnished by the instructor. Often, however, you will have to compose your own labels. With practice you will develop this skill. Keep at it. These labels are an essential aspect of the final stage of this note-taking method.
- **List vocabulary.** The left-hand column is also a great place to put content-specific vocabulary. Look again at Chapter 12. Notice that there is a glossary of terms for that chapter. This is provided so that you can immediately begin to focus on the content-specific vocabulary you will have to master for that chapter. You can create your own personal glossary of the terms used in the lecture. As you read over your notes, each time you encounter terms from the text or new terms introduced in the lecture, note the word in the left-hand column. Doing this will help you learn the needed vocabulary.
- **Expand.** Often during a lecture, you will only have time to write fragments of information. These may be meaningful at the time you write them but can be confusing later. Therefore, as you read your notes, fill in those places where there may be such gaps; otherwise, what was a small problem will become a

big one later on. It will not take long, and it will pay off. You may use the left-hand column or the lines that you left blank for adding such information.

Remember: The reworking must be done the same day as the lecture for it to be efficient and productive. The longer the interval between the lecture and this reworking, the greater the likelihood of forgetting. When you read notes the same day as the lecture, you will be able to recall almost everything said. The reworking process will only take 10 minutes or so to complete, but it will pay off in a significantly improved set of class notes. Of equal importance is the fact that the reworking process is preparation for the final, critical stage in the note-taking process.

Stage 5: Frequent, Active Review

Notes, no matter how good, need to be **studied early and often.** Learning and memory depend on rehearsal, or review, and this must be an active process. Rereading notes will improve your understanding and memory somewhat, but there is a technique you can use that will accomplish much more. This technique will help you to be an active learner and encourage frequent rehearsal. It is also efficient because it will only take you 10 to 15 minutes to completely review 2 or 3 days' worth of class notes.

When to Review. The first review of your notes should be performed within 2 days of the lecture. If the lecture has taken place on Monday, your review should occur on Tuesday or Wednesday. Do not wait more than 2 days. Studies have repeatedly shown that we forget nearly 50% of what we learn in the first 24 hours after we learn it. The reworking process will slow the forgetting process, but it will not stop it. The longer you wait to review your notes, the more time it will take and the more difficult it will be when you finally do it.

When to do a second, third, or any additional reviews depends on the success of the previous review. Review each day until you find that you remember and understand 80% or more of the material (you have to be the judge). When this is accomplished, the next review can wait for 3 or 4 days. If you find that after the first review you recall or understand only 70% of the material (an average amount), then the next review should occur within 2 or 3 days. If the amount you remember is less than 70%, you should review the material the next day. You must assess your own performance on each review to determine how soon to schedule another review. There are no hard and fast rules for this. A good review does not mean you have mastered the material forever, and what you remember clearly at one review may be the very thing you forget the next time around. **The only rule is to review frequently.** By doing this you will be well-prepared for quizzes, tests, or any other measure of your learning.

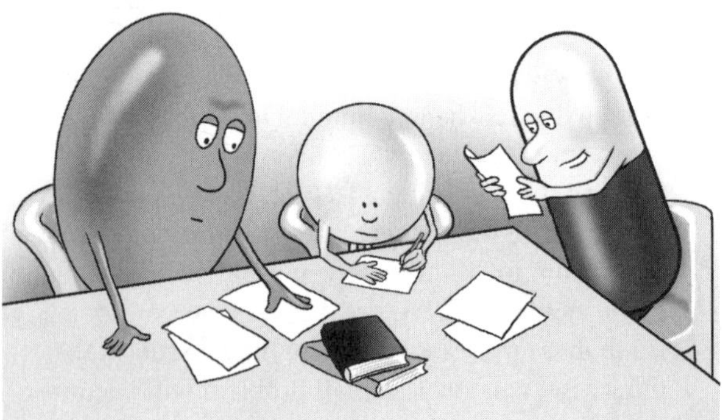

How to Review. To review your notes, **cover the right-hand column** (class notes) with a blank sheet of paper. Look at the topics, vocabulary, and further notes that you added to the left-hand column during the reworking process. These will serve as your study guide for review. Look at the first topic heading you have written. It might be something like "Hypnotics." Turn that heading into one or more questions. What are hypnotics? When are they used? What are the side effects? Are there patients for whom hypnotics are inappropriate? Ask these questions aloud; do not just think them. **Framing questions orally is what makes this review active.** Now that you have asked a question, the next step is obvious. Answer it without looking at the covered notes. Say the answer aloud. This oral question-and-answer process forces you to state the information in your own words and style. In addition, you are relying on more faculties in your learning than just the visual one of rereading. You are speaking and listening, which is more active than just looking at the words. **Recall is strongly enhanced when you express the information in your own words.**

Another benefit of this review process is that it **helps identify what you do not know.** If you ask a question and find yourself struggling to respond, then it will be clear that this is something you have not yet mastered. When this happens, uncover the class notes pertaining to that topic and read what is needed. Sometimes only three or four words will be needed to trigger recall. When this happens, immediately cover the notes and resume your oral response. Sometimes you will have to read a large portion of the notes to trigger your memory. The reading is now focused on material that you have clearly identified as unknown. This means that your review time will be much more productive. Instead of reading everything known and unknown, you will now be concentrating on reinforcing the known material and studying the unknown. **The best way to prepare for a test is to take a test.** By using the question-and-answer model, you are creating and taking your own test. You may discover that many of the questions you asked yourself also appear in some form on the classroom test covering that same material. If you have already answered the question several times for yourself, it will be easy to answer it on the test.

Two-Page Split-Note Variation. There is a variation of the split-page note paper format that some students find works better for them. If you find that the 6-inch-wide right-hand column is too narrow for taking class notes, simply take your class notes on the right-hand page in your notebook and use the left-hand page for the reworking process. This allows more room for the charts, diagrams, or complex formulas that are often part of the lecture material in courses such as pharmacology. This two-page method will also allow you to incorporate text notes. To do this, divide the left-hand page into two columns of equal width. Use the right-hand column for the reworking of class notes and the left-hand column for text notes on the same topic.

On-the-Run Action. Record the information you find to be most difficult to remember on 3" × 5" cards and carry them with you in your pocket or purse. When you are waiting in traffic or for an appointment, just pull out the cards and review again. This "found" time may add points to your test scores that you have lost in the past.

CHOOSE TO MASTER YOUR TEXTBOOKS

Many students find themselves falling asleep while reading their textbooks. Text material can be long, complex, sometimes confusing, and often highly technical. It can seem as though the more you read, the more there is to learn and the less you understand. Close the book and everything you have just read evaporates from your memory. If you feel like this, just remember—you are not alone. Every student feels this way. However, there are effective ways to maximize your learning and memory and maybe even reduce the time it takes to do this.

Many different study systems have been devised to aid in the mastery of textbook material, and each has worked for some students. The model presented here is a combination of the best elements of this multitude of systems and the best one for dealing with the subject matter in this pharmacology text.

Getting the most from a lecture requires active listening. The same active process applies to the reading of a textbook. Several techniques promote active reading. A good study system such as the PURR method presented in the textbook is one part of the process, but a good study system can be enhanced by reading with a pencil. Making text notations will help you concentrate and also make future review of the material more productive.

There are three notation systems:

- Highlighting-underlining
- Marginal notation
- Written text notes

Each of these notation systems has certain advantages and disadvantages. No single one will work perfectly all the time. Just as you must use different techniques to meet the different needs of your patients, you also need to use different techniques of text notation to meet the different needs you have as a learner. First, though, let's discuss two general guidelines that apply to the different systems of text notation.

General Guidelines

1. **Read first.** Before you begin to make any text notations, you must first read the material. The objective of text notations is to identify the important ideas, facts, and terms just as this is the objective of listening during a lecture. If you attempt to mark text while reading it for the first time, everything will seem important and you will find yourself making far too many notations or highlighting far too much material.

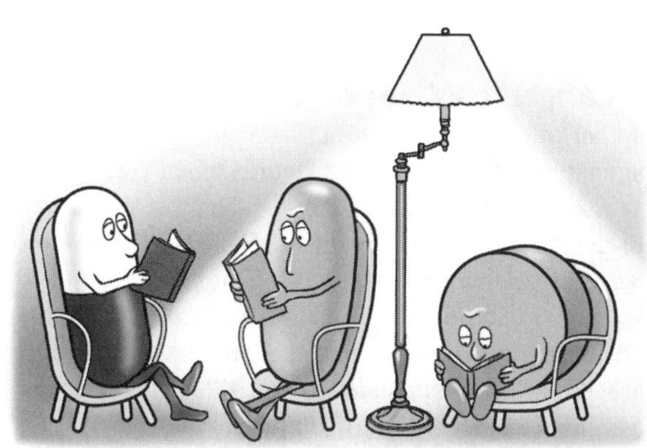

2. **Be selective.** Be very selective. The objective of text notation is much like that of taking notes during a lecture—to pick out the important ideas for immediate learning and for future review. If you have ever looked at a used textbook, you are sure to have seen that the previous owner has highlighted nearly every line on some pages. Excessive marking means the reader was not discerning the important ideas as he or she was reading. If you are taking separate handwritten notes, you should **limit what you write down** to the major headings and subheadings, important and unfamiliar vocabulary, and no more than two sentences of personal notes for each paragraph. The object is not to rewrite the chapter but to distill the important information. If you are highlighting, limit the material marked to no more than 20% to 25% of the total material. This is not to say that you must impose this limit on every paragraph, but it should be an overall goal.

Text Notation Systems

Text Conventions

As you read and prepare for making text notations, be aware of certain conventions used throughout the text. These help the reader focus on what the authors consider important. By now you have noticed the use of headings in this study tips chapter. Look back at some of them and you will also notice that they are styled differently—some are all capitals; others have only the first letter of each word capitalized. These represent main topics and subtopics. Now look at a chapter in your text. Examine the way headings and boldfacing draw your eyes to certain words, phrases, and portions of the page. These are text conventions provided by the authors to help you understand the organization of the material and the relationships within the text content. Other text conventions that you should note are numbered lists, bulleted lists, special display material, and the like.

Language Conventions

Another important aspect of text notation is to become language-sensitive. In a class lecture, when you hear a professor say, for instance, "One of the most important first-generation anesthetics was …," the words *most important* are a direct cue that this is a significant point for your notes. The same type of cueing often occurs in the text. The authors want to make certain that their important ideas are communicated to you, the reader. Because the authors cannot speak to you face to face, however, they must rely on a certain written style to get important points across. This means that you must become aware of that style so that you can identify these important ideas. For example, in a sentence saying "Opioids can be classified into four main categories," the phrase *four main categories* is the author's way of telling you not only what is coming but also what you should be taking note of.

Pay attention if a paragraph begins with the phrase "The most significant effects..." Whenever an author uses words or phrases such as these, it tells you that something important is being discussed. When you highlight text, phrases such as *most important, four main categories, and most significant* are the cues you should look for to help identify the most important information. The combination of text conventions and language conventions helps make the reading and marking of text more successful.

How to Highlight and Underline

Text marking is done to help in future review. This means that text marking is a personal process and should be used to point out only the most important information. The previous two sections on conventions gave you some concrete ideas on what to mark in your textbook. The main point is **read before you mark.**

It is essential that you read meaningful blocks of text before you do any marking. A meaningful block may be as little as a single paragraph but never less. It may be as much as an entire chapter. In a text such as *Pharmacology and the Nursing Process*, in which the material is highly technical and challenging, it is unlikely that you will want to read more than a section of the chapter at a time before going back to highlight.

Look at Chapter 13. The first paragraph mentions the boldfaced terms *sedatives* and *hypnotics*. As you read this paragraph the first time, do not mark anything. Instead **read for a general understanding of the content.** After this, go back to the beginning of the section about Sleep and note the following language conventions: *two basic elements, different stages, summarized,and is known as.* These are all words and phrases that point out important information that should be highlighted. You may not actually need to highlight all the information flagged by these words and phrases. Some of it is probably already familiar to you because of earlier courses you have taken or earlier chapters you have read in this text. Avoid highlighting information you have already mastered.

Review

When

How soon after you have done some form of text notation should you review what you have highlighted? Ideally review should begin within 24 to 48 hours after the initial learning has occurred. Psychologists have studied learning, memory, and forgetting and have found that we forget approximately 50% of what we learn after the first day or two. Therefore, the sooner you begin to review, the easier it is to move learning from short-term memory (quickly learned and quickly forgotten) to long-term memory.

How

The process for reviewing any text notations follows the same general principles that apply to lecture notes. The intent is to make your review an active process in which real learning takes place. For example, if you have written questions in the text's margins, try to answer these questions without rereading the text. If you are able to answer the question to your satisfaction, then move on to the next question. If you have highlighted terms and definitions, cover the definition and try to define the term without looking at the text. If you are able to do this, you have effectively moved material into long-term memory. If you cannot define the term, then read the text definition. As you read, think about the meaning and think about strategies you might use to help you remember the term and definition the next time. You will find additional memory strategies in the later section on studying for exams. The key is always to focus on being an active learner.

How Often

How often you review is a personal matter. The best way to judge is to be aware of your success, or lack of it, in the current review session. If you do very well at recalling information, then you can probably wait 3 to 4 days for the next review. If the review goes okay, then the next session should take place within 2 days. If you find yourself reviewing your own notations with little understanding and limited memory, then the next review should take place the following day. Each time you review, it will get easier and faster, and as you practice this approach to reviewing your text notations, you will gradually acquire a good sense of how often you need to review to maintain mastery of the material.

CHOOSE TO PASS EXAMS

You can pass your exams by **applying the recommendations and strategies** offered in this section. Start by following the dozen basic rules of exam success.

Rules for Success on Exams

1. Accept your anxiety as normal. Tests are important, both in the short-term, from the standpoint of grades and successful completion of this course, and also in the long-term, from the standpoint of completing the program and getting your degree and eventually the job you want. This fact can cause stress.
2. Reduce your stress by **studying often, not long.** The most important rule in preparing for exams is simple—spend at least 15 minutes every day (Saturdays, Sundays, and holidays included) in reviewing the "old" material. The more time you can find for this each day, the better, but spend at least 15 minutes. This one action will do more to reduce test anxiety than anything else you do. The more time you devote to reviewing past material learned, the more confident you will feel about your knowledge of the topic. This confidence will accompany you into the classroom on the exam day, and it will help you get the test score you want and of which you are capable. Just remember—**start the review process on the first day of the semester** and do some review every single day until the final exam.
3. Balance your review time between your lecture notes, textbook notes or highlighting, and any handouts you may have been given.
4. Ask your instructor about the exam. If he or she says the test is mostly on the lecture, then you may want to spend more time reviewing your class notes. Ask about the type of questions that will be on the exam. Will the test consist entirely of multiple-choice questions? Will it have true-or-false items? Will there be matching, short-answer, or essay questions? You should not study any differently for a multiple-choice exam than you should for a short-answer or essay exam. However, knowing the type or types of questions that will be on the test will help you develop a strategy for quizzing yourself.
5. Work with your study group to create practice tests. For example, if you know the test will consist of multiple-choice questions, then as you do your review, think of the kinds of questions you would ask if you were composing the test. Consider what would be a good question, what would be the right answer, and what would be other answers that would appear right but would in fact be incorrect.
6. Take the practice tests in each chapter and on the Evolve website for the text. Practice writing out the answers of short-answer or essay questions. **The best way to prepare for a test is to take one.**
7. **Study wisely, not hard.** Use the study strategies offered in this guide so you can save time and be able to get a good night's sleep the night before your exam. Cramming is not smart, and it is hard work that increases stress while reducing learning. When you cram, your mind is more likely to go blank during a test. When you cram, the information is in your short-term memory so you will need to relearn it before a comprehensive exam. Relearning takes more time. The stress caused by cramming may interfere with your sleep. Your brain needs sleep to function at its best.
8. Prepare for exams when and where you are most alert and able to concentrate. **Use your personal prime time,** which was discussed earlier in the time management section. If you are most alert at night, study at night. If you are most alert at 2 AM, study in the early morning hours. Study where you can focus your attention and avoid distractions. This may be in the library or in a quiet corner of your home. The key point is to keep on doing what is working for you. If you are distracted or falling asleep, you may want to change when and where you are studying.
9. **Relax the last hour before an exam.** Your brain needs some recovery time to function effectively.
10. Survey the test before you start answering the questions. Plan how to complete the exam in the time allowed. Read the directions carefully and answer the questions you know for sure first.
11. Before turning in the exam, make sure that you have answered all of the questions. If you are to fill in the boxes on an answer sheet that will be read electronically, be sure you have put only one answer per line and that you have answered each question. If you must make a correction, be sure to erase carefully and thoroughly.
12. Celebrate your success. Congratulate yourself for choosing to pass your exam by applying the exam preparation and exam-taking skills that have been proven to work.

Strategies for Reviewing Class Notes

Look at your class notes. If you have been using the split-page model described earlier, you have made your own topic headings in the left-hand column beside the class notes. Cover the class notes and turn each heading into one or more questions. Think carefully about the answers and then answer aloud. By answering questions aloud, you are forcing yourself to think about what you know and organizing that knowledge in the way that is most meaningful to you. If you can answer your questions, then you have demonstrated that you know the material, and there is no immediate need to reread that section of notes. If you cannot answer one of your questions, then you know you need to review that material more intensively. Uncover the notes and read the pertinent ones. You are now using your review time effectively, because instead of just rereading everything, which invites boredom—or, worse yet, daydreaming—the rereading is directed at the material of which you are unsure. The result is more efficient use of your time and more effective learning.

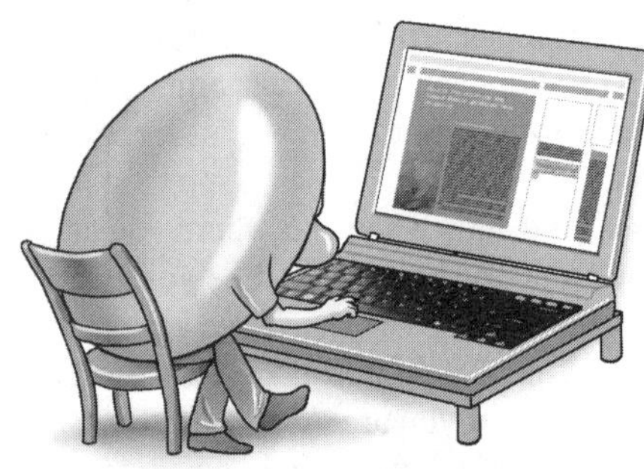

Strategies for Reviewing the Textbook

The technique you used for studying your class notes will also work for studying text material. As mentioned, in this book the authors have provided you with a variety of features that can help enormously. First, look at the objectives at the beginning of each chapter to be studied. Even if you have been assigned only small portions of the chapter, it is important to consider the objectives for the chapter as a whole. Ask yourself whether you have met these objectives. This is a quick way of assessing how much review may be necessary. If you feel confident that you have accomplished most of the objectives, then the review should go quickly. If you feel uncertain about many of them, then the review is going to take more time.

The next task is to consider the topic headings and language conventions. Use them in the same way as you have used the labels in your notes. Turn them into questions and answer these questions aloud. If you can answer them, then there is no need to reread. If you cannot, then you will need to reread the pertinent text.

Again, this way of reviewing is focusing your time and energy mostly where it is needed—on the material you have not yet mastered. Each time you review the text (or class notes), the sections of material you reread may differ. This is to be expected. You cannot remember everything forever, but if you spend time each day doing this type of review, you will remember more and for longer periods of time.

Strategies for Reviewing Terminology

One aspect of nursing that can seem overwhelming is the terminology. It is highly technical and specialized. Learning it poses the same kind of challenge as learning a foreign language. In fact, it almost is a foreign language. However, for the concepts and ideas to be mastered, the terms must be mastered. One of the best ways to go about doing this is to use a technique you probably learned in grade school—flash cards. Put each term on one side of a 3" × 5" note card and the definition or other essential information about the term on the back. Group together cards containing terms that have common word elements (e.g., terms beginning with *cardio*) or that concern common concepts (e.g., terms to do with renal function). The more relationships you can establish between words, the easier it will be to learn and remember them.

On-the-Run Action

Get in the habit of carrying a deck of 10 to 15 of these cards with you. When you have a few minutes, review as many cards as time allows. Sometimes start with the term side of the card and try to recall what is written on the back. Other times look at the definition on the back of the card and try to recall the term. Do not focus exclusively on term-to-definition learning because you may be given definitions or some variation on the exam and be asked to provide the terms.

Exam Time

This is it. The culmination of all your work—lectures, notes, flash cards, textbook readings, and handouts. **It is time to relax.** Test anxiety interferes with test performance. If you have put to use the learning techniques described in this chapter, you are ready for the exam. You have mastered the material, and you can do well on the exam. If you continue to experience test anxiety in spite of preparing thoroughly for the exam, it might be a good idea to visit a professional counselor on your campus.

Avoid cramming and remain confident in the learning techniques you have chosen to apply. This can usually control normal nervousness. Besides these learning techniques, however, techniques are also available for dealing with the various types of exam questions, and these are discussed in this section. None of these strategies can guarantee a 10-point jump in your test score. Only the degree to which you have mastered the material can make that sort of difference. However, each of the strategies described in this section may help you answer one or two questions correctly that you might otherwise have missed. **These test-taking strategies are not intended to replace regular study** and mastery; however, they are intended to enhance your test performance. If you use these strategies, you will see a positive gain in your test performance.

When the teacher passes out the exam, all your work and preparation are about to pay off, but do not just leap into the test. Take a couple of minutes to put yourself in a frame of mind for doing well on the test. At this point, you have a perfect test score—you have not answered any questions incorrectly yet. It is likely that you will get some answers wrong, but do not start out by making mistakes that cost you points which you should not have lost.

First, look over the entire test. Do not read it, but turn the pages and look at a question here and a question there. How many items are there on the test? Are all the questions of one type, or is there a mixture of types? Knowing in advance the length of the test and the types of questions helps you plan your strategy for taking the test.

Second, read the directions. This is the first opportunity you have to make a mistake that could cost points. Some directions for true-or-false questions may ask you to correct the statement and make it true. Others may ask you to justify your answer. When you respond with just a T or an F, you have lost important points because you did not read the directions.

Third, create a plan to complete the test in the time allowed. For example, if the test has 50 multiple-choice questions and the time limit is 40 minutes, then you know you will have to average a little better than one item per minute. Obviously you will need to allocate more time to essay questions if they are on the exam. Plan to glance at your watch or the classroom clock occasionally during the exam to make sure you are not losing time or going too quickly. Pace yourself. If you are answering questions quickly and are confident that the answers are right, do not worry about being ahead of schedule. If you spend too much time on individual questions, you may try to decide the answers to the last questions quickly, and this increases your chances of making errors. Planning a strategy for finishing the test within the time allowed helps you maintain a sharp focus on the task and enables you to do the best job possible.

Fourth, start answering the questions. If the test consists of only one type of question, then start with the first question. However, if the test has multiple-choice, true-or-false, and short-essay questions, for example, you must decide where it is best for you to start. If you find essay questions easy to do, then perhaps you should start with these. There is no reason you have to begin with the multiple-choice questions. On the other hand, if you find essay questions a challenge, then do not start with them. Begin the test in a way that will give you confidence.

Tips for Answering the Questions

- Start with the first question or with those types of questions you feel most confident answering. Wherever you choose to start, there is a strategy you can use that can improve your test performance.
- Read the question carefully, and if you know the answer, indicate it and move on to the next question. If you cannot immediately think of the answer, give it a few seconds of thought. If the answer comes, indicate it and move on. If the answer still does not come or if the question is confusing, then skip to the next question.
- In the first pass through the exam, answer what you know and skip what you do not know. Answering the questions you are sure of increases your confidence and saves time. This is buying you time to devote to the questions with which you have more difficulty.
- Notice that the subjects of the questions on a particular exam are related, that the answers to questions you have skipped may be provided by other questions on the test, or that a later question may trigger recall of the correct answer. Skipping questions of which you are unsure offers one more opportunity to get the correct answer.
- After you have gone through the entire test completing the questions to which you are confident you know the answers, go back to the items you skipped. First check the time, however, so you know how much time you have left to answer these questions. On this second pass through the exam, you will often be surprised at how many questions you now can answer that drew a complete blank before.
- Answer every question. A question without an answer is the same as a wrong answer. Go *ahead and guess*. You have studied for the test and you know the material well. You are not making a random guess based on no information. You are guessing based on what you have learned and your best assessment of the question.
- When you have answered all the questions on a page, put a check in the upper right corner of this page. Avoid going back and second-guessing yourself. There is nothing worse than changing right answers to wrong ones. Have confidence in your own knowledge and let go of the test. If you are the first person to complete a test but are sure of what you did, then turn it in. At the same time, do not let what others in the class are doing affect your test strategy. If you are the last person to turn the test in, it does not mean you know less than those who were faster. It simply means that you are a careful, thoughtful test-taker.

Strategies for Specific Types of Questions

For each type of question there are particular strategies you can use that can help prevent incorrect responses. Many times students miss questions not because of a lack of information but because of a poor strategy. Sometimes the error stems from misreading a question, for instance, overlooking a key word such as *not*, or from choosing an answer that does not quite fit the question asked. Errors like these can be costly. Expect to find some questions on a test to which you do not remember the answer or that are worded in a confusing way. A perfect test score is a great goal, but be realistic and accept the fact that perfect scores may be few and far between. At the same time, do not lose points because of careless and preventable errors.

Strategy for Multiple-Choice Questions

Multiple-choice questions can be challenging, because students think that they will recognize the right answer when they see it or that the right answer will somehow stand out from the other choices. This is a dangerous misconception. The more carefully the question is constructed, the more each of the choices will seem like the correct response. The successful student can do several things to improve performance on multiple-choice questions.

Before the strategies for analyzing multiple-choice questions are discussed, it is important to understand each part of a question and its purpose. There are three parts to a multiple-choice question: stem, distractors, and the correct choice.

First, there is the **question stem.** This is the complete question that one, or more, of the response choices will answer.

EXAMPLE:
If excessive amounts of water-soluble vitamins are ingested, what usually happens?

Notice that this could just as easily be a short-answer question. In this case, the stem is a complete sentence that should be answered by one of the response choices. The stem can also be an incomplete statement that one or more of the response choices completes correctly.

EXAMPLE:
The likelihood that a drug will have therapeutic effects increases dramatically when:

This statement is incomplete, and you must pick out the response choice that best completes it.

The second part of multiple-choice questions is the **distractors.** These are the response choices that do not best answer or complete the stem. They are known as *distractors* because that is their purpose, to distract you from the best choice. Good distractors are usually very similar to the **best choice.** If you have not studied enough, a good distractor will be a very tempting choice, but you must reduce the allure of distractors.

The third and final part of all multiple-choice questions is the best choice. This is the choice you want to pick. Notice that it is the "best" choice. In many multiple-choice questions there may be more than one response choice that appears to answer the stem, and the differences between the responses may be slight. Your task is therefore to identify the option that **best** answers the stem, not necessarily the only right choice.

Recall. The most reliable way to ensure that you select the correct response to a multiple-choice question is to recall it. Depend on your learning and memory to furnish the answer to the question. To do this, read the stem, and then *stop*! Do not look at the response options yet. Try to recall what you know and, based on this, what you would give as the answer. After you have taken a few seconds to do this, then look at all of the choices and select the one that most nearly matches the answer you recalled. It is important that you consider all the choices and not just choose the first option that seems to fit the answer you recall. Remember the distractors. Choice B may look okay, but choice D may be worded in a way that makes D a slightly better choice. If you do not weigh all the choices, you are not maximizing your chances of correctly answering each question.

Once you have decided on an answer, there is one more important step before you mark it. Look at the stem again. Does your choice answer the question that was asked? If the question stem asks "why," be sure the response you have chosen is a reason. If the question stem is singular, then be sure the option is singular, and the same for plural stems and plural responses. Many times, checking to make sure that the choice makes sense in relation to the stem will reveal the correct answer.

This is the most reliable technique to use for answering multiple-choice questions. If you do this for every multiple-choice question on the test, your accuracy rate will be very high, and you will not need any further strategy. Unfortunately, however, recall does not always work, and when it does not, there are some additional strategies you can apply to improve your chances of picking the correct answer.

Recognition and Elimination. Read each of the answer options carefully. Usually at least one of them will be clearly wrong. Eliminate this one from consideration. Now you have reduced the number of response choices by one and improved the odds. Continue to analyze the options. If you can eliminate one more choice in a four-option question, you have reduced the odds to 50/50, the same as the odds of correct random guessing for true-or-false questions. There are still some strategies that will help you pick the best choice. In addition, while you are eliminating the wrong choices, recall often occurs. One of the options may serve as a trigger that causes you to remember what a few seconds ago had seemed completely forgotten.

Look-Alike Answers. After you have eliminated one or more choices, you may discover that two of the options are very similar. This can be very helpful, because it may mean that one of these look-alike answers is the best choice and the other is a very good distractor. Test both of these options against the stem. Ask yourself which one completes the incomplete statement grammatically and which one answers the question more fully and completely. The option that best completes or answers the stem is the one you should choose. Here, too, pause for a few seconds, give your brain time to reflect, and recall may occur.

Absolutes. The presence of absolute words and phrases can also help you determine the correct answer to a multiple-choice item. If an answer choice contains an absolute (e.g., *none, never, must, cannot*), be very cautious. Remember that there are not many things in this world that are absolute, and in an area as complex as pharmacology, an absolute in an option may be reason to eliminate it from consideration as the best choice. This is only a guideline and should not be taken to be true 100% of the time; however, it can help you reduce the number of choices.

Negatives and Exceptions. In the stem "A drug reaction could include all but which of these symptoms?" the phrase *all but* tells you to choose the response that is an exception. *All but one* of the choice options is a symptom. In this case, the option that is *not* a symptom is the best choice. If you look at the options and see several that seem correct, look at the stem again. It may be that you have overlooked an exception phrase such as *all but* or *all but one.* A similar stem wording that can throw you off is a negative or negative prefix. The stem "It is generally not a good idea to administer adult dosages to…" is asking you to select the answer that names the inappropriate, not appropriate, recipient of a medication. The word *not* helps identify the answer.

All these strategies can help you analyze the response choices so that you have the best possible chance of selecting the correct choice. When you are ready to mark the answer, keep in mind that the final step is always to test your response against the stem.

If, after you have tried all of these strategies, you find yourself still unable to choose a response, there is one final strategy. Ask the instructor for clarification of the question. There is nothing to lose by asking and everything to gain. The worst that can happen is that the instructor will tell you that he or she cannot answer your question. The best that can happen is that the instructor will rephrase the question in a way that resolves the problem for you.

When asking for such clarification, try to phrase your question in a way that encourages a response. Do not simply state that you do not understand the question. This is generally not the approach that invites an answer. If you are having trouble with a term in the stem or response choices, ask for a definition. If there is a phrase that is unclear or a response choice that is confusing, ask for clarification. Anything you do to make your question more specific increases the likelihood that the instructor will answer it.

After all other avenues have been exhausted, remember the final rule. **Never leave a question unanswered.** Even if answering is no more than an educated guess on your part, go ahead and mark an answer. You might be right, but if you leave it blank, you will certainly be wrong and lose precious points.

Strategy for Short-Answer and Essay Questions

Notice that this strategy applies to both short-answer and essay questions. Both types of questions require careful thought and planning before you write an answer. It is helpful to get into the habit of regarding short-answer questions as short-essay questions. Too often students lose points on short-answer questions by being too brief. A short answer should usually consist of three or four sentences, but frequently students interpret "short answer" to mean four or five words.

Start answering these questions by analyzing the question carefully and then framing a response that will fully answer it. Assume that the reader—in this case, the course instructor—does not know anything and that you have to explain it all. Short-answer and essay questions require you to show what you know. Do not assume that the instructor can read your mind or read between the lines of your response to discern what you knew but did not include. It is better to have a little more than was needed in your answer than not enough. Extra information will not hurt, but missing information will always cost points. Once again, remember that the idea is to gain a point here and there throughout the test, which will result in a higher score and a better grade for the course.

Two Key Issues

1. In writing answers to short-answer and essay questions, it is essential to answer exactly the question that is asked. This means that you must understand the question before you do any writing. Unlike with true-or-false and multiple-choice questions, which you should try to answer using every possible strategy before seeking help, with these questions you

should ask for help before doing anything. The first opportunity you have to lose points in an essay question occurs with the first reading of the question. If you misread the question, you may write an excellent answer but not the right one. Such a mistake can be costly.

2. A good answer must be organized so that it is clear and logical to the reader. Do not read a question and start writing down whatever ideas spring to mind. Spend a minute or two thinking and planning the structure of the answer so that your ideas are clearly stated and the supporting details relate directly to each idea. Your instructor, the reader, will have a difficult time grading your essay if he or she has to read it two or three times to figure out what you were trying to say. Organization and clarity of expression really pay off in essay exams.

Five Steps to Good Essay Answers

1. **Read the questions carefully.** As was discussed earlier, misreading the question can result in a high-quality answer that does not address the question asked. Read and think about the question's major focus. Do not jump on the first familiar phrase or term and start writing without further thought.
2. **Decide on an approach.** Telling you to read the question carefully is good advice, but without some strategy to apply to the reading it might be difficult advice to carry out. Here is a strategy to help you read carefully and begin to plan your answer. Look at the question as you read, and identify the words and phrases that tell you what to do. Some standard "what-to-do" words and phrases are used consistently in essay questions, such as *discuss, compare, contrast, explain, tell why,* and *analyze.* Circle each of these words or phrases as you read the question. The second part of the decision step is to underline what you are to write about. This circling and underlining will force a careful reading of the question and help you begin the process of organizing the answer. The sample question that follows is marked to show the circle and underline strategy.

   SAMPLE QUESTION:

   Discuss the ways in which pediatric and elderly patients are alike in determining appropriate dosage. Explain why adult dosage may be inappropriate and the dangers in using adult dosage in these special populations.

3. **Compile a brief written outline.** Before you start writing your answer, take a few minutes to organize the points you want to cover. This should not be an elaborate outline with roman numerals, capital letters, and arabic numbers, but rather a quick sketch of the question and the points you want to make in the answer. The circle-and-underline step described earlier will help make this easy to do.

SAMPLE OUTLINE*:

Discuss

- Pediatric and elderly patients' similarity with regard to drug dosage
  - Body weight factor
  - Organ function

Explain

- Reasons adult dosage inappropriate
  - Drugs not tested on pediatric and elderly population
- Dangers of adult dosage
  - Possible organ damage
  - Increased absorption and possible side effects

Sketching out an outline like this will organize your ideas, speed your writing, and ensure that you are answering the question asked.

4. **Write an answer.** With the question analyzed and a quick outline in place, it is time to put your answer on paper. The basic structure of an exam essay or answer to a short-answer question is the same as that for an in-class composition on an assigned topic. Every rule on which composition teachers insist for writing assignments should be followed in writing essay answers.

Any answer of more than four or five sentences should follow the basic three-part essay structure of introduction, body, and conclusion.

The **introduction** should be only one or two sentences long. It tells the reader what you are going to present in your answer. There is a relatively simple way to write an essay introduction. State the question positively and add a few words that show the main points you intend to make in your answer.

SAMPLE INTRODUCTION:

Pediatric and elderly patients have a number of similarities that must be considered in determining drug dosage. Two of the most important are body weight and organ function, and these factors can make adult dosages inappropriate for these two populations.

---

*This is a model of the process of the Decision and Outline Steps. It is not to be viewed as an accurate outline of pharmacologic content.

These two sentences tell the reader exactly what you plan to discuss. From this point on, it becomes your task to explain why those two are important and how they affect drug dosage. You have told the reader what to expect, and you have begun to organize your answer.

The **body** is the most important part of any essay answer. In it you want to state the ideas, concepts, and points that you believe answer the question. These should be stated clearly and positively. Do not ramble on trying to cover all the possible variations that might fit into an answer. Decide on the most important, most significant points you have to make. Then state them and support and explain with relevant details that show how and why your points answer the question. For short-answer questions where three to five sentences are expected, drop the introduction and conclusion, and put all of your energy into a clear, concise body.

For the **conclusion,** there should be a concluding sentence or two to let the reader know that you have finished. Like the introduction, it should be brief and direct. Restate the question, and summarize the key points made in your answer.

SAMPLE CONCLUSION:

It is evident that elderly and pediatric patients are very similar in their responses to drug dosages. Clearly the factors of body weight and organ function will play a major role in determining the appropriate dosages for these two groups.

5. **Read the answer.** The writing has been completed. Before you turn in the paper, take another minute or two and read over what you have written. Look for errors that would make the reader pause, question what you have said, or be unable to read a word or phrase. Sometimes the mind works much faster than the pen, and a word or phrase is left out in writing. Use a caret (^) and insert the word or phrase where it belongs. If your writing got a little sloppy and a word is hard to read, cross it out and print it clearly right above. Proofreading and correcting small errors like these will make the answer easier to read and understand. Anything that contributes to the overall quality of an answer will influence the grade in a positive manner. You will not have time to rewrite an answer, but you should correct obvious errors.

Strategy for True-or-False Questions

True-or-false items outwardly appear to be fairly simple. After all, the statement is either true or false. The odds of answering correctly are 50/50, and if all else fails, a coin toss can decide the issue. Appearances are deceiving, however, and true-or-false questions can be very challenging to answer. Good test strategy should be applied to answer all types of questions, because the object is to get the best score you can, and this represents the total points for all correct answers.

Read the Question. Reading the question may seem like such an obvious part of all test-taking strategies that it may appear absurd even to be told to do this. If you do not pay careful attention to the wording of true-or-false statements, however, then you are increasing the odds of making an otherwise avoidable error. Take the time to read and understand the statement. Read it all the way through to the end. Do not jump to conclusions based on half of the statement.

Assume That the Statement Is True. As you read each true-or-false statement, begin with the assumption that the statement is true. The idea behind this strategy is that it will cause you to read the statement carefully, which will result in your choosing the correct answer. This approach to reading the statement makes the reading an active process, because you are then reading to confirm the truth in the statement. You will be analyzing the statement as you read, looking for any information that would contradict or change the statement from true to false. You will also be choosing your answer as you read rather than waiting to the end to decide whether the statement was true or false. Obviously not every statement will be true, but this step makes you a much more thoughtful reader, and that encourages better test performance.

Remember one other important rule when analyzing true-or-false statements**. If any part of the statement is false, then the entire statement is false.** There may be only one altered word or prefix (such as *un-* or *anti-*) that changes a statement from true to false, but that is all that is required.

Strategies for Analysis. Sometimes, no matter how carefully you have read the question, the answer is not immediately obvious. When that happens, there are a number of strategies you can use to analyze the question. Using these strategies will not guarantee that you will get the correct answer, but they will often help you see something about the statement you might have overlooked and assist you in identifying the correct answer.

Absolutes and Qualifiers. Absolutes are words such as *none, never, all,* or *always.* These words mean that there are absolutely no exceptions to the statement. For instance, the statement "All birds fly" means just that. Every bird, past, present, and future, has flown or does fly. If there is or has been just one bird that has not flown or does not fly, then the statement is false. "All" in this statement is an absolute. True-or-false statements that contain such absolutes are usually false. In an area as complex as pharmacology, it is unlikely that there are many absolutes. If you are struggling with a question that has you stumped, look for absolute words. They may help you determine the answer.

On the other hand, there are words that suggest the possibility of exceptions. Such words or phrases are called *qualifiers*; examples of these are *some, possibly, in most cases,* and *will generally.* "Most birds can fly" is an example of a qualified statement. The word *most* tells you that some not precisely specified number of all birds can fly. This makes it more probable that the statement is true.

Stated in the Negative. A true-or-false statement that is rendered in the negative can be very difficult to answer. To draw on the earlier example, "It is not true that all birds can fly" is such a statement. The word *not* in this statement can make it much more complex to read and answer. There is a relatively simple way to deal with this type of statement. Read it as though the negative were not included, so that it becomes "It is true that all birds can fly." This statement is clearly false. Because the word *not* reverses the meaning of the statement, this makes the statement "It is not true that all birds can fly" true. Simply put, if the statement is true without the negative, then it becomes false with the negative. Similarly, if it is false without the negative, then it is true with the negative.

Strings. A string is a true-or-false statement that requires careful attention. It is a statement that contains a list of several words or phrases, but often one or more of the words or phrases is false. It is easy to read the statement and see that the first two or three words or phrases are true but then to overlook the one that is incorrect, with the consequence that you mark the answer as true when it is actually false. An example of a string is "Many warm-weather crops, such as tomatoes, can be grown year-round in southern California, southern Florida, South America, and South Dakota." As you read this statement, it is easy to be lured by the words *southern* and *South* into thinking that the statement is true without noting the fact that South Dakota is a northern state with fairly harsh winters and that there are parts of South America where the climate is very cold. The statement is false, but the string can trick you into thinking that the statement is true.

These strategies for analyzing true-or-false items can help you increase the number of correct answers, but they are not intended to replace study and learning. The best way to perform well on any test is to know the answers based on your own learning. When the answer does not immediately come to mind, however, apply these strategies. Although they will not necessarily lead to a 10-point difference in your score, they may help you add 2 points to your score. Better scores mean better course grades, and of course, this results in improved self-confidence and improved chances of success.

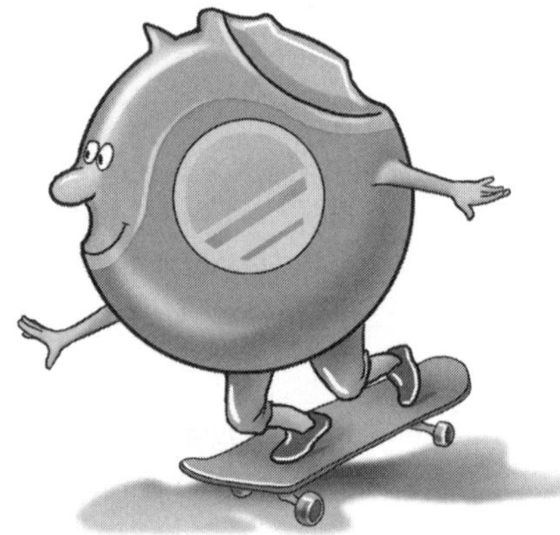

CONCLUSION

Remember: These study tips are only as valuable as you make them!

CHAPTER 1

The Nursing Process and Drug Therapy

Chapter Review and NCLEX® Examination Preparation

Select the best answer for each question.

1. Which phase of the nursing process requires the nurse to establish a comprehensive baseline of data concerning a particular patient?
   a. Assessment
   b. Planning
   c. Implementation
   d. Evaluation

2. The nurse monitors the fulfillment of goals, and may revise them, during which phase of the nursing process?
   a. Assessment
   b. Planning
   c. Implementation
   d. Evaluation

3. The nurse prepares and administers prescribed medications during which phase of the nursing process?
   a. Assessment
   b. Planning
   c. Implementation
   d. Evaluation

4. When developing a plan of care, which nursing action ensures the goal statement is patient-centered?
   a. Considering family input
   b. Involving the patient
   c. Developing the goal first, and then sharing it with the patient
   d. Including the physician

5. The nurse includes which information as part of a complete medication history?
   a. Use of "street" drugs
   b. Current laboratory work
   c. History of surgeries
   d. Family history

6. During which phase of the nursing process does the nurse prioritize the nursing diagnoses?
   a. Assessment
   b. Planning
   c. Implementation
   d. Evaluation

7. The nurse is administering a medication and the order reads: Give 250 mcg PO now. The tablets in the medication dispensing cabinet are in milligram strength. What is the right dose of the drug in milligrams? ________________

8. Place the steps of the nursing process in order, with (1) being the first step and (5) being the last step.
   ____ a. Implementation
   ____ b. Planning
   ____ c. Evaluation
   ____ d. Assessment
   ____ e. Formulation of nursing diagnoses

Critical Thinking and Application

Answer the following questions on a separate sheet of paper.

9. Below is a list of data gathered during an assessment of Ms. B., a young woman visiting an outpatient clinic with what she describes as "maybe an ulcer." Label each item as either objective data (O) or subjective data (S).
   ____ Ms. B. tells the nurse that she smokes a pack of cigarettes a day.
   ____ She is 5 feet 5 inches tall and weighs 135 pounds.
   ____ The nurse finds that her pulse rate is 68 beats/min and her blood pressure is 128/72 mm Hg.
   ____ Her stool was tested for occult blood by a laboratory technician; the results were negative.

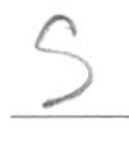
Ms. B. says that she does not experience nausea, but she reports pain and heartburn, especially after eating popcorn—something she and her husband have always done while watching TV before bedtime.

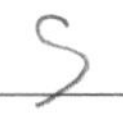
She experiences occasional increases in stomach pain, a "feeling of heat" in her abdomen and chest at night when she lies down, and increased incidents of heartburn.

10. Identify the "Six Rights" of drug administration and specify ways to ensure that each of these rights is addressed. right drug, dose, time, route patient, documentation
11. The following items will help in reviewing the nursing process:

Data are collected during the (a) assesment phase of the nursing process.

Data can be classified as (b) objective or (c) subjective.

To formulate the nursing diagnosis, the nurse must first (d) analyze the information collected.

The planning phase includes identification of (e) goals and (f) outcome criteria.

The (g) implementation phase consists of initiation and completion of the nursing care plan.

The (h) evaluation phase is ongoing and includes monitoring the patient's response to medication and determining the status of goals.

Case Study

Read the scenario and answer the following questions on a separate sheet of paper.

A 75-year-old woman has been admitted to the hospital due to nausea and vomiting. She also has a diagnosis of hepatitis C. She says she stopped drinking 3 years ago but has had increasing problems with peripheral edema and shortness of breath and has had trouble getting out of bed or a chair by herself. Laboratory results show that her liver enzyme levels are elevated; her sodium and potassium levels are decreased. Her blood pressure is 160/98 mm Hg, her pulse rate is 98 beats/min, and her respiratory rate is 24 breaths/min. She is afebrile and states that she is having slight abdominal pain.

1. From the brief facts given, what information will be important to consider when obtaining a drug history?
2. From the nursing diagnoses in Box 1-3, choose at least two current and two "risk for" nursing diagnoses for this patient. What priority would you assign to your nursing diagnoses?
3. The physician wrote the following drug order:

   November 4, 2009

   Give Lasix now.

   Charles Simmons, MD

Patient's Name: Jane Dow	F	Age: 75
Medical Record No: 1234567		Date of Birth: 1/16/34

   What elements, if any, are missing from the medication order? What will you do next? dosage + route
4. After the order is clarified, the pharmacy sends up furosemide (Lasix), 80-mg tablets, but the patient is unable to swallow them because of her nausea. Your colleague suggests giving the furosemide to her as an intravenous injection. What will you do next?
5. After the patient receives the dose of furosemide, what will you do?

CHAPTER 2

Pharmacologic Principles

Chapter Review and NCLEX® Examination Preparation

Select the best answer for each question.

1. Number the following drug forms in order of speed of dissolution and absorption, with (1) being the fastest and (4) being the slowest:
   ____ a. Capsules
   ____ b. Enteric-coated tablets
   ____ c. Elixirs
   ____ d. Powders

2. When considering the various routes of drug elimination, the nurse is aware that elimination occurs mainly by which routes?
   a. Renal tubules and skin
   b. Skin and lungs
   c. Bowel and renal tubules
   d. Lungs and gastrointestinal tract

3. The nurse is aware that excessive drug dosages, poor circulation, impaired metabolism, or inadequate excretion may result in which drug effect?
   a. Tolerance
   b. Cumulative effect
   c. Incompatibility
   d. Antagonistic effect

4. Drug half-life is defined as the amount of time required for 50% of a drug to:
   a. be absorbed by the body.
   b. reach a therapeutic level.
   c. exert a response.
   d. be removed by the body.

5. The nurse recognizes that drugs given by which route will be altered by the first-pass effect?
   a. Oral
   b. Sublingual
   c. Subcutaneous
   d. Intravenous

6. If a drug binds with an enzyme and thereby prevents the enzyme from binding to its normal target cell, it will produce which effect?
   a. Receptor interaction
   b. Enzyme affinity
   c. Enzyme interaction
   d. Nonspecific interaction

7. A drug has a half-life of 4 hours. If at 0800 the drug level is measured as 200 mg/L, at what time would the drug level be 50 mg/L? ____________

Match each field of study with the corresponding job description of a person working in that field.

8. ____ Pharmaceutics
9. ____ Pharmacokinetics
10. ____ Pharmacodynamics
11. ____ Pharmacogenetics
12. ____ Pharmacotherapeutics
13. ____ Pharmacognosy
14. ____ Toxicology
15. ____ Pharmacoeconomics

a. Lisa is researching botanical and zoologic sources of drugs to treat multiple sclerosis. She is part of a university research team that is currently experimenting with varying the biochemical composition and therapeutic effects of several possible new drugs.
b. Jeffrey works for a pharmaceutical corporation. One of its new drugs looks very promising, and Jeffrey's company is experimenting with dosage forms for this investigational new drug. He is responsible for measuring the relationship between the physiochemical properties of the dosage form and the clinical therapeutic response.
c. Micah is performing a cost-benefit analysis to compare the effectiveness of two blood pressure medications for a health insurance company.
d. Devon researches various poisons and is particularly concerned with the detection and treatment of

the effects of drugs and other chemicals in certain mammals.

e. Diane and Phil have spent the last 3 years gathering family histories, legal case reports, and current clinical data to identify possible genetic factors that influence individuals' responses to meperidine and related drugs.
f. David works on a study that is gathering data on the use of two different drugs for the treatment of rheumatoid arthritis.
g. Michelle's research has taken her to Southeast Asia and Australia to participate in worldwide research on the treatment of a neoplastic disease that is more prevalent in the populations of those two regions.
h. Leslie's laboratory monitors drug distribution rates between various body compartments, from absorption through excretion. Recently, her laboratory was able to suggest a positive change in the dosage regimen for an injectable drug, bringing her firm a prestigious award.
i. Gregory's research unit recently recommended two new contraindications for the use of a newly marketed drug after discovering previously unknown biochemical and physiologic interactions of this drug with another unrelated drug.

Critical Thinking and Application

Answer the following questions on a separate sheet of paper.

16. Mr. C. is to receive a drug that can be given intramuscularly or subcutaneously. The order is written for the nurse to choose the route; however, Mr. C.'s condition dictates that the drug needs to be absorbed quickly. Which route of administration will the nurse choose? How can the nurse further increase absorption?

17. Ms. D. has had ovarian cancer for over a year. She is now in the late stages of her illness and is in severe pain. She has been admitted to a hospice unit and is receiving morphine through a patient-controlled analgesia pump. This is an example of which type of drug therapy: acute, maintenance, supplemental, or palliative? Explain your answer.

Case Study

Read the scenario and answer the following questions on a separate sheet of paper.

A 65-year-old man with liver cirrhosis is admitted to the medical-surgical unit with nausea and vomiting. He also has a diagnosis of heart failure. You note that his serum albumin (protein) level is low. The physician has written admission orders, and you are trying to make the patient comfortable. He is to take nothing by mouth except for clear liquids. An intravenous infusion of dextrose 5% in water at 50 mL/hr has been ordered, and the nurses have had difficulty inserting his intravenous (IV) line.

1. One of the drugs ordered is known to reach a maximum level in the body of 200 mg/L and has a half-life of 2 hours. If this maximum level of 200 mg/L is reached at 4 PM, then what will the drug's level in the body be at 10 PM?

2. Describe how factors identified in the patient's history would affect the following:
   a. Absorption
   b. Distribution
   c. Metabolism
   d. Excretion

3. Placement of a peripherally inserted central catheter is ordered. The physician writes an order for a dose of an IV antibiotic to be given as soon as IV access is established. What is the reason for this order?

4. This patient is also receiving digoxin (Lanoxin) for heart failure. This drug is known to have a low therapeutic index. Explain this concept.

CHAPTER 3

Life Span Considerations

Chapter Review and NCLEX® Examination Preparation

Select the best answer for each question.

1. Which physiologic factor is most responsible for the differences in the pharmacokinetic and pharmacodynamic behavior of drugs in neonates and adults?
   a. Infant's stature
   b. Infant's smaller weight
   c. Immaturity of neonatal organs
   d. Adult's longer exposure to toxins

2. A woman who has just discovered that she is pregnant is asking the nurse about taking medications. The nurse keeps in mind that the greatest risk for drug-induced developmental defects occurs during which trimester of pregnancy?
   a. First trimester
   b. Second trimester
   c. Third trimester
   d. The risk is the same throughout pregnancy.

3. Most drug references provide recommended pediatric dosages based on which of the following?
   a. Total body water content
   b. Fat-to-lean mass ratio
   c. Height
   d. Body weight

4. When considering drug dosages in older patients, the nurse recognizes that drug dosages in older adults should be based on which factor?
   a. More on age than on height or weight
   b. On body weight and organ function
   c. On the total body water content
   d. The strength of the drug

5. When giving medications to older adults, the nurse should keep in mind the changes that occur due to aging. Which statements regarding changes in the older patient are true? *(Select all that apply.)*
   a. Total body water content increases as body composition changes.
   b. Gastric pH is less acidic because of reduced hydrochloric acid production.
   c. Protein albumin binding sites are reduced because of decreased protein.
   d. Fat content is increased because of decreased lean body mass.
   e. The absorptive surface area of the gastrointestinal tract is increased due to flattening and blunting of the villi.

6. A child is to receive a medication that is dosed as 8 mg/kg. The child weighs 40 kg. What is the dose of medication that the nurse will administer to this child? ____________

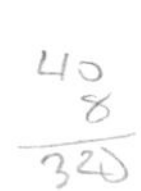

Match each pregnancy safety category with its corresponding description.

7. ______ Category A
8. ______ Category B
9. ______ Category C
10. ______ Category D
11. ______ Category X

a. Possible fetal risk in humans is reported; however, consideration of potential benefit versus risk may, in selected cases, warrant use of these drugs in pregnant women.
b. Studies indicate no risk to animal fetuses; information for humans is not available.
c. Fetal abnormalities are reported, and positive evidence of fetal risk in humans is available from animal and/or human studies.
d. Studies indicate no risk to the human fetus.
e. Adverse effects are reported in animal fetuses; information for humans is not available.

Critical Thinking and Application

Answer the following questions on a separate sheet of paper.

12. The nurse works at a community clinic frequented by a number of older patients. Mrs. M. comes to the clinic complaining of dizziness and nausea. As the nurse takes her medication history, she shows the nurse her "pill box." Inside the nurse sees almost a dozen different pills, all to be taken at noon. How could this happen? How could she possibly need so many medications at the same time?

13. The physician confirms that Mrs. M.'s "new symptoms," as she refers to them, are a result of polypharmacy. She protests, telling the nurse, "Honey, I've got news for the doctor. I've had to take lots of drugs at the same time all my life. It never bothered me before. Why would it now when I'm even more used to it?" Explain at least three physiologic changes that occur with aging and the way in which these changes affect pharmacokinetics and pharmacodynamics.

Case Study

Read the scenario and answer the following questions on a separate sheet of paper.

You are performing telephone triage in a pediatric clinic. A mother calls about her 28-month-old toddler, who has had chickenpox for 2 days. She wants to give aspirin because the toddler's fever is 101° F (38.3° C) but is unsure because her toddler "hates to take pills."

1. Should the mother use aspirin for this fever? Check a drug reference, if needed, for developmental considerations in this situation.

2. The mother states that her husband is going to the drugstore for some medicine. What advice will you give her regarding the dosage form of an antipyretic for her toddler?

3. When the husband returns from the store, he shows the mother the bottle of generic acetaminophen liquid suspension formula for children that was recommended by the store's pharmacist. He wonders, though, why the pharmacist would need to know the toddler's weight before suggesting this medication. Explain.

4. The toddler receives a dose of 1 teaspoon per the directions for a child of his weight of 28 pounds. Later, when his 5-year-old sister needs a dose, she receives 1.5 teaspoons because she weighs 45 pounds. If the drug contains 160 mg per teaspoon, then how many milligrams of medication did the 5-year-old receive in her dose?

5. What should the parents look for when evaluating the children's response to a dose of acetaminophen?

CHAPTER 4

Cultural, Legal, and Ethical Considerations

Chapter Review and NCLEX® Examination Preparation

Select the best answer for each question.

1. When reviewing drug classifications, the nurse knows that drugs classed as category C-I, which are to be dispensed "only with an approved protocol," include which drugs?
   a. Codeine, cocaine, and meperidine (Demerol)
   b. Heroin, LSD, and marijuana
   c. Phenobarbital, chloral hydrate, and benzodiazepines
   d. Cough preparations and diarrhea control drugs

2. When a health care provider is writing a prescription for a drug, he or she is not permitted to mark a refill on the prescription if the drug falls into which category?
   a. C-II
   b. C-III
   c. C-IV
   d. C-V

3. The nurse is aware that the ethical principle of "Do no harm" is known by which name?
   a. Autonomy
   b. Beneficence
   c. Confidentiality
   d. Nonmaleficence

4. Which legal act required drug manufacturers to establish the safety and efficacy of a new drug before its approval for use?
   a. Federal Food and Drugs Act of 1906
   b. Federal Food, Drug, and Cosmetic Act of 1938
   c. Kefauver-Harris Amendment of 1962
   d. Durham-Humphrey Amendment of 1951

5. Which is the correct definition for *placebo*?
   a. An investigational drug used in a new drug study
   b. An inert substance that is not a drug
   c. A legend drug that requires a prescription
   d. A substance that is not approved as a drug but is used as an herbal product

6. The nurse is performing an admission assessment. Which finding is considered part of the cultural assessment?
   a. The patient uses aspirin as needed for pain.
   b. The patient has a history of hypertension.
   c. The patient is allergic to shellfish.
   d. The patient does not eat pork products for religious reasons.

7. While reviewing a newsletter about medications, the nurse notices that one drug has a new black box warning from the Food and Drug Administration (FDA). What does this warning entail? *(Select all that apply.)*
   a. The drug is about to be recalled by the FDA.
   b. Serious adverse effects have been reported with the use of this drug.
   c. The drug can still be prescribed, but the warning is present to make sure that the prescriber is aware of the potential risks.
   d. The drug manufacturer has refused to recall the medication, despite documented problems.
   e. The drug cannot be prescribed.

8. The nurse is to administer ranitidine (Zantac) 150 mg IV. The available medication is ranitidine 25 mg/mL. How many mL will the nurse administer?

   ____6 mL____

Match each investigational drug study phase with its corresponding description.

9. __d__ Phase I
10. __a__ Phase II
11. __c__ Phase III
12. __b__ Phase IV

a. A study using small numbers of volunteers who have the disease or disorder that the drug is meant to diagnose or treat. Subjects are monitored for drug effectiveness and adverse effects.
b. Postmarketing studies conducted by drug companies to obtain further proof of the drug's therapeutic and adverse effects.
c. A study that involves a large number of patients at research centers designed to monitor for infrequent adverse effects and to identify any associated risks. Double-blind, placebo-controlled studies eliminate patient and researcher bias.
d. A study that uses small numbers of healthy volunteers, as opposed to volunteers with the target ailment, to determine dosage range and pharmacokinetics.

Match each cultural group with its corresponding cultural practice.

13. __c__ Asian
14. __a__ Hispanic
15. __d__ Native American
16. __b__ African

a. Some may seek a balance between the body and mind through the use of "cold" remedies or foods for "hot" illnesses, and vice versa.
b. Some may use folk medicine, protective bracelets, and laying on of hands.
c. Some believe that opposing forces lead to illness or health, depending on which force is dominant in the individual and whether the forces are balanced. Balance produces healthy states.
d. Some believe in the need for a balance among body, mind, and environment to maintain health and harmony with nature.

Critical Thinking and Application

Answer the following questions on a separate sheet of paper.

17. Identify a cultural group in the area in which you live and explore the health belief practices for that group.
    a. Are there any barriers to adequate health care?
    b. What is the attitude toward Western medicines and health treatments?
    c. What questions should you ask in your cultural assessment?

Case Study

Read the scenario and answer the following questions on a separate sheet of paper.

You work in an outpatient treatment clinic for patients with human immunodeficiency virus (HIV) infection. During a recent staff meeting, the medical director discussed a new drug that has shown good results in clinical trials in another country. This drug has not yet been tested in the United States. She stated that she hopes to start clinical trials of that drug in the HIV clinic.

The following week, you are asked to start a new drug regimen for four patients with HIV infection. One of the drugs is new to you, and when you ask about it, the medical director replies, "Oh, that's the new drug I mentioned last week! One of my colleagues in that country sent me some samples, so we're going to try it here. The Food and Drug Administration has already started trials here in the United States. We will be comparing how these four patients do compared with four other patients who are in the same stages of HIV infection. The patients won't even know about this change."

1. Should you give the drugs as requested? If not, what should be done to correct the situation?

2. What ethical principle(s) guide your decision?

3. One of the potential study patients, brought in by his brother, seems reluctant to answer questions and says he "doesn't need any drugs." Upon further questioning, you find out that he would prefer to take some home remedies that his mother has made for him. How will you handle this situation?

4. When you meet with potential study patients, several mention that they fear others will find out about their illness if they participate in the study. What will you tell these patients?

CHAPTER 5

Gene Therapy and Pharmacogenetics

Chapter Review and NCLEX® Examination Preparation

Match each definition with its corresponding term. (Note: Not all terms will be used.)

1. g A structure in the nucleus that contains a linear thread of DNA that transmits genetic information
2. f A term for all of the chromosomal material within a cell
3. b The biologic unit of heredity
4. c The complete set of genetic material of any organism
5. d The study of genomes, including the way genes and their products work in both health and disease

a. Allele
b. Gene
c. Genome
d. Genomics
e. Genetics
f. Chromatin
g. Chromosome

Critical Thinking and Application

Answer the following questions on a separate sheet of paper.

6. What is DNA, and what is its primary purpose?
7. What was the goal of the Human Genome Project?
8. Name two effects of the Human Genome Project.
9. What is recombinant DNA, and how is this technology useful in pharmacology?
10. Explain the purpose of gene therapy. Has it been approved in the United States for routine treatment of disease?

Case Study

Read the scenario and answer the following questions on a separate sheet of paper.

Dale, a 32-year-old construction worker, fell off a roof 2 months ago and, as a result, needs to have surgery on his ankle. The nurse is preparing him for the surgery and begins the admission process. During the interview, Dale mentions that he is a bit nervous because his cousin had surgery and had a "terrible reaction" to the medications.

1. Is this information about his cousin significant? Explain.
2. What further questions will the nurse ask?
3. When obtaining a genetic history, how many generations back should the nurse ask about?
4. What will be done about Dale's surgery?

CHAPTER 6

Medication Errors: Preventing and Responding

Chapter Review and NCLEX® Examination Preparation

Provide the best answer for each question.

1. A(n) medication error is defined as any preventable adverse drug event that involves inappropriate medication use by a patient or health care professional. It may or may not cause harm to the patient.

2. A(n) idiosyncratic reaction is defined as any abnormal and unexpected response to a medication, other than an allergic reaction, that is peculiar to an individual patient.

3. A(n) allergic reaction is an immunologic hypersensitivity reaction resulting from an unusual sensitivity of a patient to a particular medication.

4. A(n) adverse drug reaction is a type of adverse drug event that is defined as any unexpected, unintended, undesired, or excessive response to a medication given at therapeutic dosages.

5. A(n) adverse drug event is an undesirable occurrence related to administration of or failure to administer a prescribed medication.

6. True or (false): High-alert medications are involved in more errors than other drugs.

7. True or (false): All adverse drug events are caused by medication errors.

8. Identify six ways to avoid medication errors.

9. Name at least four of the classes of medications that are considered "high alert" drugs.

10. The National Coordinating Council for Medication Error Reporting and Prevention recommends that certain terms be written out in full instead of being abbreviated. Write out the full meaning of each abbreviated word or phrase that appears in bold in the following list.

Digoxin 125 **mcg** PO now	micrograms
Lasix 40 mg IV **qd**	every day
d/c all meds	discontinue
NPH insulin 12 **u** subcut **ac** breakfast **qAM**	unit every morning
Floxin Otic 1 **gtt AD** bid	drop right ear
Zolpidem 5 mg PO at **HS** as needed	bedtime

11. The medication order reads: "Metoprolol 25 mg PO twice a day for high blood pressure. Hold if systolic blood pressure is less than 95 mm Hg." Today the pharmacy supplied 50-mg tablets because there were no 25-mg tablets in stock.

    a. How many tablets will the nurse administer per dose? 1/2

    b. The nurse gives the patient the entire tablet. How many mg does the patient receive? 50mg

    c. What will the nurse do next? call the doctor

Case Study

Read the scenario and answer the following questions on a separate sheet of paper.

A nursing student discovers that she has given her patient two aspirin tablets instead of the one-tablet daily dose that was ordered for antiplatelet effects. She is upset and talks to her fellow students, who tell her to keep quiet about it. "One extra aspirin won't hurt your patient," they tell her.

1. What should the nursing student do first? Describe other appropriate actions after this.

2. How could the student have prevented this error?

3. Should the patient be told about it? Explain your answer.

4. If the patient was not hurt by this incident, then is it considered a medication error? Explain.

5. The student has decided to inform her instructor. The instructor helps the student complete a report to the U.S. Pharmacopeia Medication Errors Reporting Program. Explain the reason for this report. Will the student's name be reported?

CHAPTER 7

Patient Education and Drug Therapy

Chapter Review and NCLEX® Examination Preparation

1. A nurse is preparing for an education session on safe medication administration. Which is the best example of a learning activity that involves the cognitive domain?
   a. Teaching a patient how to self-administer nasal spray
   b. Teaching a patient how to measure the pulse before taking digoxin
   c. Discussing which foods to avoid while taking oral anticoagulants
   d. Teaching a family member how to give an injection

2. The nurse is developing a discharge plan regarding a patient's medications. When is the most ideal time to begin discharge planning?
   a. When family members are present
   b. Just before the patient leaves the hospital
   c. When the patient has been medicated for pain
   d. As soon as possible when the patient is ready

Critical Thinking and Application

Answer the following questions on a separate sheet of paper.

3. The nurse is to present information regarding antihypertensive drug therapy to two patients, a 40-year-old and a 78-year-old. Describe the differences in interventions the nurse would use in his or her teaching strategies related to possible alterations in thought processes and sensory-perceptual status in these two patients.

4. The nurse is to present information to a young mother on how to help her 8-year-old child use a metered-dose inhaler. Neither the mother nor her child speaks English. Discuss strategies the nurse will use in developing a teaching plan for them.

5. The patient has been taking oral hypoglycemics for 1 month, and her blood glucose readings are still very high. On assessment, the nurse discovers a possible reason for these high readings. Develop a nursing diagnosis for this patient based on the following:
   a. The patient says that no-one has ever told her about required dietary restrictions.
   b. The patient tells the nurse that she only takes the medication if she feels ill.

6. For each of the following medications, develop a measurable goal and specific outcome criteria related to teaching a patient about the medication therapy. Use later chapters in the textbook for reference.
   a. Oral contraceptives
   b. Diuretic therapy with furosemide (Lasix)
   c. metformin (Glucophage)
   d. Transdermal nitroglycerin patches
   e. indomethacin (Indocin)

7. Develop a patient teaching plan for a 55-year-old patient who will be receiving warfarin (Coumadin) therapy after discharge. Refer to the appropriate chapter in the text for information. Include the following:
   a. Assessment—the objective and subjective data that would be needed
   b. Nursing diagnosis
   c. Planning—a measurable goal and outcome criteria
   d. Implementation—specific educational strategies
   e. Evaluation—means for validating that learning has occurred

8. A patient has been instructed to take 25 mg of diphenhydramine (Benadryl) oral syrup twice a day as treatment for a severe case of poison ivy. The medication comes in a bottle that contains 12.5 mg/5 mL. The nurse will be teaching the patient how to measure a dose of the medication. How many mL will he measure for each dose? 10 mL

Case Study

Read the scenario and answer the following questions on a separate sheet of paper.

A 77-year-old male, accompanied by his wife, visits the office for a 3-month checkup. He has been treated for hypertension and has a history of angina. While in the office, he pulls a small bottle of sublingual nitroglycerin tablets from his pants pocket and states, "I never go anywhere without these." He says he "gets along okay" with his medicines at home and that it "doesn't hurt anything" if he misses a day or two of his medications. His blood pressure today is 130/92 mm Hg, pulse rate is 88 beats/min, and respiratory rate is 12 breaths/min. Previously, his blood pressure readings have been 160/98, 152/92, and 148/94 mm Hg.

After the patient is evaluated by the physician, new medication orders are written as follows:

- HCTZ, 25-mg tablet, once a day
- potassium chloride (K-Dur), 20 mEq tablet, once a day
- diltiazem (Cardizem), 60-mg tablet, three times a day
- lansoprazole (Prevacid), 15-mg capsule, before breakfast and dinner
- nitroglycerin sublingual tablets, as needed for chest pain

1. Based on your assessment, what nursing diagnosis would you suggest for this situation?
2. State a goal and outcome criteria for your nursing diagnosis.
3. Describe the teaching strategies you would use when teaching this patient about how to take his medications correctly.
4. How would you evaluate the effectiveness of the education process in this situation?

CHAPTER 8

Over-the-Counter Drugs and Herbal and Dietary Supplements

Critical Thinking Crossword

Each statement refers to an herbal product that is described in this text. For reference, see "Herbal Therapies and Dietary Supplements" on the inside back cover of your text.

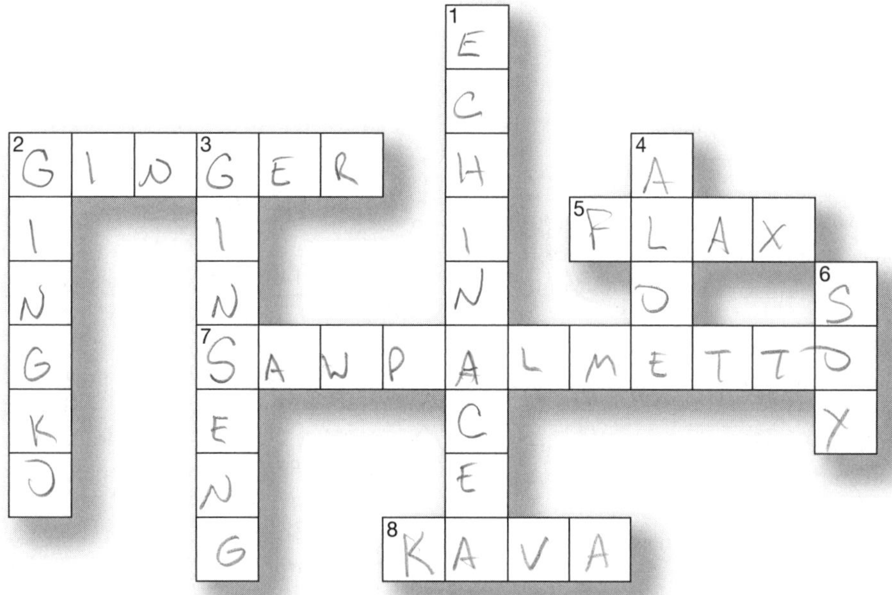

Across

2. Used for relief of nausea and vomiting induced by cancer chemotherapy, morning sickness, and motion sickness.
5. Both the seed and the oil of this plant are used to reduce high cholesterol levels.
7. Used to relieve the symptoms of benign prostatic hyperplasia (two words).
8. Used to help promote relaxation or sleep. However, prolonged use may cause yellow discoloration of nails and skin and a risk of liver toxicity.

Down

1. Used for its immunostimulant effect to reduce cold symptoms and recovery time when taken early in the illness.
2. The dried leaf of this plant is used by some to prevent organic brain syndrome.
3. Has been used for over 5000 years to improve physical endurance and concentration, and reduce stress.
4. The topical application of this plant has been known for years to aid in wound healing.
6. Used by women for relief of menopause symptoms, as an alternative to hormonal therapy.

Chapter Review and NCLEX® Examination Preparation

Select the best answer for each question.

1. Which drug classes are commonly used as over-the-counter (OTC) remedies? *(Select all that apply.)*
   a. Nonsteroidal antiinflammatory drugs
   b. Cold remedies
   c. Antibiotics
   d. Smoking deterrent systems
   e. Antihypertensive drugs
   f. Histamine-2 (H_2) blockers

2. Which is an advantage of OTC remedies?
   a. Third-party health insurance payers usually cover the costs.
   b. Patients can feel better faster when self-medicating.
   c. There are fewer drug interactions.
   d. Patients can self-treat minor ailments and reduce physician visits.

3. A patient is discussing his wish to use herbal products instead of medications and exclaims, "They are safe! The government tests them!" How will the nurse respond?
   a. "The U.S. Food and Drug Administration does enforce standards of herbal product quality and safety."
   b. "The U.S. Food and Drug Administration does require the manufacturers of herbal products to prove that the herbals are effective."
   c. "The U.S. government sets standards for quality control of herbal products."
   d. "In the U.S., herbal products are classified as dietary supplements and do not undergo testing for safety or effectiveness."

4. A patient is asking about taking omega-3 fatty acids to reduce his cholesterol levels because he has a family history of coronary artery disease. Which nursing diagnosis is most appropriate for this patient?
   a. Noncompliance
   b. Health-seeking behavior
   c. Decreased cardiac output
   d. Risk for constipation

5. The nurse is admitting a patient who has a diagnosis of right lower lobe pneumonia. Upon assessment, the nurse learns that the patient is wearing an herbal pack on her chest. What will the nurse do first?
   a. Remove the pack immediately.
   b. Report the pack to the physician.
   c. Ask the patient about the herbal pack.
   d. Document the presence of the herbal pack.

6. A construction worker is treating himself with acetaminophen after an injury on the job. After 2 days, he comes to the urgent care facility because he thinks his hand is broken. He tells the nurse that he has been taking two "extra-strength" acetaminophen tablets six times a day but he still has pain. Each tablet is 1000 mg. How many mg per day has he taken?
   12,000 mg per day

7. Is there a concern regarding the construction worker's acetaminophen intake (see question 6)? Explain.
   toxic to the liver

Critical Thinking and Application

Answer the following questions on a separate sheet of paper.

8. Review the herbal boxes for garlic, ginger, ginseng, flax, saw palmetto, ginkgo, and valerian in the appropriate chapters. (See "Herbal Therapies and Dietary Supplements" located inside the back cover of the textbook.) Which of these herbal products may have serious interactions with anticoagulants such as warfarin (Coumadin) and heparin?

9. List the types of individuals who may have more frequent adverse reactions to OTC drugs.

10. Identify an OTC product or herbal or dietary supplement that you (or a family member) take and review the indications, drug interactions, contraindications, and adverse effects. Did you find any concerns?

Case Study

Read the scenario and answer the following questions on a separate sheet of paper. You may need to refer to "Herbal Therapies and Dietary Supplements" on the inside back cover of your text.

A 30-year-old woman is in the clinic for her yearly gynecologic checkup. She is not pregnant but would like to have children soon and states that she and her husband are trying to conceive. She says that she is "very concerned" about her health, and watches her diet and exercises regularly to stay in shape. She has a family history of heart disease but no other health concerns. Her physical assessment reveals no abnormalities or health problems.

On her medical history sheet, she writes that she takes several drug and herbal products as follows:

- Echinacea, from September to March, to prevent the flu
- Adult aspirin, one tablet every day, to prevent a heart attack
- Garlic tablets twice a day for my heart
- Kava tea, as needed for relaxation
- One glass of red wine with dinner
- Valerian capsules for sleep, as needed (usually three or four times a week)

1. Does the patient's regimen of drugs and herbal products pose any risk for drug or herbal interactions?

2. Do any of these products have a potential for problems if used long-term?

3. Is there any specific information on which you should focus in taking the patient's history or performing an assessment, given that she is using these drugs and herbal products?

4. She tells you that she thinks the herbal products are "safe" because the government would not allow them to be sold if they were not. Is this true?

5. What would you emphasize when teaching her about the use of herbal products and OTC drugs?

CHAPTER 9

Substance Abuse

Chapter Review and NCLEX® Examination Preparation

Match each drug with its corresponding description.

1. ______ cocaine
2. ______ ecstasy
3. ______ flumazenil (Romazicon)
4. ______ heroin
5. ______ disulfiram (Antabuse)
6. ______ nicotine
7. ______ naltrexone (ReVia)
8. ______ bupropion (Zyban)
9. ______ opium
10. ______ "roofies"

a. A nicotine-free treatment for nicotine dependence
b. Known as the "date rape" drug
c. The source plant for heroin
d. The addictive chemical in tobacco products
e. An opioid that is injected by "mainlining" or "skin popping"
f. Used to antagonize the action of benzodiazepines and reverse sedation
g. Used to deter the use of alcohol during alcohol abuse treatment
h. A stimulant that is either "snorted" through the nasal passages or injected intravenously
i. A stimulant that is popular at "raves" with college-age students
j. An opioid antagonist used for opioid abuse or dependence

Select the best answer for each question.

11. A patient who has been taking disulfiram (Antabuse) therapy for 3 months has been off the therapy for 2 days. He decides to go out with friends to have a beer. What effects may he experience?
    a. No ill effects
    b. Diarrhea
    c. Vomiting
    d. Euphoria

12. During an information session about drug abuse, the nurse relates that the most common drug effects that lead to abuse of opioids include:
    a. hallucinations.
    b. sleep.
    c. stimulation.
    d. relaxation and euphoria.

13. The nurse is assisting a patient who is experiencing opioid withdrawal and anticipates the possible use of which medications? *(Select all that apply.)*
    a. disulfiram (Antabuse)
    b. clonidine (Catapres)
    c. methadone
    d. bupropion (Zyban)
    e. naltrexone (ReVia)

14. When teaching a patient about drug interactions, the nurse is aware that combining benzodiazepines with ethanol or barbiturates may lead to death due to:
    a. cardiac dysrhythmia.
    b. convulsions.
    c. respiratory arrest.
    d. stroke.

15. A patient with a known history of chronic excessive ingestion of ethanol has developed memory problems and comes to the health clinic with hard-to-believe stories of what has happened to him. The nurse recognizes that these symptoms are associated with which disorder?
    a. Cerebrovascular accident
    b. Korsakoff's psychosis
    c. Narcolepsy
    d. Bipolar disorder

Critical Thinking and Application

Answer the following questions on a separate sheet of paper.

16. Describe how nicotine is used to ease withdrawal from nicotine use. Compare the use of bupropion (Zyban) and varenicline (Chantix) in smoking cessation programs.

17. How is medication therapy different for mild, moderate, and severe alcohol withdrawal?

18. A woman brings her teenage daughter into the emergency department. The teen is lethargic, dizzy, and has been vomiting. While the teen is being examined and stabilized, the mother tells the nurse that her daughter told her that she and her friends used cough syrup to get high. The mother states, "How could cough syrup do this?" What is the nurse's best answer?

Case Study

Read the scenario and answer the following questions on a separate sheet of paper.

A 19-year-old male, Mr. C., is admitted to the emergency department after he collapsed at a fraternity party. The paramedics state that there were beer-drinking contests at the party, and it is unknown how much Mr. C. had to drink. His friend says that Mr. C. was upset over breaking up with a girlfriend and he was worried about how heavily Mr. C. has been drinking in the past 2 weeks.

Mr. C. is semiconscious but unable to answer questions coherently, and his speech is slurred. His blood pressure is 100/58 mm Hg, his pulse rate is 110 beats/min, and his breathing is heavy with a respiratory rate of 16 breaths/min. He vomited on the way to the hospital.

1. Is ethanol considered a central nervous system stimulant or depressant?

2. What are the effects of severe alcoholic intoxication on the cardiovascular and respiratory systems?

3. The patient is admitted to the medical unit for observation. For what should the nurse be observant at this time?

4. The next evening, Mr. C. is more alert but still unsteady in his gait. He says he wants to go home, but you notice fine tremors of his hands. Should he be discharged at this time? Explain.

5. If Mr. C. continues the pattern of heavy drinking, what effects could the chronic ingestion of ethanol have on his body?

CHAPTER 10

Photo Atlas of Drug Administration

Chapter Review and NCLEX® Examination Preparation

Select the best answer for each question.

1. When giving intradermal injections, what will the nurse remember to do?
   a. Massage the site lightly after the injection.
   b. Have the patient massage the site until the pain diminishes.
   c. Avoid massaging the site.
   d. Apply heat to the site after the injection.

2. When giving a medication via intravenous push, how will the nurse correctly occlude the intravenous line?
   a. By pinching or clamping the tubing just above the injection port
   b. By pinching the tubing at least 2 inches above the injection port
   c. By folding the tubing just above the injection port
   d. It is not necessary to occlude the tubing for this procedure.

3. The nurse is adding more than one medication to a solution. What action is most important at this time?
   a. Use an equal volume of each medication.
   b. Assess the two drugs for compatibility.
   c. Add the drugs at least 1 hour apart.
   d. Use the same needle for both medications.

4. When administering oral medications, the nurse will follow which correct procedure?
   a. If a patient cannot swallow medications, crush all the medications together and administer with applesauce.
   b. Give oral medications with meals to avoid gastrointestinal upset.
   c. Stay with the patient until each medication has been swallowed.
   d. Give all medications on an empty stomach to facilitate absorption.

5. When administering eardrops, which action by the nurse is correct?
   a. Press a cotton ball firmly into the ear canal after giving the drops.
   b. Have the patient sit up and tilt the head for 2 to 3 minutes.
   c. Gently massage the tragus of the ear.
   d. Have the patient remain in the side-lying position for 20 minutes.

6. Which position is correct when the nurse administers nasal drops for the frontal or maxillary sinuses?
   a. Tilt the patient's head backward and facing toward the left side.
   b. Tilt the patient's head back over the edge of the bed with the head turned toward the side treated.
   c. Place a pillow under the patient's shoulders and tilt the head back.
   d. Tilt the patient's head to the side opposite the side treated.

7. Which action by the nurse is most correct when administering drugs via a nasogastric tube?
   a. Allow the fluid to flow via gravity.
   b. Use gentle but consistent pressure when forcing the fluid into the tube.
   c. Shake the tube gently to facilitate the movement of fluid in the tube.
   d. Confirm placement of the tube after the medication is given.

8. Z-track intramuscular injections are indicated in which situation?
   a. When there is insufficient muscle mass in the landmarked area
   b. Whenever massaging the area after medication administration is contraindicated
   c. With medications that are known to be irritating, painful, and/or staining to tissues
   d. With any injection that is given into the dorsogluteal muscle

9. When giving sublingual medications, the nurse recalls that medications given by this route have which advantage?
   a. They are immediately absorbed.
   b. They are excreted rapidly.
   c. They are metabolized immediately.
   d. They are distributed equally.

10. The prochlorperazine (Compazine) rectal suppository is twice the strength of what has actually been ordered. Which is the nurse's best action?
    a. Cut the suppository in half.
    b. Call the physician for clarification.
    c. Administer another type of suppository.
    d. Instruct the patient to retain the suppository for only 5 minutes.

11. During medication administration, which will the nurse consider to be a contraindication to the administration of rectal suppositories?
    a. Vomiting
    b. Fever
    c. Constipation
    d. Rectal bleeding

12. The nurse will apply a transdermal patch to a site that is:
    a. hairy.
    b. nonhairy.
    c. moist.
    d. within a skinfold.

13. Which is important for the nurse to teach the patient about the instillation of nasal drops?
    a. Clear the nasal passages by blowing the nose gently before administering the medication.
    b. Clear the nasal passages by blowing the nose gently after administering the medication.
    c. Sit in a semi-Fowler's position for 5 minutes after the instillation of the medication.
    d. Place the nose dropper approximately 1/2 inch into the nostril when instilling drops.

14. The nurse is administering ophthalmic medications. Which interventions are correct regarding the administration of ophthalmic medications? *(Select all that apply.)*
    a. Have the patient look upward while instilling the medication.
    b. Instill the prescribed number of drops into the conjunctival sac.
    c. Have the patient close his or her eyes tightly after the drop has been instilled.
    d. Apply gentle pressure to the patient's nasolacrimal duct for 30 to 60 seconds after instilling the drops.
    e. Apply ointment to the conjunctival sac starting at the outer canthus and working toward the inner canthus.

15. When withdrawing medication from a vial, the nurse needs to remove 1 mL for the medication dosage. How much air will the nurse inject into the vial before removing the medication? 1 mL

Critical Thinking and Application

Answer the following questions on a separate sheet of paper.

16. Describe how to assess injection sites for each of the following:
    a. Subcutaneous injections
    b. Intramuscular injections
    c. Intradermal injections

17. Describe the proper technique of needle insertion for each of the following:
    a. Subcutaneous injections
    b. Intramuscular injections
    c. Intradermal injections

18. You are administering an intramuscular injection to your patient. After the needle enters the site, you grasp the lower end of the syringe barrel with your nondominant hand and slowly pull back on the plunger to aspirate the drug. Blood appears in the syringe. What is the best action at this time?

19. You are preparing an oral liquid medication for a patient. How does the usual procedure change when the volume of medication required is less than 5 mL?

20. A patient has been given a new inhaler that contains 100 doses of medication. The order specifies that the patient is to take "one puff four times a day." How many days will this inhaler last before it becomes empty?

Case Study

Read the scenario and answer the following questions on a separate sheet of paper.

A mother comes to a family practice office with her 2-year-old daughter and 8-month-old son. She is planning a trip abroad and needs to obtain immunizations for herself and her children before she leaves.

1. The mother and the infant each need to be given an intramuscular immunization. Describe the differences in choosing sites and giving an intramuscular injection in the mother and the infant.

2. The 2-year-old daughter has an ear infection and the physician has prescribed eardrops. What should you teach the mother about giving these eardrops to her child?

3. Two days later, the mother brings the infant back to the office because she has developed a high fever. You prepare to give the infant a liquid oral antipyretic and note that the dose is 4 mL. How do you measure this medication?

4. The mother wants to add the medication to her baby's bottle. What is the best method for administering this liquid medication to the infant?

CHAPTER 11

Analgesic Drugs

Critical Thinking Crossword

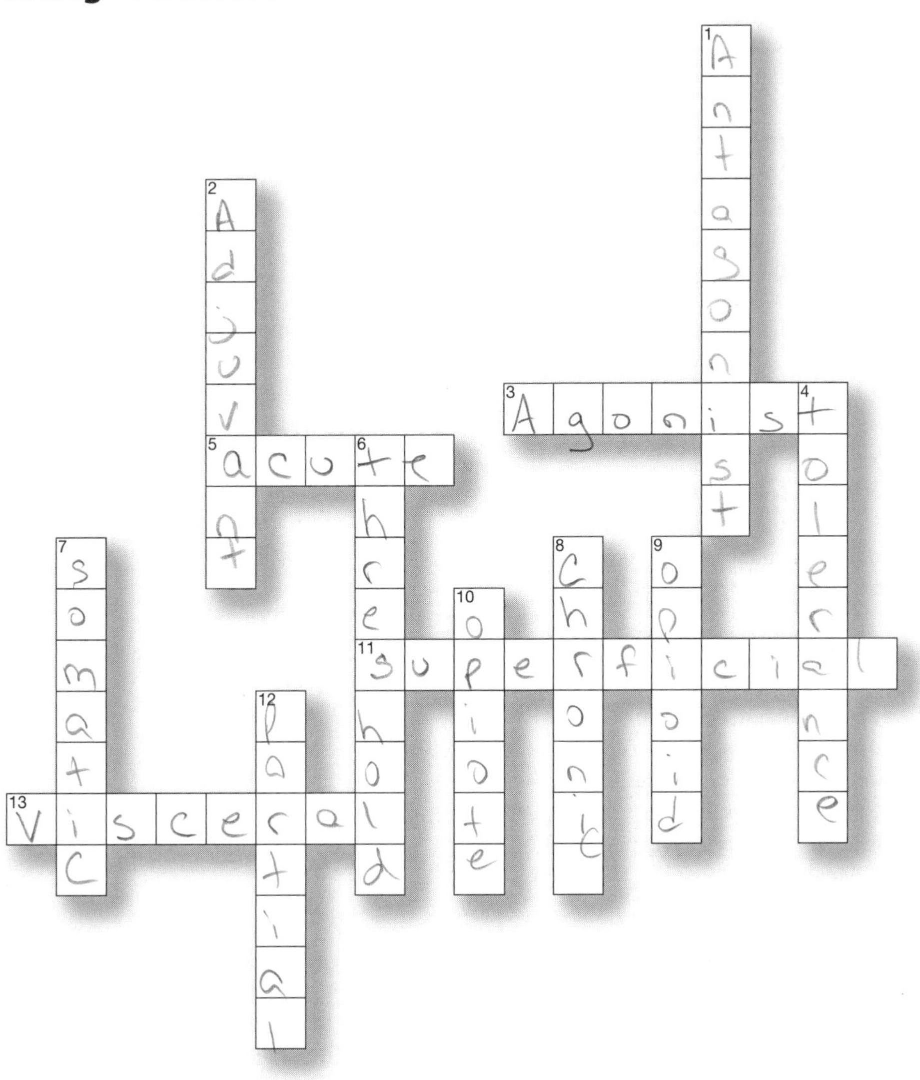

Across

3. Any drug that binds to a receptor and causes a response has __________ properties.
5. Mrs. M. had breast reduction surgery yesterday and is complaining of pain around her incisions. Mrs. M. is experiencing ___________ pain.
11. Mrs. G. is experiencing pain and itching due to a severe case of poison ivy on the skin of her arms and legs. She is experiencing __________ pain.
13. Mr. E. paces the floor all night, holding his side. The pain is so severe that he is sick to his stomach. His wife brings him to the emergency department, where it is quickly discovered that Mr. E. has a kidney stone. The type of pain he has been experiencing is __________ pain.

Down

1. Mr. D.'s drug binds to a receptor but causes an effect opposite to that of the type of drug discussed in 3 Across. He is taking a drug with __________ properties.
2. Mr. V. has been taking an opioid pain reliever for a week. When his pain level increases, the drug is not as effective. He is given a second analgesic drug in addition to the first drug. "Two pain killers?" he asks you. "Is that safe?" You explain that the second drug is not a primary analgesic but has properties that will add to the analgesic effects of the opioid. It is being used, then, as a(n) __________ drug.
4. Mr. R., described in 9 Down, is recovering. He requires continued pain management and has found that he needs more medication for the same pain relief. Mr. R. is describing his level of pain __________.
6. Ms. L. was in an auto accident and injured her leg. In assessing the level of a stimulus applied to her toe that results in a perception of pain, you are testing her pain __________.
7. Mr. J. has injured his ankle in a friendly basketball game with his peers after work. His wife brings him to the urgent care center several hours later because of the pain. Mr. J. is probably experiencing __________ pain.
8. Mrs. H. has experienced back pain "for years." She says that it is worse in the late afternoon and at night but that "really, even when it lessens somewhat, it is there all the time in some form." Mrs. H. is experiencing __________ pain.
9. Mr. R. is brought to the emergency department in tremendous pain. The emergency department team recognizes the need to immediately bring the pain under some control to make assessment, diagnosis, and treatment more manageable. After assessing that it is not contraindicated, the attending physician initiates administration of a very strong and addicting pain reliever. This is no doubt a(n) __________ analgesic.
10. This word is often used interchangeably with the term *opioid.*
12. Ms. T. is taking a drug that binds to part of a receptor and causes effects that are not as strong as those of a pure agonist. She is taking a(n) __________ agonist.

Chapter Review and NCLEX® Examination Preparation

Select the best answer for each question.

1. During a marathon, a runner had to drop out after 16 miles because of severe muscle spasms. Which type of pain is the runner experiencing?
   a. Chronic pain
   b. Somatic pain
   c. Visceral pain
   d. Superficial pain

2. A young man has been taken to the emergency department because of a suspected overdose of morphine tablets. The nurse prepares to administer which drug?
   a. meperidine (Demerol)
   b. naproxen (Naprosyn)
   c. aspirin
   d. naloxone (Narcan)

3. An anticonvulsant drug has been ordered as part of a patient's pain management program. The nurse explains to the patient that the purpose of the anticonvulsant is to:
   a. produce sleep.
   b. prevent seizures.
   c. relieve neuropathic pain.
   d. reduce anxiety.

4. Moderate to severe pain is best treated with which medication(s)?
   a. acetaminophen (Tylenol)
   b. naloxone (Narcan)
   c. alprazolam (Xanax)
   d. fentanyl (Duragesic)

5. The nurse is preparing to administer an opioid analgesic. Which factors should be assessed before the dose is given? *(Select all that apply.)*
   a. Blood clotting times
   b. The level of pain rated on a scale
   c. Prior analgesic use (time, type, amount, and effectiveness)
   d. Dietary history
   e. Allergies

6. A postoperative patient is complaining of pain at a level of 7 on a 1–10 scale. The nurse checks the medication administration sheet and sees that the patient can receive morphine oral solution (Roxanol) 6 mg PO every 4 hours, and the patient has not had a dose for 8 hours. The medication comes in a 5-mL unit dose container that is labeled 10 mg per 5 mL. How many mL will the nurse administer to the patient? ______3 mL______

Match each type of pain with its corresponding description.

7. F Acute pain
8. E Chronic pain
9. H Somatic pain
10. G Visceral pain
11. C Superficial pain
12. A Vascular pain
13. I Neuropathic pain
14. B Phantom pain
15. D Central pain

a. Pain that is thought to account for most migraine headaches
b. Pain that relates to a body part that has been removed
c. Pain that originates from the skin or mucous membranes
d. Pain that occurs with tumors, trauma, or inflammation of the brain
e. Persistent or recurring pain that is often difficult to treat
f. Pain that is sudden and usually subsides when treated
g. Pain that originates from the organs or smooth muscles
h. Pain that originates from the skeletal muscles, ligaments, or joints
i. Pain that results from injury or damage to the peripheral nerve fibers

Case Study

Read the scenario and answer the following questions on a separate sheet of paper.

A 58-year-old woman has been admitted for surgery to remove a small growth from her lower back, just under the skin. That evening she asks for pain medication. Upon assessment, you find that she rates her pain level as an "8" on a scale from 1–10 and states that her pain is located mainly in the immediate area around her incision. You prepare to give her an intravenous dose of morphine sulfate.

1. What type of pain is she experiencing?
2. What nonpharmacologic intervention may be used to reduce her pain?
3. Within an hour of receiving the morphine, the patient complains that her skin feels "itchy" but she cannot see any hives. What do you tell her?
4. What serious adverse effect is possible if she receives too much morphine sulfate? What, if anything, can be given to treat this?
5. Two days later she is ready to be discharged home. Her physician writes a prescription for hydrocodone/acetaminophen (Vicodin). The patient sees the generic label and asks why the medication contains Tylenol. Explain the purpose of the acetaminophen (Tylenol) in this medication and for her pain treatment.

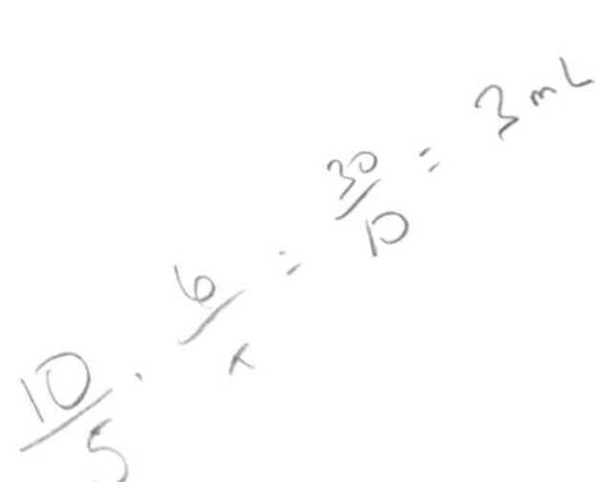

CHAPTER 12

General and Local Anesthetics

Critical Thinking Crossword

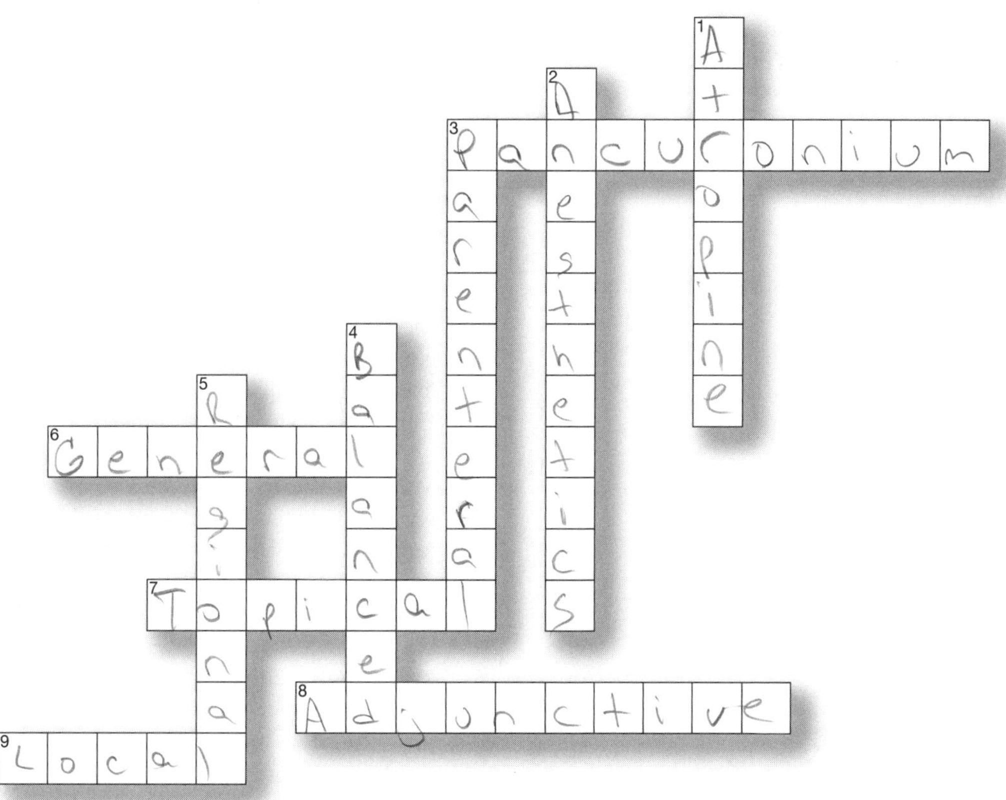

Across

3. A commonly used, long-acting, nondepolarizing neuromuscular blocking drug (NMBD).
6. Anesthetic drugs that alter the central nervous system (CNS), resulting in loss of consciousness and deep muscle relaxation, are termed __________ anesthetics
7. __________ anesthetics are applied directly to the skin and mucous membranes.
8. Drugs used in combination with anesthetics for anesthesia initiation (induction), sedation, reduction of anxiety, and amnesia
9. Drugs that reduce pain sensations at the level of peripheral nerves are called __________ anesthetics

Down

1. An anticholinergic drug given preoperatively to dry secretions
2. A broad term for drugs that depress the CNS
3. Anesthetic drugs that are given intravenously are also called __________ drugs.
4. The practice of using combinations of drugs to produce general anesthesia rather than using a single drug
5. Another name for 9 Across

Chapter Review and NCLEX® Examination Preparation

Select the best answer for each question.

1. Which drug classes are used as adjunctive drugs with anesthesia? *(Select all that apply.)*
   a. Sedative-hypnotics
   b. Anticonvulsants
   c. Anticholinergics
   d. Inhaled gas
   e. Opioid analgesics

2. While assisting with a procedure in the emergency department, the nurse prepares lidocaine (Xylocaine) for use with which type of anesthesia?
   a. Spinal
   b. Local
   c. Intravenous
   d. General

3. The nurse monitoring a patient after surgery keeps in mind that the primary concern with use of a neuromuscular blocking drug is which adverse effect?
   a. Respiratory arrest
   b. Headache
   c. Bradycardia
   d. Hypertension

4. To decrease the possibility of a headache after spinal anesthesia, the nurse will provide which instruction to the patient?
   a. Sit in high Fowler's position.
   b. Maintain strict bedrest.
   c. Limit fluids.
   d. Ambulate in the hall several times a day.

5. The nurse is reviewing a policy for local anesthesia. Local anesthesia is indicated for which procedures? *(Select all that apply.)*
   a. Cardioversions
   b. Suturing a skin laceration
   c. Diagnostic procedures
   d. Long-duration surgery
   e. Dental procedures

6. A patient who has just returned from surgery has suddenly developed a severe elevation in body temperature. The nurse recognizes that this change may indicate which condition?
   a. A normal temperature change after surgery
   b. Malignant hypertension
   c. Malignant hyperthermia
   d. Fever

7. A patient is receiving a neuromuscular blocking drug. Indicate the order in which the following areas become paralyzed once this drug is given (1 = first, 3 = last).
   ______ a. Limbs, neck, trunk muscles
   ______ b. Intercostal muscles and diaphragm
   ______ c. Small, rapidly moving muscles, such as those of the fingers and eyes

8. A patient has an order to receive atropine sulfate, 0.4 mg IM, as a preoperative medication. The vial contains atropine sulfate, 1 mg/mL. How many mL of medication will the nurse draw up for this injection?
   ____

Critical Thinking and Application

Answer the following questions on a separate sheet of paper.

9. Henry is a student nurse who has assisted the nurse anesthetist in surgery on prior occasions. Today, however, he is nervous because it is a child who will undergo general anesthesia. Why might this make Henry more nervous than usual?

10. Mr. S. is being administered a neuromuscular blocking drug while he is receiving mechanical ventilation. What is the most important thing the nurse needs to remember when working with him during this therapy?

11. Mrs. E. will undergo cardioversion this afternoon, and the nurse anesthetist has explained to her that she will not be asleep but that she will not remember the procedure. Mrs. E. asks, "How can this be?" What is the nurse anesthetist's explanation?

Case Study

Read the scenario and answer the following questions on a separate sheet of paper.

You are a nursing student, and today you are assigned to an observation day in the operating room, with a certified registered nurse anesthetist (CRNA) as your contact for the day. The first case is a patient undergoing a right lower lung lobectomy due to lung cancer. The patient has a history of paraplegia from an old automobile accident. The patient's blood pressure has been maintained at 120/72 mm Hg, and the pulse has ranged from 100 to 110 beats/min during the surgery. The patient's body temperature has lowered to 96.2° F (35.7° C) after surgery. The patient's respiration has been maintained by ventilator.

1. Before the surgery, the CRNA explained that the patient will undergo “balanced anesthesia.” What is meant by this term?

2. What is the purpose of administering the drug succinylcholine (Anectine) during anesthesia?

3. As your patient goes to the postanesthesia care unit (PACU), the CRNA asks you to monitor for signs of succinylcholine toxicity. Why would this be of concern at this time?

4. What can be done if the patient has received too much succinylcholine?

5. Another patient is undergoing a procedure performed using local anesthesia. Are there advantages of this type of anesthesia over general anesthesia?

6. In the PACU, what are the main concerns of the nurse monitoring the patient recovering from anesthesia?

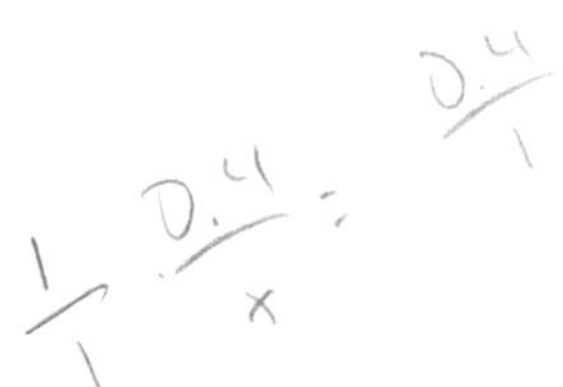

1. Before the surgery, the CRNA explained that the patient will undergo “balanced anesthesia.” What is meant by this term?

2. What is the purpose of administering the drug succinylcholine (Anectine) during anesthesia?

3. As your patient goes to the postanesthesia care unit (PACU), the CRNA asks you to monitor for signs of succinylcholine toxicity. Why would this be of concern at this time?

4. What can be done if the patient has received too much succinylcholine?

5. Another patient is undergoing a procedure performed using local anesthesia. Are there advantages of this type of anesthesia over general anesthesia?

6. In the PACU, what are the main concerns of the nurse monitoring the patient recovering from anesthesia?

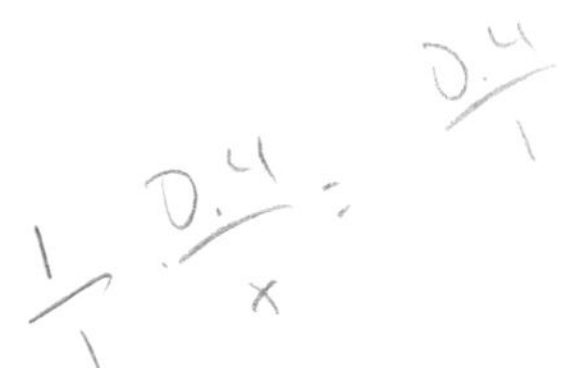

CHAPTER 13

Central Nervous System Depressants and Muscle Relaxants

Chapter Review and NCLEX® Examination Preparation

Select the best answer for each question.

1. When reviewing actions of drugs, the nurse recognizes that a hypnotic is a drug that performs which action?
   a. Produces sleep
   b. Stops seizures
   c. Prevents nausea and vomiting
   d. Relieves pain

2. A patient who has been taking a benzodiazepine for 5 weeks has been instructed to stop the medication. Which instruction will the nurse provide to the patient on how to discontinue the medication?
   a. Stop taking the drug immediately.
   b. Plan a gradual reduction in dosage.
   c. Overlap this medication with another drug.
   d. Take the medication every other day for a number of weeks.

3. A patient will be undergoing a brief surgical procedure to obtain a biopsy from a superficial mass on his arm. The nurse expects that which type of barbiturate will be used at this time?
   a. Ultrashort
   b. Short
   c. Intermediate
   d. Long

4. While monitoring a patient who took an overdose of barbiturates, the nurse keeps in mind that the cause of death would be which of the following?
   a. Tachycardia
   b. Hypertension
   c. Dyspnea
   d. Respiratory arrest

5. A patient with back muscle spasms is being treated with a skeletal muscle relaxant. In order to ensure that these drugs are most effective, the nurse will make sure what other treatment is ordered?
   a. Benzodiazepines
   b. Moist heat
   c. Physical therapy
   d. Aspirin

6. The nurse is providing care for a patient who has accidentally taken an overdose of benzodiazepines. Which drug would be used to treat this patient?
   a. methamphetamine
   b. theophylline
   c. flumazenil
   d. naloxone (Narcan)

7. A child will be receiving PO midazolam (Versed) as preoperative sedation. The child weighs 33 pounds. The dose ordered is 0.5 mg/kg, and the medication is available as a syrup, with a concentration of 2 mg/mL.
   a. What will be the dosage for this child? 7.5 mg
   b. How much is the PO dose for this child in mL? 3.75 mL

Critical Thinking and Application

Answer the following questions on a separate sheet of paper.

8. A 19-year-old college freshman is brought into the emergency department with a suspected barbiturate overdose. What symptoms would you expect to see? How is overdose treated?

9. Jackie is taking benzodiazepines to treat her insomnia. Today she visits your clinic and states that she is going to Europe for 2 months and wants a prescription that will allow her to take enough medication along for her entire stay. The physician declines. She

is a little insulted and asks you why the physician refused her request. "Does my doctor think I'm an addict or something?" What do you explain to her? What other options are possible for her?

10. Mrs. A., who is 81 years of age, weighs significantly more than her 47-year-old daughter, yet she is given a lower dosage of medication for insomnia of a similar degree. Why? Is this a dosage calculation error?

11. You have been asked to take a patient history for William, who will be given a benzodiazepine.
    a. What conditions or disorders should you ask about?
    b. What drug intake should you be most concerned about?
    c. What if William were an infant? A great-grandfather? Would this additional information matter? Why or why not?

12. Mr. P. is recovering from an automobile accident and has received a prescription for cyclobenzaprine for painful muscle spasms.
    a. What patient teaching should he receive about this medication?
    b. What other measures should be included in addition to this drug therapy?

Case Study

Read the scenario and answer the following questions on a separate sheet of paper.

A 54-year-old woman has had problems with insomnia "off and on for a few years" and has tried over-the-counter medications, herbal remedies, and prescription drugs. She likes to drink a glass of wine each night before going to bed. Today she is visiting the clinic for a checkup and asks for a prescription for secobarbital (Seconal) because that was the last drug she tried several years ago. She says she can't understand why the pharmacy won't refill her prescriptions for Seconal. The physician prescribes zaleplon (Sonata) instead.

1. Why did the physician change her prescription?

2. What are the consequences of long-term use of barbiturates?

3. What interactions should she be cautioned about while she is taking zaleplon?

4. What other patient teaching is important for this patient?

CHAPTER 14

Central Nervous System Stimulants and Related Drugs

Chapter Review and NCLEX® Examination Preparation

Select the best answer for each question.

1. The nurse is reviewing a patient's medication administration record. Which best describes a common use for doxapram (Dopram)?
   a. To control increased respiration caused by other drugs
   b. To treat respiratory insufficiency associated with chronic obstructive pulmonary disease
   c. To treat postoperative respiratory excitation
   d. To stimulate respirations in patients with head injury

2. The nurse is administering a stimulant drug. Which are results of stimulation of the central nervous system (CNS) by these drugs? *(Select all that apply.)*
   a. Increased fatigue
   b. Decreased drowsiness
   c. Increased respiration
   d. Bradycardia
   e. Euphoria

3. A patient has asked for a cup of coffee. The nurse keeps in mind that caffeine should be avoided by patients who have a history of which condition?
   a. Cardiac dysrhythmias
   b. Asthma
   c. Diabetes mellitus
   d. Gallbladder disease

4. The physician has ordered orlistat (Xenical). The nurse recognizes that this drug is used to treat which condition?
   a. Anorexia
   b. Malnutrition
   c. Narcolepsy
   d. Obesity

5. When a child is taking drugs for attention deficit hyperactivity disorder (ADHD), what will the nurse instruct the caregivers to closely monitor in the child?
   a. Blood glucose levels
   b. Physical growth, especially weight
   c. Grades at school
   d. Respiratory rates

6. A patient with migraine headaches is being evaluated. One potential treatment is ergotamine tablets. The nurse notes that the patient has the following conditions. Which would be a contraindication to the use of ergotamine?
   a. Asthma
   b. Hypertension
   c. Pregnancy
   d. Hypothyroidism

7. A 14-year-old boy will be taking atomoxetine (Strattera) for ADHD. He weighs 110 pounds, and the dose ordered is 1.2 mg/kg daily. How many mg will the nurse administer with each dose?

   ____

Critical Thinking and Application

Answer the following questions on a separate sheet of paper.

8. Stacey, age 35, reports that she falls asleep unexpectedly at work, in class, and even while singing in her city's choir.
   a. Which condition might Stacey have?
   b. What might be the drug of choice for Stacey?
   c. Describe the therapeutic effects of such drugs.
   d. Draw up a patient teaching plan for Stacey. Offer guidelines for substances she might be wise to avoid.

9. Five-year-old Jeffrey is taking atomoxetine (Strattera) for ADHD. What specific precautions must be taken with children who are taking ADHD drugs? Why?

10. What nutritional counseling is needed for patients taking orlistat (Xenical)?

11. Sadie experiences migraine headaches about four times a year and has a new prescription for a triptan antimigraine medication. She tells you that she hopes that the medication will prevent her "awful headaches." What is the best response to Sadie's comments?

Case Study

Read the scenario and answer the following questions on a separate sheet of paper.

Nancy, a 44-year-old accountant, has had an increasing number of headaches in the past year. When she has these headaches, she often is nauseated and vomits. She has been to her physician, who has ordered several diagnostic tests. As a result, Nancy has been diagnosed with migraine headaches and will be given a prescription for a serotonin agonist.

1. How do serotonin agonists work in the treatment of migraine headaches?

2. What dosage form(s) would be helpful for Nancy's situation?

3. If the physician decides to write a prescription for sumatriptan (Imitrex), Nancy's history should be assessed for which conditions?

4. What foods may be associated with the development of migraine headaches?

5. What else should be included in the treatment regimen for Nancy's migraine headaches?

CHAPTER 15

Antiepileptic Drugs

Critical Thinking Crossword

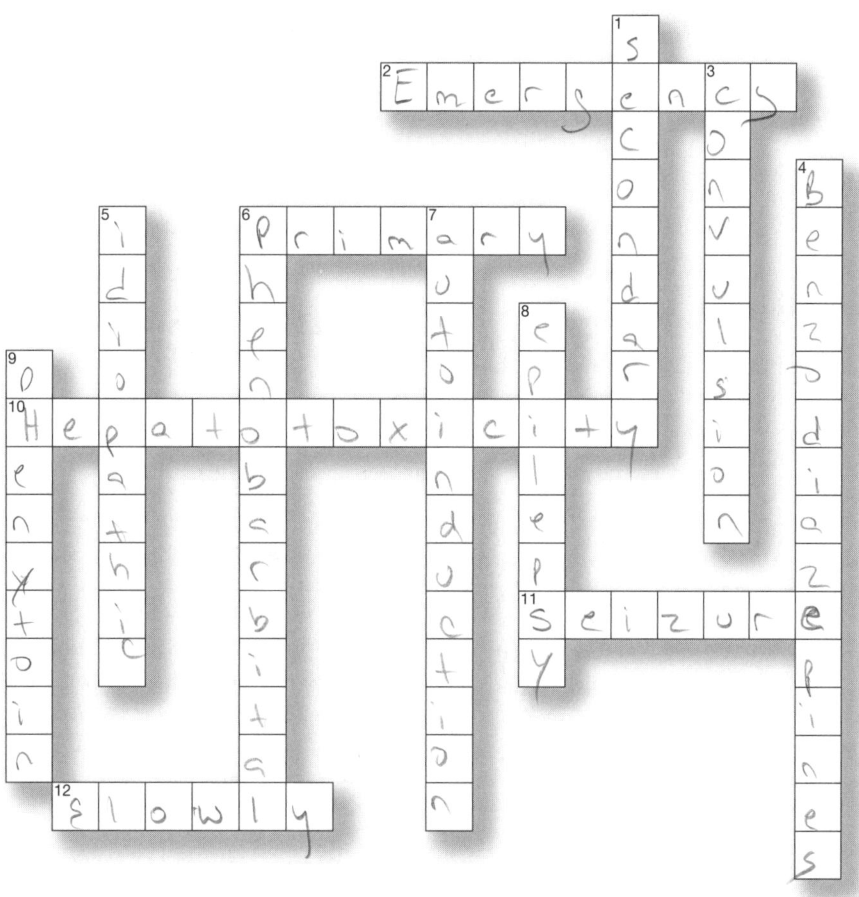

Across

2. Status epilepticus is considered a life-threatening medical __________.
6. A type of epilepsy with an unknown cause
10. A potential adverse effect of valproic acid
11. A brief episode of abnormal electrical activity in the nerve cells of the brain
12. Intravenously administered antiepileptic drugs should be delivered this way to avoid serious adverse effects

Down

1. A type of epilepsy with a distinct cause
3. An involuntary spasmodic contraction of voluntary muscles throughout the body
4. This class of drugs is one of the first-line drugs used to treat status epilepticus.
5. Another term for 6 Across
6. A barbiturate used primarily to control tonic-clonic and partial seizures
7. The metabolic process that occurs when the metabolism of a drug increases over time, which leads to lower-than-expected drug concentrations
8. Recurrent episodes of convulsive seizures
9. A first-line antiepileptic drug, the long-term use of which can cause gingival hyperplasia

Chapter Review and NCLEX® Examination Preparation

Select the best answer for each question.

1. A patient has been taking antiepileptic drugs for a year. The nurse is reviewing his recent history and will monitor for which condition that may develop during this time?
   a. Loss of appetite
   b. Jaundice
   c. Weight loss
   d. Suicidal thoughts or behavior

2. A patient is experiencing a seizure that has lasted for several minutes and he has not regained consciousness. The nurse recognizes that this is a life-threatening emergency known as:
   a. status epilepticus.
   b. tonic-clonic convulsion.
   c. epilepsy.
   d. secondary epilepsy.

3. The nurse is giving an intravenous dose of phenytoin (Dilantin). Which guidelines will the nurse follow for administration? *(Select all that apply.)*
   a. Phenytoin should be injected quickly.
   b. Phenytoin should be injected slowly.
   c. Phenytoin should be followed by an injection of sterile saline.
   d. Continuous infusion should be avoided.

4. The nurse is administering phenobarbital (Luminal) and will monitor the patient for which possible adverse effect?
   a. Constipation
   b. Gingival hyperplasia
   c. Drowsiness
   d. Dysrhythmias

5. A patient has been admitted to the emergency department with status epilepticus. The nurse knows that which drug is considered the first choice for this condition?
   a. phenobarbital (Luminal)
   b. diazepam (Valium)
   c. valproic acid
   d. phenytoin (Dilantin)

6. A patient who is experiencing neuropathic pain tells the nurse that the physician is going to start him on a new medication that is generally used to treat seizures. The nurse anticipates that which drug will be ordered?
   a. phenobarbital (Luminal)
   b. phenytoin (Dilantin)
   c. gabapentin (Neurontin)
   d. tiagabine (Gabitril)

7. A patient is unable to take oral medications and has received a loading dose of phenytoin (Dilantin) intravenously. The orders call for him to receive phenytoin, 5 mg/kg/day in three divided doses. The medication comes in a vial with 50 mg/mL. The patient weighs 90 kg.
   a. How many mg will the patient receive each day? For each dose?
   b. How many mL of medication will be drawn up for each dose? ______

Critical Thinking and Application

Answer the following questions on a separate sheet of paper.

8. What is meant by *autoinduction* in a drug? Identify at least one antiepileptic drug that undergoes autoinduction.

9. Jeremy, an 8-year-old boy, has resisted his oral doses of topiramate (Topamax), which has made compliance with the drug regimen difficult. His mother calls and says that she has found a way to get him to take it: she crushes the tablet and sprinkles it on flavored gelatin. She is delighted. How will the nurse respond?

Case Study

Read the scenario and answer the following questions on a separate sheet of paper.

Four-year-old Mattie has started preschool. Today the teacher called Mattie's mother to tell her that she noticed that Mattie seems to have a problem with "daydreaming." She explained that Mattie seemed inattentive during group work and was staring out into space several times a day. She was also worried because she saw Mattie's eyes move back and forth rapidly during these episodes. These "spells" lasted a minute or two, and then Mattie seemed fine. The mother has brought Mattie to the pediatric office to have her checked. The physician suspects that Mattie is experiencing a type of seizure disorder and has ordered some diagnostic testing.

1. What type of seizure is Mattie experiencing?

2. Mattie's mother is given a prescription for a liquid antiepileptic drug for Mattie. What is important to teach the mother regarding administration of this type of medication?

3. What should the mother be taught to monitor while Mattie is taking this medication?

4. After a year, Mattie's mother is pleased that the seizures have "disappeared" and wants to take Mattie off the medication. What is the best response in this situation by the nurse?

CHAPTER 16

Antiparkinsonian Drugs

Chapter Review and NCLEX® Examination Preparation

Select the best answer for each question.

1. A patient with Parkinson's disease has difficulty performing voluntary movements. What is the correct term for this symptom?
   a. Akinesia
   b. Dyskinesia
   c. Chorea
   d. Dystonia

2. Which drug may be used early in the treatment of Parkinson's disease but eventually loses effectiveness and must be replaced by another drug?
   a. amantadine (Symmetrel)
   b. levodopa (Larodopa)
   c. selegiline (Eldepryl)
   d. tolcapone (Tasmar)

3. The nurse is reviewing an order for apomorphine (Apokyn). What is the most important guideline when administering this drug?
   a. Observe the patient for severe diarrhea that may occur.
   b. Prepare the patient for problems with insomnia.
   c. The drug should be prescribed in milliliters, not milligrams.
   d. It is given in extended-release, PO forms only.

4. A patient who is newly diagnosed with Parkinson's disease and beginning medication therapy with entacapone (Comtan), a COMT inhibitor, asks the nurse, "How soon will improvement occur?" What is the nurse's best response?
   a. "That varies from patient to patient."
   b. "You should discuss that with your physician."
   c. "You should notice a difference right away."
   d. "It may take several weeks before you notice any degree of improvement."

5. A patient asks the nurse why a second drug is given with his drugs for Parkinson's disease. The nurse notes that this drug, an anticholinergic, is given to control or minimize which symptoms? *(Select all that apply.)*
   a. Drooling
   b. Constipation
   c. Muscle rigidity
   d. Bradykinesia
   e. Dry mouth

6. The nurse is providing teaching on COMT inhibitors to a patient with a new prescription. The nurse will be sure to educate the patient on the possibility of which adverse effect?
   a. Dizziness
   b. Urine discoloration
   c. Leg edema
   d. Visual changes

7. The medication order reads: "Give apomorphine (Apokyn), 0.2 mL now, subcutaneously." The injection solution is 10 mg/mL. How much apomorphine will the nurse administer? 0.2 mL ____________

Critical Thinking and Application

Answer the following questions on a separate sheet of paper.

8. Mr. H. is about to have levodopa added to his carbidopa treatment regimen.
   a. Why must dopamine be administered in the form of levodopa?
   b. What problems are avoided when carbidopa is given with levodopa?
   c. How does the carbidopa work when given with levodopa?

9. Mrs. R., a 35-year-old new mother, has experienced slowing movements, cogwheel rigidity, and pill-rolling tremor. She has been diagnosed with Parkinson's disease, a somewhat rare occurrence in someone her age. In addition to the usual history questions, what must you ask in anticipation of dopaminergic therapy in Mrs. R.'s specific situation?

10. Jane, age 45, is taking benztropine in addition to a dopaminergic drug for Parkinson's disease. Her 76-year-old neighbor comments that he cannot take benztropine because it is too risky for him. Jane calls and asks why this is not a concern in her case. What do you say?

Case Study

Read the scenario and answer the following questions on a separate sheet of paper.

Alexander, a 54-year-old man, has been diagnosed with Parkinson's disease and is about to start drug therapy. His symptoms are mild, yet he has some akinesia that interferes with his ability to type at work. The physician explains that Alexander may have to take a variety of drugs as the disease progresses.

1. What is the underlying pathologic defect in Parkinson's disease?

2. What is the aim of drug therapy for Parkinson's disease?

3. The first drugs prescribed for Alexander are amantadine (Symmetrel) along with levodopa-carbidopa (Sinemet CR). What is the purpose of taking the amantadine at this time?

4. The physician tells Alexander that the amantadine may be helpful in the early stages but will need to be changed at a later date. Why is this true?

5. What is the "on-off phenomenon" that may occur with the use of levodopa? How does the carbidopa affect this phenomenon?

CHAPTER 17

Psychotherapeutic Drugs

Chapter Review and NCLEX® Examination Preparation

Select the best answer for each question.

1. The nurse is administering the antipsychotic drug clozapine (Clozaril) and should monitor the patient for what long-term problem associated with this drug? *(Select all that apply.)*
   a. Mood swings
   b. Agranulocytosis
   c. Weight gain
   d. Anorexia
   e. Increased appetite

2. During therapy for depression with a selective serotonin reuptake inhibitor (SSRI), it is most important for the nurse to instruct the family to monitor for which adverse effect?
   a. Suicidal thoughts
   b. Visual disturbances
   c. Tardive dyskinesia
   d. Bleeding tendencies

3. The wife of a patient who has started taking antidepressant therapy asks, "How long will it take for him to feel better?" What is the nurse's best response?
   a. "Well, depression rarely responds to medication therapy."
   b. "He should be feeling better in a few days."
   c. "It may take 4 to 6 weeks before you see an improvement."
   d. "You may not see any effects for several months."

4. When administering certain antipsychotic drugs, the nurse monitors for extrapyramidal effects such as: *(Select all that apply.)*
   a. tremors.
   b. elation and a sense of well-being.
   c. painful muscle spasms.
   d. motor restlessness.
   e. bradycardia.

5. The nurse instructs a patient who is undergoing therapy with monoamine oxidase inhibitors (MAOIs) to avoid tyramine-containing foods. What medical emergency may occur if the patient eats these foods while taking MAOIs?
   a. Gastric hemorrhage
   b. Toxic shock
   c. Cardiac arrest
   d. Severe hypertensive crisis

6. A patient will be receiving benztropine (Cogentin) 1.5 mg PO daily. The medication comes in 0.5-mg tablets. How many tablets will the nurse administer per dose? ______ 3 tablets ______

Match each term with its corresponding definition or description.

7. __L__ buspirone (BuSpar)
8. __F__ tyramine
9. __G__ Tricyclics
10. __N__ Psychosis
11. __B__ Mania
12. __I__ diazepam (Valium)
13. __J__ amitriptyline (Elavil)
14. __K__ risperidone (Risperdal)
15. __C__ Benzodiazepines
16. __M__ lithium (Eskalith)
17. __A__ Anxiety
18. __D__ Affective disorders
19. __H__ Depression
20. __E__ Bipolar affective disorder

a. The unpleasant state of mind in which real or imagined dangers are anticipated and/or exaggerated
b. A state characterized by an expansive emotional state (including symptoms of extreme excitement and elation) and hyperactivity
c. A group of psychotropic drugs prescribed to alleviate anxiety

d. Emotional disorders characterized by changes in mood
e. A major psychologic disorder characterized by episodes of mania or hypomania, cycling with depression
f. Patients taking MAOIs need to be taught to avoid foods that contain this substance.
g. An older class of antidepressant drugs
h. An abnormal emotional state characterized by exaggerated feelings of sadness, melancholy, and worthlessness out of proportion to reality
i. A frequently prescribed benzodiazepine
j. The most widely used tricyclic antidepressant
k. An atypical antipsychotic drug used to treat schizophrenia
l. A non-benzodiazepine drug used to treat anxiety
m. Used to treat mania
n. A type of serious mental illness that can take several different forms and is associated with being truly out of touch with reality

Critical Thinking and Application

Answer the following questions on a separate sheet of paper.

21. Carl, a 26-year-old unemployed electrician, is brought to the emergency department by his sister. He is extremely drowsy and confused, his breathing is slow and shallow, and he smells strongly of whiskey. The sister tells you that Carl has been seeing a psychiatrist for his "anxiety."
    a. What do you suspect might be wrong with Carl?
    b. How will he likely be treated?

22. Mr. D., a 49-year-old restaurant owner, has been prescribed the MAOI phenelzine (Nardil). After the physician leaves the room but before you have a chance to discuss Mr. D.'s medication regimen with him, he turns to his wife and says, "I'm sure this medicine will work. Let's have a bottle of wine tonight to celebrate our anniversary."
    a. What should you say?
    b. A few weeks later, Mr. D. is brought to the emergency department with a severe headache, stiff neck, sweating, and elevated blood pressure. His wife says his symptoms started a few minutes after they ate at their favorite restaurant. What is wrong with Mr. D., and what probably caused it?

23. Beth has been diagnosed with depression. Why might the physician prescribe a second-generation antidepressant instead of a first-generation antidepressant?

24. A young adult has been admitted to the emergency department with a suspected overdose of an antidepressant. The physicians are monitoring his cardiac status closely. Why is this?

Case Study

Read the scenario and answer the following questions on a separate sheet of paper.

Gene, a 38-year-old businessman, mentions during a checkup that he has felt very anxious and upset over the past few months. He discusses the pressures of his business and states that he has had trouble sleeping at night, which makes him more irritable. Lately he has been very worried over a contract proposal presentation that will take place in a few months. The physician gives him a prescription for alprazolam (Xanax), 0.25 mg three times a day.

1. Gene is concerned about potential adverse effects of this medication. What will you tell him?

2. What other measures will be taken for Gene at this time?

3. After 3 months, Gene is back in the office for a follow-up appointment. He is upset because a friend told him about another friend who was taking that same medication but died due to an overdose. Gene wants to stop taking the alprazolam immediately. Is this recommended? If not, why not?

4. What are the symptoms of alprazolam overdose, and what is the antidote, if any?

5. Six months later, Gene is no longer taking alprazolam but comes back to the office because he still feels anxious. The physician gives him a prescription for buspirone (BuSpar), 15 mg twice a day. Gene questions why he is given a different drug. What are the advantages, if any, of taking buspirone instead of alprazolam?

CHAPTER 18

Adrenergic Drugs

Chapter Review and NCLEX® Examination Preparation

Select the best answer for each question.

1. What is another name for an adrenergic drug?
   a. Anticholinergic drug
   b. Parasympathetic drug
   c. Central nervous system drug
   d. Sympathomimetic drug

2. The nurse is administering an adrenergic drug and will monitor for which possible effect?
   a. Urinary retention
   b. Hypotension
   c. Decreased respiratory rate
   d. Increased heart rate

3. The nurse is aware that adrenergic drugs may be used to treat which conditions? *(Select all that apply.)*
   a. Asthma
   b. Glaucoma
   c. Hypertension
   d. Nasal congestion
   e. Seizures
   f. Nausea and vomiting

4. A woman who is allergic to bees has just been stung while out in her garden. She reaches for her bee-sting kit, which would most likely contain which drug?
   a. epinephrine (EpiPen)
   b. methylphenidate HCl (Ritalin)
   c. dopamine
   d. norepinephrine (Levophed)

5. A 13-year-old girl was diagnosed with asthma 2 years ago. Today her physician wants to start her on salmeterol (Serevent) administered via inhaler. The nurse needs to remember to include which statement when teaching the girl and her family about this drug?
   a. "It should be taken at the first sign of an asthma attack."
   b. "The dosage is two puffs every 4 hours or any time needed for asthma attacks."
   c. "This inhaler is for prevention of asthma attacks, not for an acute attack."
   d. "Be sure to take your steroid inhaler first."

6. The nurse is to administer epinephrine 0.5 mg subcutaneously. The ampule contains 1 mL of medication and is labeled "Epinephrine 1:1000." How many mL of epinephrine will the nurse give? 0.5 mL

Critical Thinking and Application

Answer the following questions on a separate sheet of paper.

7. The mother of 3-year-old Kyle is giving him phenylephrine drops as a nasal decongestant.
   a. How does this medication help with nasal congestion?
   b. Kyle's mother comes back to the clinic and complains that after a week his congestion is worse, not better. What possible explanation can the nurse offer?

8. Mr. D., who has had a history of problems with a hormonal imbalance, has been admitted for septic shock, and the physician prescribes dopamine. However, something tells the nurse that she should double-check whether he should take this drug. What makes the nurse think to do this?

9. Mr. G. and Mr. C. are both on dopamine infusions. Mr. G.'s infusion is being administered at a low rate, and Mr. C.'s at a high rate. Why might these infusion rates be different?

10. A patient in the intensive care unit has received too high a dose of epinephrine. For what will the nurse monitor, and what will the nurse expect to do for this patient?

11. Greg, a 49-year-old construction worker, is in the urgent care center for treatment of a leg laceration. Just after receiving an intravenous antibiotic, he starts to wheeze and says, "Oh, I just remembered. I'm allergic to penicillin!"
    a. What is happening?
    b. What will the nurse do first?
    c. What drug will be given in this situation?

Case Study

Read the scenario and answer the following questions on a separate sheet of paper.

Sixteen-year-old Maureen, who plays soccer on her high school team, has been treated for asthma for a year. Her symptoms have been controlled with an inhaled steroid and occasional use of an albuterol metered-dose inhaler. This afternoon, though, her mother brings her into the urgent care center because Maureen has had trouble "getting her breath" after a particularly rough game. Maureen complains of a feeling of "tightness" in her chest and wants to sit up. She appears anxious and has a nonproductive cough. Her respiratory rate is 28 breaths/min, and her peak expiratory flow is 70% of normal. Chest auscultation reveals a short inspiratory period with prolonged expiratory wheezes in both lungs.

1. The physician orders albuterol (Ventolin) to be given through a nebulizer. What should the nurse assess before giving this medication? During and after administration?

2. Why is the albuterol given via inhalation rather than orally?

3. After the nebulizer medication treatment is completed, Maureen complains of feeling "shaky and jittery." What do you tell her?

4. The physician gives Maureen a prescription for a salmeterol (Serevent) inhaler. What is important to teach Maureen and her mother about this medication?

CHAPTER 19

Adrenergic-Blocking Drugs

Chapter Review and NCLEX® Examination Preparation

Select the best answer for each question.

1. Adrenergic blockade at the alpha-adrenergic receptors leads to which of the following effects? *(Select all that apply.)*
   a. Vasodilation
   b. Decreased blood pressure
   c. Increased blood pressure
   d. Constriction of the pupil
   e. Tachycardia

2. The nurse discovers that the intravenous infusion of a patient who has been receiving an intravenous vasopressor has infiltrated. The nurse will expect which drug to be used to reverse the effects of the vasopressor in the infiltrated area?
   a. phentolamine
   b. prazosin (Minipress)
   c. ergotamine
   d. metoprolol (Lopressor)

3. A patient has a new prescription for a beta-blocker as part of treatment for hypertension. The nurse is reviewing the patient's current medications and notes that there may be a concern regarding interactions with which medication?
   a. Thyroid hormone supplement
   b. Antibiotic for a sinus infection
   c. Oral hypoglycemic for type II diabetes mellitus
   d. Oral contraceptive

4. A patient has been given an alpha-blocker as treatment for benign prostatic hyperplasia. Which instruction is important to include when the nurse is teaching him about the effects of this medication?
   a. Avoid foods and drinks that contain caffeine.
   b. Change positions slowly to avoid orthostatic blood pressure changes.
   c. Watch for weight loss of 2 pounds within a week.
   d. Take extra supplements of calcium.

5. A patient who has been taking a beta-blocker for 6 months tells the nurse during a follow-up visit that she wants to stop taking this medication. She is wondering if there is any problem with stopping the medication all at once. What is the nurse's best response?
   a. "No, there are no ill effects if this medication is stopped."
   b. "There should be only minimal effects if you stop this medication."
   c. "You may experience orthostatic hypotension if you stop this medication abruptly."
   d. "If you stop this medication suddenly, there is a possibility you may experience chest pain or rebound hypertension."

6. An admission order reads, "Start IV of 0.9% normal saline and infuse 1 L over the next 12 hours." At what rate will the nurse set the infusion pump?

   ____

Critical Thinking and Application

Answer the following questions on a separate sheet of paper.

7. Mrs. W., a patient on the nurse's hospital floor, is receiving a dopamine intravenous infusion. When the nurse first comes on the late-night shift, she seems just fine. However, the next time the nurse checks on her, the intravenous line has dislodged and the infusion has infiltrated. What could happen as a result? Is this serious? What kind of treatment will the nurse expect to see ordered? Describe the procedure and provide the rationale.

8. Mr. C. has had a myocardial infarction (MI). He is told that he will be prescribed a "cardioprotective drug." He asks the nurse to explain. How can some beta-blockers be said to "protect" the heart?

9. Ms. M. has been prescribed a beta-blocker. She is about to be released from the hospital, but first her nurse gives her instructions about taking her apical

pulse for 1 full minute, as well as her blood pressure. Why? What should she be looking for? Is there anything she should be instructed to report to her physician?

10. Mr. S., a 78-year-old widower, has a new prescription for tamsulosin (Flomax) because of a new diagnosis of benign prostatic hyperplasia. What concern, if any, is there with this drug? What teaching will he need?

Case Study

Read the scenario and answer the following questions on a separate sheet of paper.

Bruce, a 58-year-old accountant, is in the hospital after having an MI. The physician has told him that damage to his heart was minimal and the patient has started post-MI rehabilitation and education. The patient has discussed having to "mend his ways," because in addition to the MI he has had asthma for years that has been managed poorly. The physician discusses starting Bruce on a beta-blocker to "protect his heart" and gives him a prescription for atenolol (Tenormin).

1. What type of beta-blocker is appropriate for Bruce, and why?

2. Discuss how atenolol helps in this situation.

3. What adverse effects should Bruce be taught about when he starts this medication?

4. At his 3-month checkup, Bruce tells you that he wants to stop taking this medication. Should this medication be stopped abruptly?

CHAPTER 20

Cholinergic Drugs

Chapter Review and NCLEX® Examination Preparation

Match each definition with its corresponding term. (Note: Not all terms will be used.)

1. _____ Antidote for overdose of a cholinergic drug
2. _____ Cholinergic drugs that act by making more acetylcholine (ACh) available at the receptor site, which thus allows ACh to bind to and stimulate the receptor
3. _____ Cholinergic drugs that bind to cholinergic receptors and activate them
4. _____ Receptors located postsynaptically in the effector organs (smooth muscle, cardiac muscle, the glands) supplied by the parasympathetic fibers
5. _____ Receptors located in the ganglia of the parasympathetic nervous system (PSNS) and the sympathetic nervous system (SNS)
6. _____ A description of the action of the PSNS
7. _____ The neurotransmitter responsible for the transmission of nerve impulses to the effector cells in the PSNS
8. _____ The enzyme responsible for breaking down ACh

a. Cholinesterase
b. Muscarinic
c. Catecholamine
d. "Fight or flight"
e. "Rest and digest"
f. Direct-acting cholinergic drugs
g. Indirect-acting cholinergic drugs
h. Atropine
i. Acetylcholine
j. Nicotinic

Select the best answer for each question.

9. The desired effects of cholinergic drugs come from stimulation of which receptors?
   a. Cholinergic
   b. Nicotinic
   c. Muscarinic
   d. Ganglionic

10. The undesirable effects of cholinergic drugs come from stimulation of which receptors?
    a. Cholinergic
    b. Nicotinic
    c. Muscarinic
    d. Ganglionic

11. When a patient mentions bethanechol when asked about his medication history, the nurse recognizes that this drug is used for the treatment of which condition?
    a. Diarrhea
    b. Urinary retention
    c. Urinary incontinence
    d. Bladder spasms

12. When caring for a patient with a diagnosis of myasthenia gravis, the nurse can expect to see which drug ordered for the systemic treatment?
    a. bethanechol (Urecholine)
    b. tacrine (Cognex)
    c. donepezil (Aricept)
    d. physostigmine

13. A 62-year-old woman has started taking donepezil for early-stage Alzheimer's disease. Her daughter expresses relief that "there is finally a pill to cure Alzheimer's disease." What is the nurse's best response?
    a. "She should expect reversal of symptoms within a few days."
    b. "The dosage should be increased if no improvement is noted."
    c. "This drug may help to improve symptoms, but it is not intended as a cure."
    d. "Yes, it has been a great help for many patients."

14. A patient has received an inadvertent overdose of a cholinergic drug. The nurse will monitor for which early signs of a cholinergic crisis? *(Select all that apply.)*
    a. Dry mouth
    b. Salivation
    c. Flushing of the skin
    d. Abdominal cramps
    e. Constipation
    f. Dyspnea

15. The nurse will prepare to give which drug to a patient who is experiencing a cholinergic crisis?
    a. atropine
    b. tacrine (Cognex)
    c. donepezil (Aricept)
    d. physostigmine

16. An intravenous piggyback medication is ordered to infuse over 1 hour. The volume of the medication bag is 100 mL; the tubing drop factor is 10 gtt/mL. What is the rate for a gravity infusion of this medication? ______________

Critical Thinking and Application

Answer the following questions on a separate sheet of paper.

17. List the effects of cholinergic poisoning by using the acronym SLUDGE.

18. Mrs. S. has recently had abdominal surgery, and she is resting well except that she is unable to void her urine. She has some distension in her lower abdomen over the symphysis pubis.
    a. What is likely to be the drug of choice?
    b. Mrs. S. is still unable to void her urine. Her urinary retention worsens and becomes painful, and when her physician is contacted, he recommends radiography to determine whether a stone is present in her urinary tract; his suspicions are confirmed. How much can the physician increase her dosage?

19. Mr. K. has been determined to have a high potential for a negative reaction to the cholinergic prescribed to him. However, his physician believes that the potential benefits are worth the risk.
    a. For what reaction should the nurse be closely monitoring for in Mr. K.?
    b. In addition to close monitoring, what else can the nurse do to be prepared?

20. Ms. B. has recently been diagnosed with myasthenia gravis and is taking medication for the treatment of symptoms associated with the disease. She asks the nurse, "How much success can I expect?"
    a. How should the nurse respond?
    b. What kind of negative effects should Mrs. B. report to her physician?

Case Study

Read the scenario and answer the following questions on a separate sheet of paper.

Arthur, a 68-year-old retired banker, has been diagnosed with early-stage Alzheimer's disease. He has remained active in his church and likes to golf every week. He is in the office today with his son and is asking about the "new drugs that are available to reverse Alzheimer's disease." The son is concerned because Arthur was diagnosed with Parkinson's disease 6 months ago, but it has been controlled well with medications.

1. What drugs are available to "reverse Alzheimer's disease?" Explain.

2. The physician is considering either galantamine (Razadyne) or rivastigmine (Exelon) for Arthur. Is there anything in his history that may influence the choice of medication?

3. Describe the different mechanisms of action of direct-acting and indirect-acting cholinergic-blocking drugs.

4. Arthur is given a prescription for rivastigmine. What adverse effects should be expected, and what should he and his son be told regarding ways to manage these adverse effects?

CHAPTER 21

Cholinergic-Blocking Drugs

Chapter Review and NCLEX® Examination Preparation

Select the best answer for each question.

1. Before giving an anticholinergic drug, the nurse should check the patient's history for which conditions? *(Select all that apply.)*
   a. Glaucoma
   b. Osteoporosis
   c. Acute asthma
   d. Thyroid disease
   e. Diabetes mellitus
   f. Benign prostatic hyperplasia

2. The nurse will monitor for which adverse effects of anticholinergic drugs? *(Select all that apply.)*
   a. Dilated pupils
   b. Constricted pupils
   c. Dry mouth
   d. Urinary retention
   e. Urinary frequency
   f. Diarrhea

3. In reviewing the medication orders for a newly admitted patient, the nurse recognizes that which is an indication for atropine sulfate?
   a. Myasthenia gravis
   b. Reduction of secretions preoperatively
   c. Tachycardia due to sinoatrial node defects
   d. Narrow-angle glaucoma

4. During patient teaching for a 70-year-old man who will be taking an anticholinergic drug, the nurse will reinforce that this medication places the patient at higher risk for which problem?
   a. Angina
   b. Fluid overload
   c. Heatstroke
   d. Hypothermia

5. A 28-year-old woman is preparing to take a cruise and has asked for a prescription drug to prevent motion sickness. The physician orders scopolamine transdermal patches (Transderm-Scōp). The nurse should include which statement when teaching the patient about this drug?
   a. "The patch can be applied anywhere on the upper body."
   b. "Apply the patch 4 to 5 hours before travel."
   c. "Apply the patch just before boarding the ship"
   d. "Be sure to change the patch daily."

6. The preoperative orders read, "Give atropine 0.6 mg IV push, 30 minutes before the procedure." The medication comes in a 1 mg/mL vial. How much medication will the nurse administer? ____________

Critical Thinking and Application

Answer the following questions on a separate sheet of paper.

7. A patient is given atropine sulfate before surgery. Describe how this drug is helpful during the perioperative period. What other drug can be used for this purpose?

8. Mr. M. is brought into the emergency department conscious but with an overdose of a cholinergic blocker.
   a. Describe how Mr. M. will be treated.
   b. How will the nurse respond if Mr. M. begins having hallucinations related to the overdose?

9. Mr. H. is taking dicyclomine (Bentyl) for irritable bowel syndrome. He calls the clinic and tells the nurse that he would like to get his doctor's permission to take an antihistamine for his cold. What drug interactions might he expect?

10. How does atropine work in the following situations?
    a. A patient is experiencing severe bradycardia, with a heart rate of 38 beats/min, and he is losing consciousness.
    b. A crop duster pilot has been exposed to an organophosphate insecticide in an industrial accident.

Case Study

Read the scenario and answer the following questions on a separate sheet of paper.

Mrs. W., age 63, is in the outpatient clinic today for a physical. During history taking, she admits to having a "terrible problem" with her bladder. She describes having sudden urges to urinate and is "ashamed to say" that, at times, she has lost control of her bladder. She has had no other health issues except for "some eye problems" off and on for the past year. The physician is considering starting Mrs. W. on tolterodine (Detrol).

1. What are the contraindications for this medication? Are there any potential concerns given Mrs. W.'s history?
2. What are the advantages of using tolterodine rather than other drugs with similar actions?
3. Mrs. W. enjoys working outside in her yard. What special precautions should she take?
4. After a week of therapy, she calls the clinic to complain of a dry mouth. She said she didn't think this was supposed to happen with this drug. What advice do you give to her?

CHAPTER 22

Heart Failure Drugs

Chapter Review and NCLEX® Examination Preparation

Select the best answer for each question.

1. As part of treatment for early heart failure, a patient is started on an angiotensin-converting enzyme (ACE) inhibitor. The nurse will monitor the patient's laboratory work for which potential effect?
   a. Agranulocytosis
   b. Proteinuria
   c. Hyperkalemia
   d. Hypoglycemia

2. Before giving oral digoxin (Lanoxin), the nurse discovers that the patient's radial pulse is 52 beats/min. What will be the nurse's next action?
   a. Give the dose.
   b. Delay the dose until later.
   c. Hold the dose and notify the physician.
   d. Check the apical pulse for 1 minute.

3. Which statement regarding digoxin therapy and potassium levels is correct?
   a. Low potassium levels increase the chance of digoxin toxicity.
   b. High potassium levels increase the chance of digoxin toxicity.
   c. Digoxin reduces the excretion of potassium in the kidneys.
   d. Digoxin promotes the excretion of potassium in the kidneys.

4. When infusing inamrinone, the nurse should keep in mind which statement?
   a. The medication should be mixed in saline before administration.
   b. The true color of intravenous inamrinone is clear yellow.
   c. The drug may cause reddish discoloration of the extremities.
   d. Hypertension is the primary effect seen with excessive doses.

5. When caring for a patient who is taking digoxin, the nurse should monitor for which signs and symptoms of toxicity? *(Select all that apply.)*
   a. Anorexia
   b. Diarrhea
   c. Visual changes
   d. Nausea and vomiting
   e. Headache
   f. Bradycardia

6. What is 250 mcg expressed in mg? ______________

Critical Thinking and Application

Answer the following questions on a separate sheet of paper.

7. The nurse is caring for Mrs. C., who is undergoing cardiac glycoside therapy. She begins to vomit and complains of a headache and fatigue. Diagnostic studies reveal short episodes of ventricular tachycardia on the ECG and a serum potassium level of 6 mEq/L. What action might the nurse expect to be taken?

8. Mr. D. has atrial fibrillation and flutter, and the physician initially prescribes digoxin intravenously at 1.5 mg/day. What is the purpose of this dosage, and how does it compare with the dosage on which Mr. D. will be maintained?

9. Explain the limitations of nesiritide (Natrecor) therapy for heart failure.

10. While monitoring Mr. F. after oral digoxin (Lanoxin) administration, the nurse notes increased urinary output, decreased dyspnea and fatigue, and constipation. Mr. F. complains that if he were allowed to eat bran as often as he used to, he wouldn't be constipated. What do the nurse's findings indicate? How will the nurse response to Mr. F.?

11. Mr. M. is experiencing heart failure that has not responded well to diuretic and digoxin therapy. The physician changes his medication to inamrinone.
    a. What effect does inamrinone have on cardiac muscle contractility and the blood vessels?
    b. What advantage does this phosphodiesterase inhibitor have over the cardiac glycosides?
    c. What is the most worrisome adverse effect of inamrinone?

Case Study

Read the scenario and answer the following questions on a separate sheet of paper.

A 68-year-old woman is admitted to the hospital with a diagnosis of mild left-sided heart failure. At rest she is comfortable, but she has noticed that she has symptoms when she tries to get dressed or do simple housework. She becomes short of breath with activity, tires easily but cannot sleep at night, and feels "generally irritable." She also has diffuse bilateral crackles that do not clear with coughing and a third heart sound. She has slight pedal edema. The physician has ordered therapy with intravenous digoxin (Lanoxin).

1. Digoxin has several effects. Explain the meaning of each of the following:
    a. Positive inotropic effect
    b. Negative chronotropic effect
    c. Negative dromotropic effect

2. As a result of these effects, what would you expect to see with regard to each of the following?
    a. Stroke volume
    b. Venous blood pressure and vein engorgement
    c. Coronary circulation
    d. Diuresis

3. After 3 days of therapy, the patient complains of feeling nauseated and has no appetite. She also wonders why the lights are so bright and blurry. Her radial pulse rate is 52 beats/min. When you check the results of her laboratory work, you note that her digoxin level from that morning is 3.5 ng/mL. What will you do?

CHAPTER 23

Antidysrhythmic Drugs

Chapter Review and NCLEX® Examination Preparation

Select the best answer for each question.

1. The antidysrhythmic drug lidocaine is used mainly to treat which condition?
   a. Atrial fibrillation
   b. Bradycardia
   c. Complete heart block
   d. Ventricular dysrhythmias

2. When monitoring a patient who is taking quinidine (Quinidex), the nurse recognizes that which is a possible adverse effect of this drug?
   a. Weakness
   b. Tachycardia
   c. Gastrointestinal upset
   d. Hypertension

3. The nurse is administering amiodarone (Cordarone) and should monitor for which potential adverse effect?
   a. Pulmonary toxicity
   b. Hypertension
   c. Urinary retention
   d. Visual halos

4. Which condition is most appropriately treated with verapamil (Calan)?
   a. Cardiac asystole
   b. Heart block
   c. Ventricular dysrhythmia, including premature ventricular contraction
   d. Recurrent paroxysmal supraventricular tachycardia (PSVT)

5. A patient is experiencing a rapid dysrhythmia, and the nurse is preparing to administer adenosine (Adenocard). Which is the correct administration technique for this drug?
   a. It should be given as a fast intravenous push.
   b. It should be given intravenously, slowly, over at least 5 minutes.
   c. It should be taken with food or milk.
   d. It should be given as an intravenous drip infusion.

6. If a drug has a prodysrhythmic effect, then the nurse must monitor the patient for which effect?
   a. Decreased heart rate
   b. New dysrhythmias
   c. A decrease in dysrhythmias
   d. Reduced blood pressure

7. A patient with sustained ventricular tachycardia will be receiving a lidocaine infusion following a bolus dose. The order reads, "Give a bolus of 1.5 mg per kg, then start a drip at 2 mg/min." The lidocaine is available as 20 mg/mL, and the patient weighs 220 pounds. How many mg of lidocaine will be given in the bolus dose? ________________

8. Match the site to its correct intrinsic rate:

   _____ a. Sinoatrial node

   _____ b. Atrioventricular node

   _____ c. Purkinje fibers

   (1) 40 to 60 beats/min
   (2) 40 or fewer beats/min
   (3) 60 to 100 beats/min

Critical Thinking and Application

Answer the following questions on a separate sheet of paper.

9. Mr. K., who has been diagnosed with hypertension, is hospitalized after a myocardial infarction (MI).
   a. To reduce the risk of sudden cardiac death in Mr. K., the physician prescribes a drug from which class? Why?
   b. How would a history of asthma in Mr. K. affect the drug choice?

10. Mr. N. has a life-threatening ventricular tachycardia that has been resistant to treatment. What drug will the nurse expect to be used and what precautions are there with this drug?

11. Mr. M. is a 50-year-old schoolteacher being treated with lidocaine after an MI.
    a. He is very upset and says that he hates injections; he wants to know why he can't just take a pill. What will the nurse tell him?
    b. If Mr. M. has a history of cirrhosis, would the dosage of the lidocaine be affected?

12. Alicia calls the health clinic complaining of chest pain and dizziness. She says she cannot remember whether she took her quinidine (Quinidex) yesterday and wants to know whether she should take two doses today, especially because she is feeling so bad. What will the nurse tell Alicia?

Case Study

Read the scenario and answer the following questions on a separate sheet of paper.

Jack, age 39, is taking diltiazem (Cadizem) as part of his treatment for occasional PSVT. He also has a history of seizures.

1. How do calcium channel blockers such as diltiazem work?

2. What therapeutic effects are expected?

3. Is there a possible concern with drug interactions?

4. After 4 months of therapy, Jack experiences dizziness, dyspnea, and a very rapid heart rate and is taken to the emergency department. He is diagnosed with sustained PSVT, and intravenous verapamil (Calan) does not help. What do you think will be tried next?

CHAPTER 24

Antianginal Drugs

Chapter Review and NCLEX® Examination Preparation

Choose the best answer for each question.

1. What is the purpose of antianginal drug therapy?
   a. To increase myocardial oxygen demand
   b. To increase blood flow to peripheral arteries
   c. To increase blood flow to ischemic cardiac muscle
   d. To decrease blood flow to ischemic cardiac muscle

2. The nurse should teach a patient who will be taking nitroglycerin (Nitrostat) about which common adverse effect of this drug?
   a. Blurred vision
   b. Dizziness
   c. Headache
   d. Weakness

3. The nurse is reviewing dosage forms of nitroglycerin (Nitrostat). This drug can be given by which routes? *(Select all that apply.)*
   a. Continuous intravenous drip
   b. Intravenous bolus
   c. Sublingual spray
   d. Oral dosage forms
   e. Topical ointment
   f. Rectal suppository

4. For a patient using transdermal nitroglycerin patches, the nurse anticipates that the prescriber will order which procedure for preventing tolerance?
   a. Leave the old patch on for 2 hours when applying a new patch.
   b. Apply a new patch every other day.
   c. Leave the patch off for 24 hours once a week.
   d. Remove the patch at night for 8 hours and then apply a new patch in the morning.

5. Patients who are taking beta-blockers for angina need to be taught which information?
   a. These drugs are for long-term prevention of angina episodes.
   b. These drugs must be taken as soon as angina pain occurs.
   c. These drugs should be discontinued if dizziness is experienced.
   d. These drugs should be carried with the patient at all times in case angina occurs.

6. A patient with coronary artery spasms will be most effectively treated with which type of antianginal medication?
   a. Beta-blockers
   b. Calcium channel blockers
   c. Nitrates
   d. Nitrites

Critical Thinking and Application

Answer the following questions on a separate sheet of paper.

7. The order reads "Nitroglycerin transdermal patch, 0.2 mg/hr; apply one patch in the morning and remove every evening at 10 PM." The pharmacy has supplied a transdermal patch that supplies 0.4 mg/hr. What will the nurse do in order to administer this drug?

8. The nurse is playing racquetball at a community center when he notices a commotion at a gathering of senior citizens in a nearby room. The nurse rushes in to find a man lying unconscious on the floor. Several people say that he is having a "heart attack." One man hands the nurse a pill bottle and asks, "Would it help to give him one of my heart pills?" A woman agrees, saying, "Yes! Can't you put it under his tongue?" The nurse sees that the medication bottle is labeled Isordil (isosorbide dinitrate). What does the nurse know about this medication and what will he do?

9. Ms. V. is a 70-year-old patient seen in the emergency department for a laceration to her thumb. During the assessment, Ms. V. tells the nurse that she has been "tired and depressed" and has been having "nightmares" since her physician prescribed heart medicine for her angina. Which drug does the nurse suspect Ms. V. is taking and why?

10. During a home visit with Theresa, she shows the nurse a journal entry describing the duration, time of onset, and severity of a recent angina attack. She reports no adverse effects to her nitroglycerin and shows the nurse where she keeps the tablets, in a clear plastic pillbox on the kitchen windowsill. What will the nurse discuss with Theresa?

Case Study

Read the scenario and answer the following questions on a separate sheet of paper.

While playing handball, 59-year-old Gideon experiences chest pain. He has had angina before and has sublingual nitroglycerin (Nitro-Bid) in his gym bag.

1. What type of angina is he experiencing?

2. What should he do to treat this episode of angina?

3. After he takes the nitroglycerin tablet, the chest pain does not subside. He wants his handball partner to drive him to the hospital. Is this what he should do at this time?

4. Other than nitroglycerin, which class of drugs is typically used for this type of angina?

CHAPTER 25

Antihypertensive Drugs

Critical Thinking Crossword

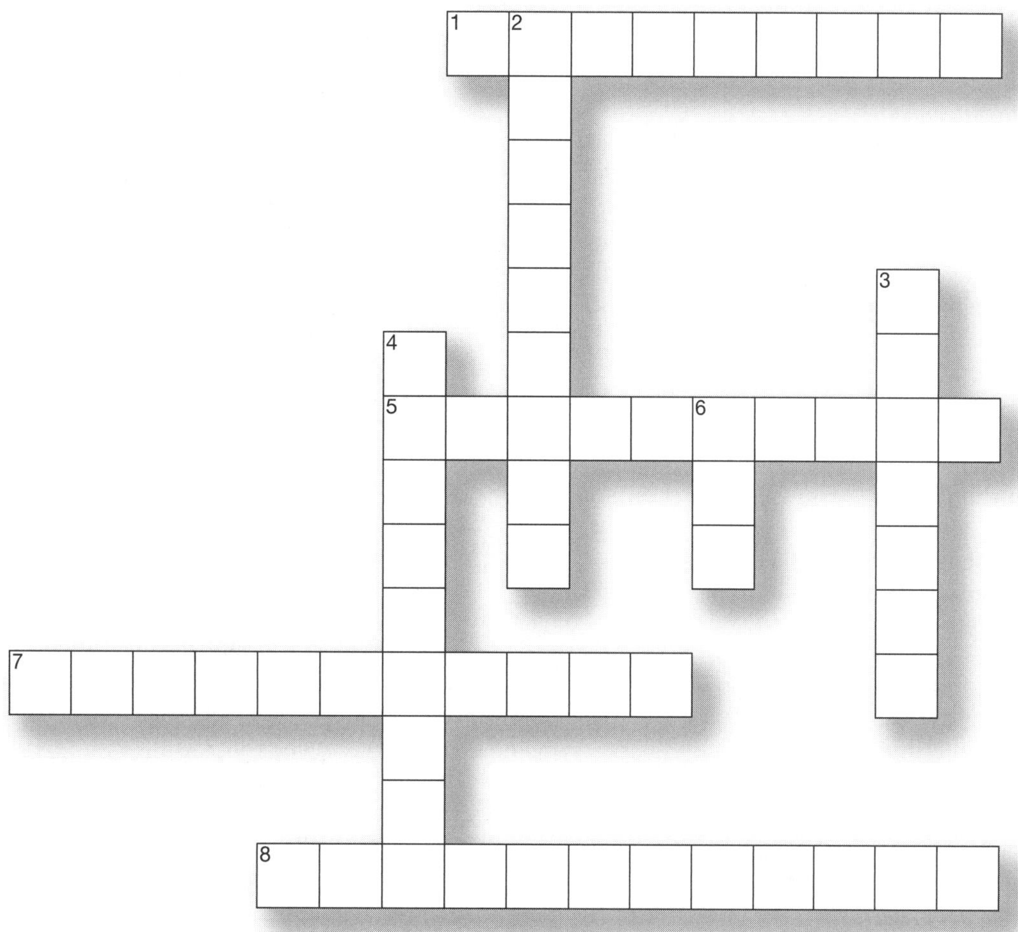

Across

1. High blood pressure associated with diseases such as renal, pulmonary, endocrine, and vascular diseases is known as __________ hypertension.
5. Another term for 3 Down.
7. A common adverse effect of adrenergic drugs involving a sudden drop in blood pressure when patients change position is known as __________ hypotension.
8. These drugs are used in the management of hypertensive emergencies.

Down

2. Another term for 3 Down.
3. Elevated systemic arterial pressure for which no cause can be found is known as __________ hypertension.
4. The primary effect of these drugs is to decrease plasma and extracellular fluid volumes.
6. Drugs that are often used as first-line drugs in the treatment of both heart failure and hypertension are known by the acronym __________ inhibitors.

Chapter Review and NCLEX® Examination Preparation

Select the best answer for each question.

1. A 46-year-old man has been taking clonidine for 5 months. For the last 2 months, his blood pressure has been normal. During this office visit, he tells the nurse that he would like to stop taking the drug. What is the nurse's best response?
   a. "I'm sure the doctor will stop it—your blood pressure is normal now."
   b. "Your doctor will probably have you stop taking the drug for a month, and then we'll see how you do."
   c. "This drug should not be stopped suddenly; let's talk to your doctor."
   d. "It's likely that you can stop the drug if you exercise and avoid salty foods."

2. When administering angiotensin-converting enzyme (ACE) inhibitors, the nurse keeps in mind that which are possible adverse effects? *(Select all that apply.)*
   a. Diarrhea
   b. Fatigue
   c. Restlessness
   d. Headaches
   e. A dry cough
   f. Tremors

3. A patient with type 2 diabetes mellitus has developed hypertension. What is the blood pressure goal for this patient?
   a. Less than 110/80 mm Hg
   b. Less than 130/80 mm Hg
   c. Less than 130/84 mm Hg
   d. Less than 140/90 mm Hg

4. A patient is being treated for a hypertensive emergency. The nurse expects which drug to be used?
   a. sodium nitroprusside (Nitropress)
   b. losartan (Cozaar)
   c. captopril (Capoten)
   d. prazosin (Minipress)

5. A patient in her eighth month of pregnancy has preeclampsia. Her blood pressure is 210/100 mm Hg this morning. This type of hypertension is classified as which of the following?
   a. Primary
   b. Idiopathic
   c. Essential
   d. Secondary

6. The order reads, "Give captopril 25 mg PO every 8 hours." The available tablets are 12.5-mg strength. How many tablets will the nurse administer per dose? ____________________

Critical Thinking and Application

Answer the following questions on a separate sheet of paper.

7. Mr. Q., 61 years of age, comes to the emergency department at night with symptoms of severe hypertensive emergency. The emergency department resident on call initiates therapy with sodium nitroprusside (Nitropress). The patient is transferred to the intensive care unit and monitored. Hours later, his blood pressure falls to 100/60 mm Hg, and he is lethargic and complaining of feeling dizzy. What will the nurse do?

8. Indicate which ACE inhibitor would be best for the following patients. Explain your answers.
   a. Irene, who has liver dysfunction, has high blood pressure, and is seriously ill
   b. Kory, who has a history of poor compliance with his medication regimen

9. Mr. B. will be starting prazosin (Minipress) for hypertension. What will he be taught before he takes even the first dose of this medication?

10. White and African-American patients are known to react differently to antihypertensive agents.
    a. Which antihypertensives are considered more effective in white patients than in African-American patients?
    b. Which antihypertensives are considered more effective in African-American patients than in white patients?

Case Study

Read the scenario and answer the following questions on a separate sheet of paper.

John, a 44-year-old African-American man, has been seen twice in the last month for "blood pressure problems." At the first visit, his blood pressure was 144/90 mm Hg; at the second visit, his blood pressure was 154/96 mm Hg. The physician is preparing to start antihypertensive therapy. John has no other medical conditions.

1. What initial drug therapy would be appropriate for him? What factors are considered when choosing which drug to use?

2. John tells you that he hopes this medication will not "slow him down" because he likes to "jump out of bed and get started" with his day. What teaching will you provide for him to help him adjust to his blood pressure medication?

3. John also mentions that he likes to go the gym three times a week and visit with his friends in the sauna after a good workout. What teaching will you emphasize for this patient?

CHAPTER 26

Diuretic Drugs

Chapter Review and NCLEX® Examination Preparation

Match each term with its corresponding definition.

1. _____ Diuretics
2. _____ Potassium-sparing diuretics
3. _____ Loop of Henle
4. _____ Osmotic diuretics
5. _____ Thiazides
6. _____ Ascites
7. _____ CAIs
8. _____ Loop diuretics
9. _____ Nephron
10. _____ GFR

a. Potent diuretics that act along the ascending limb of the loop of Henle; furosemide is an example
b. Abbreviation for the term that describes a gauge of how well the kidneys are functioning as filters
c. A general term for drugs that accelerate the rate of urine formation
d. The main structural unit of the kidney
e. Part of the kidney structure located between the proximal and distal convoluted tubules
f. Diuretics that result in the diuresis of sodium and water and the retention of potassium; spironolactone is an example.
g. Diuretics that act on the distal convoluted tubule, where they inhibit sodium and water resorption; hydrochlorothiazide (HCTZ) is an example.
h. Abbreviation for a class of diuretics that inhibit the enzyme carbonic anhydrase; acetazolamide is an example.
i. Drugs that induce diuresis by increasing the osmotic pressure of the glomerular filtrate, which results in rapid diuresis; mannitol is an example.
j. An abnormal intraperitoneal accumulation of fluid

Select the best answer for each question.

11. Which are indications for the use of diuretics? *(Select all that apply.)*
    a. To increase urine output
    b. To reduce uric acid levels
    c. To treat hypertension
    d. To treat open-angle glaucoma
    e. To treat edema associated with heart failure

12. When providing patient teaching to a patient who is taking a potassium-sparing diuretic such as spironolactone (Aldactone), the nurse will include which dietary guidelines?
    a. There are no dietary restrictions with this medication.
    b. The patient should consume foods high in potassium, such as bananas and orange juice.
    c. The patient should avoid foods high in potassium.
    d. The patient should drink 1 to 2 liters of fluid per day.

13. When teaching a patient about diuretic therapy, which time would the nurse indicate as the best time of day to take these medications?
    a. Morning
    b. Midday
    c. Bedtime
    d. Time of day does not matter.

14. When monitoring a patient for hypokalemia related to diuretic use, the nurse looks for which possible symptoms?
    a. Nausea, vomiting, and anorexia
    b. Diarrhea and abdominal pain
    c. Orthostatic hypotension
    d. Muscle weakness and lethargy

15. A patient with severe heart failure has been started on therapy with a carbonic anhydrase inhibitor (CAI), but the nurse mentions that this medication may be stopped in a few days. What is the reason for this short treatment?
    a. CAIs are not the first choice for treatment of heart failure.
    b. CAIs lose their diuretic effect in 2 to 4 days because metabolic acidosis develops.
    c. It is expected that the CAIs will dramatically reduce the fluid overload related to the heart failure.
    d. Allergic reactions to the CAIs are common.

16. A patient is to receive 30 g of mannitol (Osmitrol) intravenously. The medication on hand is mannitol 20% in a 500-mL bag. How many mL will the patient receive? ________________

Critical Thinking and Application

Answer the following questions on a separate sheet of paper.

17. Ms. A. is a 62-year-old retired teacher who is being treated for diabetes and open-angle glaucoma. The physician has prescribed a diuretic as an adjunct drug in the management of Ms. A.'s glaucoma.
    a. Which diuretic drug was probably prescribed?
    b. What undesirable effect of the drug does the physician need to consider?

18. The nurse is about to administer mannitol (Osmitrol) to Arthur, who is in early acute renal failure.
    a. What is the significance of Arthur's renal blood flow and glomerular filtration in this situation?
    b. By what means will the nurse administer the mannitol? What special guidelines will be followed?
    c. Arthur later complains of a headache and chills. Should the mannitol therapy be ended? Explain your answer.

19. Mr. F. has been admitted for treatment of ascites. He also has some renal impairment and a history of heavy drinking.
    a. Which diuretic drug will the nurse expect to be administered to Mr. F.?
    b. What monitoring will be performed frequently? Why?

20. Brendan, a 39-year-old bricklayer, is taking thiazide for hypertension. During a follow-up visit, he tells the nurse that he thinks the drug is affecting his "love life."
    a. To what adverse effect of thiazide therapy is Brendan probably referring?
    b. While the nurse is talking, she notices a package of licorice in Brendan's coat pocket. He tells her that he eats the candy "for energy," especially because he has been feeling so tired the past couple of days. What will the nurse tell Brendan?

21. The nurse receives a call from Mrs. H., who recently started diuretic therapy for hypertension. Mrs. H. is concerned because her neighbor, who also takes medication for hypertension, has told her not to eat a lot of bananas or other foods containing potassium. "But you told me to eat foods high in potassium," Mrs. H. says to the nurse, "What's going on?" What will the nurse respond to Mrs. H.?

Case Study

Read the scenario and answer the following questions on a separate sheet of paper.

Lily has been taking furosemide (Lasix) for 3 months as part of her treatment for heart failure. At this time, she is complaining that she is feeling tired and has muscle weakness and no appetite; her blood pressure is 100/50 mm Hg.

1. What do her symptoms suggest? How did this happen?

2. What dietary measures could she have taken to prevent this problem?

The physician switches her medication to spironolactone (Aldactone).

3. How does this drug differ from furosemide?

4. For what drug interactions should you check before she begins taking spironolactone?

CHAPTER 27

Fluids and Electrolytes

Chapter Review and NCLEX® Examination Preparation

Select the best answer for each question.

1. Which are common uses of crystalloids? *(Select all that apply.)*
   a. Fluid replacement
   b. Promotion of urinary flow
   c. Transport of oxygen to cells
   d. Replacement of electrolytes
   e. As maintenance fluids
   f. Replacement of clotting factors

2. The intravenous order for a newly admitted patient calls for "Normal saline to run at 100 mL/hr." The nurse will choose which concentration of normal saline?
   a. 0.33%
   b. 0.45%
   c. 0.9%
   d. 3.0%

3. A patient has been admitted with severe dehydration after working outside on a very hot day. The nurse expects which intravenous fluid to be ordered for rapid fluid replacement?
   a. Albumin
   b. Hetastarch
   c. Fresh frozen plasma
   d. 3% sodium chloride

4. When giving intravenous potassium, which is important for the nurse to remember?
   a. Intravenous doses are preferred over oral dosage forms.
   b. Intravenous solutions should contain at least 50 mEq/L.
   c. Potassium must always be given in diluted form.
   d. It should be given by slow intravenous bolus.

5. When a patient is receiving blood products, the nurse monitors for which signs of a possible transfusion reaction?
   a. Subnormal temperature and hypertension
   b. Apprehension, restlessness, fever, and chills
   c. Decreased pulse and respirations and fever
   d. Headache, nausea, and lethargy

6. A patient with a demonstrated deficiency in clotting factors needs a replacement product that will not increase his fluid levels. The nurse expects which product to be given?
   a. Plasma protein fraction
   b. Fresh frozen plasma
   c. Packed red blood cells
   d. Albumin

7. The following IV is to be given: 1000 mL D_5W with 20 mEq potassium chloride (KCl) over the next 24 hours. The tubing drop factor is 15.
   a. At what rate will the KCl be administered? ______________
   b. What will the gtt/min be? ______________

Critical Thinking and Application

Answer the following questions on a separate sheet of paper.

8. Name advantages and disadvantages of using crystalloids to replace fluid in patients with dehydration.

9. Some fluids are known as *oxygen-carrying resuscitation fluids*.
   a. Which class of fluids is given this designation?
   b. Why are these fluids able to carry oxygen?
   c. Why are they the most expensive of the three types of fluids and why is their origin a potential problem for a recipient?

10. Tanya, a 16-year-old student, is brought to the clinic by her mother, who says that Tanya has been on "some sort of fad diet." The mother is concerned because Tanya is tired and weak. During the nurse's assessment, Tanya admits that she has been using laxatives and eating very little during the past few weeks.
    a. What electrolyte imbalance is Tanya probably experiencing?
    b. Assuming that laboratory studies show the problem to be mild, how can it be corrected?

11. Mr. S., a 45-year-old mail carrier, has come to the emergency department sweating profusely and complaining of stomach cramps and diarrhea. He says that he has been "miserable" from the heat the past few days. His serum sodium level is 128 mEq/L.
    a. What electrolyte imbalance will the nurse suspect?
    b. The physician prescribes an oral medication and then asks the nurse to discuss dietary considerations with Mr. S.. What will the nurse tell Mr. S.?
    c. What adverse effect of sodium may be of special concern for Mr. S.?

12. Victor is receiving a transfusion of a blood product.
    a. The nurse observes Victor, knowing that an adverse reaction to the transfusion may be manifested by what signs and symptoms?
    b. Victor's wife is crying and says, "People get AIDS from transfusions. What happens if Victor gets AIDS?" What will the nurse tell her?
    c. The transfusion for Victor seems to be progressing smoothly. How often will the nurse check Victor's vital signs while he is receiving the transfusion?
    d. After 45 minutes, Victor is restless and his pulse rate has increased. What will the nurse do?

Case Study

Read the scenario and answer the following questions on a separate sheet of paper.

An older man was admitted to the unit with hypoproteinemia caused by chronic malnutrition. You note that he has some edema over his body, and his total protein level is 4.8 g/dL.

1. What is the relationship between his serum total protein level and the edema you have noted?

2. You are preparing to give him 1 unit of 5% albumin. How does albumin work in this situation?

3. What advantages does albumin have over crystalloids in this situation?

4. For what adverse effects will you monitor while he is receiving albumin?

CHAPTER 28

Coagulation Modifier Drugs

Chapter Review and NCLEX® Examination Preparation

Match each definition with its corresponding term. (Note: Not all terms will be used; terms may be used more than once.)

1. _____ A drug that prevents the lysis of fibrin, thereby promoting clot formation
2. _____ The termination of bleeding by mechanical or chemical means
3. _____ A substance that prevents platelet plugs from forming
4. _____ The general term for a drug that dissolves thrombi
5. _____ The general term for a substance that prevents or delays coagulation of the blood
6. _____ A laboratory test used to measure the effectiveness of heparin therapy
7. _____ Two tests used to monitor the effects of drug therapy with warfarin sodium.
8. _____ A standardized measure of the degree of coagulation achieved by drug therapy with warfarin sodium
9. _____ A substance that reverses the effect of heparin
10. _____ A substance that reverses the effect of warfarin sodium
11. _____ Naturally occurring tissue plasminogen activator secreted by vascular endothelial cells
12. _____ A blood clot that dislodges and travels through the bloodstream

a. Prothrombin time (PT)
b. Activated partial thromboplastin time (APTT)
c. International normalized ratio (INR)
d. streptokinase (Streptase)
e. alteplase (Activase)
f. Thrombus
g. Embolus
h. Vitamin K
i. protamine sulfate
j. Antiplatelet drug
k. Antifibrinolytic
l. Thrombolytic drug
m. Anticoagulant
n. Hemostasis

Select the best answer for each question.

13. The nurse is reviewing the use of anticoagulants. Anticoagulant therapy is appropriate for which conditions? *(Select all that apply.)*
    a. Atrial fibrillation
    b. Thrombocytopenia
    c. Myocardial infarction
    d. Presence of mechanical heart valve
    e. Aneurysm
    f. Leukemia

14. During teaching of a patient who will be taking warfarin sodium (Coumadin) at home, which statement by the nurse is correct regarding over-the-counter drug use?
    a. "Choose nonsteroidal antiinflammatory drugs as needed for pain relief."
    b. "Aspirin products may result in increased anticoagulant effect."
    c. "Vitamin E therapy is recommended to improve the effect of the warfarin."
    d. "Mineral oil is the laxative of choice while taking anticoagulants."

15. A patient is at risk for a stroke. Which drug is recommended to prevent platelet aggregation for stroke prevention by the American Stroke Society?
    a. aspirin
    b. warfarin sodium (Coumadin)
    c. heparin
    d. alteplase (Activase)

16. When administering subcutaneous heparin, the nurse will remember to perform which action?
    a. Use the same sites for injection to reduce trauma.
    b. Use a 1-inch needle for subcutaneous injections.
    c. Inject the medication without aspirating for blood return.
    d. Massage the site after the injection to increase absorption.

17. During thrombolytic therapy, the nurse monitors for bleeding. Which symptoms may indicate a serious bleeding problem? *(Select all that apply.)*
    a. Hypertension
    b. Hypotension
    c. Decreased level of consciousness
    d. Increased pulse rate
    e. Restlessness

18. Which drug is often used after major orthopedic surgery, even when the patient is home?
    a. Antiplatelet drugs, such as aspirin
    b. Adenosine diphosphate (ADP) inhibitors, such as clopidogrel (Plavix)
    c. Anticoagulants, such as warfarin sodium (Coumadin)
    d. Low-molecular-weight heparins, such as enoxaparin (Lovenox)

19. A patient is to receive a bolus dose of heparin 8,000 units via IV push. The vial contains heparin, 10,000 units per mL. How many mL of medication will the nurse draw up to administer the ordered dose?

    ____

Critical Thinking and Application

Answer the following questions on a separate sheet of paper.

20. Mrs. W., a 60-year-old homemaker, is receiving subcutaneous heparin therapy for prevention of deep vein thrombosis. After the nurse gives Mrs. W. her injection, she complains of pain and begins to rub the site. What will the nurse do?

21. During cardiopulmonary bypass for heart surgery, Mr. J. was intentionally given a large dose of heparin. The surgeon then determines that the effects of the heparin need to be reversed quickly.
    a. How will this be done?
    b. How will the amount of antidote be determined?
    c. What is the most commonly used test for determining the effects of heparin therapy?

22. A patient is experiencing warfarin toxicity from accidentally taking too many warfarin tablets.
    a. What will be used as an antidote?
    b. How will the dose of the antidote be determined?
    c. After 4 days, the patient requires anticoagulation again. What drug will be ordered?

23. Following surgery, Mr. T. has a chest tube in place. The site has been bleeding excessively. What type of drug might the physician prescribe in this situation and why?

24. William, a 38-year-old writer who has von Willebrand's disease, has undergone emergency surgery after an automobile accident. What drug is used in the management of bleeding in patients like William? What is its effect?

25. Tobias has been given alteplase (Activase) during his treatment for acute myocardial infarction.
    a. Do you expect Tobias to have an allergic reaction to the drug? Explain your answer.
    b. A few minutes later, Tobias suffers a reinfarction. What drug should Tobias receive now?

26. Ursula, an inpatient on the nurse's unit, is on anticoagulant therapy. The nurse enters her room to find that she is restless and confused.
    a. Why are these findings significant?
    b. In this case, what other problems might the nurse expect to find?
    c. What will the nurse do?

27. Sara is receiving heparin, 5000 units, twice a day for deep vein thrombosis (DVT) prevention. Will her anticoagulation be monitored by laboratory work? Explain.

Case Study

Read the scenario and answer the following questions on a separate sheet of paper.

After experiencing transient ischemic attacks, Doug has been started on clopidogrel (Plavix). He has had a history of atherosclerotic heart disease and has had problems with peptic ulcer disease.

1. He asks, "Why am I taking this fancy medicine? Why can't I just take an aspirin a day, like they say on television?" What do you tell him?
2. What should he be taught to report to his health care provider while he is taking this drug?
3. What precautions should he follow while he is taking this drug?
4. What herbal products should he avoid while he is taking this drug?

CHAPTER 29

Antilipemic Drugs

Chapter Review and NCLEX® Examination Preparation

Select the best answer for each question.

1. Patients taking cholestyramine (Questran) may experience which adverse effects?
   a. Blurred vision and photophobia
   b. Drowsiness and difficulty concentrating
   c. Diarrhea and abdominal cramps
   d. Belching and bloating

2. The nurse should instruct the patient who is taking antilipemic drugs about which dietary measures? *(Select all that apply.)*
   a. Taking supplements of fat-soluble vitamins
   b. Taking supplements of B vitamins
   c. Increasing fluid intake
   d. Choosing foods that are lower in cholesterol and saturated fats
   e. Increasing the intake of raw vegetables, fruit, and bran

3. In reviewing the history of a newly admitted cardiac patient, the nurse knows that the patient would have a contraindication to antilipemic therapy if which condition is present?
   a. Liver disease
   b. Renal disease
   c. Coronary artery disease
   d. Diabetes mellitus

4. A woman is being screened in the cardiac clinic for risk factors for coronary artery disease. Which would be considered a negative, or favorable, risk factor for her?
   a. High-density lipoprotein (HDL) cholesterol level of 30 mg/dL
   b. HDL cholesterol level of 75 mg/dL
   c. Low-density lipoprotein (LDL) level of 31 mg/dL
   d. LDL level of 25 mg/dL

5. A patient who has started taking niacin complains that he "hates the side effects." Which statement by the nurse is most appropriate?
   a. "You will soon build up tolerance to these side effects."
   b. "You should take the niacin on an empty stomach."
   c. "You can take the niacin every other day if the side effects are bothersome."
   d. "Try taking a small dose of ibuprofen (Advil) 30 minutes before taking the niacin."

6. A patient asks, "What is the 'good cholesterol?'" How will the nurse answer?
   a. Very-low-density lipoprotein (VLDL)
   b. Low-density lipoprotein (LDL)
   c. High-density lipoprotein (HDL)
   d. Triglycerides

7. The medication order reads, "Give lovastatin (Mevacor) 30 mg daily at bedtime, PO." The medication is available in 20-mg tablets. How many tablets will the nurse administer to the patient?

   ____

Critical Thinking and Application

Answer the following questions on a separate sheet of paper.

8. For each of the following drugs, name the antilipemic category and briefly describe how the drug lowers lipid levels.
   a. gemfibrozil (Lopid)
   b. niacin
   c. lovastatin (Mevacor)
   d. cholestyramine (Questran)

9. Mr. H. is a 46-year-old business executive who travels frequently. He is slightly overweight "from all that room service," but he did quit smoking 6 years ago. He has no history of coronary heart disease (CHD), nor family history of CHD. During a routine checkup, Mr. H. is found to have an LDL cholesterol

level of 170 mg/dL. He says, "I'm a busy man! Just give me some pills. I've got a plane to catch!" Will the physician prescribe an antilipemic for Mr. H.? Explain your answer.

10. Mr. J. is a 49-year-old farmer. During assessment, you discover the following: Mr. J.'s mother is living, but his father "dropped dead of a heart attack" at 53 years of age. Mr. J. is a smoker with mild asthma and some arthritis in his hands. His blood pressure today is 122/78 mm Hg, and laboratory studies show an HDL cholesterol level of 77 mg/dL. Discuss Mr. J.'s risk factors for high cholesterol levels.

11. Mrs. K. has been treated with cholestyramine for type IIa hyperlipidemia for the past 2 months. She tells the nurse that she "can't stand being so irregular" and that she has developed another "embarrassing problem" as well. What is wrong with Mrs. K., and how can the nurse help her?

12. Justus is a 55-year-old attorney being treated with lovastatin (Mevacor) for his hyperlipidemia. His current health status includes mild hypertension and a peptic ulcer. The nurse knows that niacin is frequently prescribed as an adjunct to other antilipemic drugs. Would niacin be helpful for Justus? Explain your answer.

13. You are visiting Mrs. N., a homebound patient who is being treated for hyperlipidemia and hypertension. During your visit, Mrs. N. takes her antihypertensive medication and then begins to mix her dose of cholestyramine into a glass of orange juice. What patient teaching does Mrs. N. require?

Case Study

Read the scenario and answer the following questions on a separate sheet of paper.

Mr. Miller has been diagnosed with type IIa hyperlipidemia and has been given a prescription for atorvastatin (Lipitor). He acts thrilled with the news, and says, "Great! Now I don't have to worry about watching my diet because I'm on this medicine!"

1. Is he right? What type of dietary guidelines should he follow while on this therapy?

2. What therapeutic effects do you hope to see as a result of his taking this medication?

3. After 2 months of therapy, you note that his liver enzyme levels are slightly elevated. Is this a concern? What other laboratory values should be monitored while Mr. M. is taking atorvastatin?

4. Mr. Miller calls the office to complain about some muscle pain. He thought he had pulled a muscle during a tennis match, but the pain has not lessened in 3 days. Is this a concern?

CHAPTER 30

Pituitary Drugs

Chapter Review and NCLEX® Examination Preparation

1. **Complete the following table.**

Hormone	Function	Mimicking Drug(s)
Adrenocorticotropic hormone (ACTH, corticotropin)	Targets adrenal gland; mediates adaptation to stressors; promotes synthesis of the following three hormones: a.	b.
Growth hormone	c.	d.
e.	Increases water resorption in distal tubules and collecting duct of nephron; concentrates urine; potent vasoconstrictor	f.
Endogenous oxytocin	g.	h.

Select the best answer for each question.

2. When administering vasopressin, which is the priority vital sign for the nurse to monitor?
   a. Temperature
   b. Pulse
   c. Respirations
   d. Blood pressure

3. A nurse is administering octreotide (Sandostatin) to a patient who has a metastatic carcinoid tumor. The patient asks about the purpose of this drug. What is the nurse's best response?
   a. "This drug helps to reduce the size of your tumor."
   b. "This drug works to prevent the spread of your tumor."
   c. "Octreotide is given to reduce the nausea and vomiting you are having from the chemotherapy."
   d. "This drug helps to control the flushing and diarrhea that you are experiencing."

4. Which nursing diagnosis is most appropriate for a patient who is receiving a pituitary drug?
   a. Constipation
   b. Disturbed body image
   c. Impaired physical mobility
   d. Impaired skin integrity

5. The nurse will instruct a patient taking desmopressin acetate as a nasal spray for the treatment of diabetes insipidus to perform which action to obtain maximum benefit from the drug?
   a. Clear the nasal passages after spraying the medication.
   b. Inhale the spray for full drug effect.
   c. Take an over-the-counter preparation to control mucus if nasal congestion occurs.
   d. Administer the nasal spray at the same time every day.

6. During vasopressin therapy, which is the priority nursing action?
   a. Check blood glucose levels regularly.
   b. Monitor the electrocardiogram for changes.
   c. Monitor the IV site for signs of infiltration.
   d. Watch for hyperthermia.

7. When assessing a patient who is receiving octreotide (Sandostatin) therapy, the nurse should monitor which assessment finding?
   a. Blood glucose levels
   b. Pulse
   c. Weight
   d. Serum potassium levels

8. A child who weighs 44 pounds experiencing growth failure is to receive growth hormone therapy. The dosage ordered is 0.3 mg/kg per week, to be given as a series of six daily injections.
   a. What is the dose per week that this child will receive? _____________
   b. What is the dose per injection? ____________

Critical Thinking and Application

Answer the following questions on a separate sheet of paper.

9. The nurse has recently begun working in a specialized endocrinology clinic. Her first patient, Patricia, a second-grader, is not growing at the expected rate. The physician has determined that Patricia is a candidate for somatropin therapy. Her parents are nervous about giving injections to Patricia. What should be emphasized when the nurse is teaching her parents about giving this drug?

Case Study

Read the scenario and answer the following questions on a separate sheet of paper.

Mr. Collins has been experiencing severe thirst, which he reports "of course makes me go to the bathroom all the time, it seems." He is also dehydrated, despite the large amounts of water he has been drinking.

1. Predict Mr. Collins' probable disorder and two likely drugs of choice for Mr. Collins.

2. How will you assess Mr. Collins before administering these drugs?

3. As a result of your assessment, it has been determined that Mr. Collins should do well with desmopressin therapy. Indicate how you would describe the treatment and its therapeutic effects (that is, how it mimics the natural hormone) to the patient.

4. Following your explanation, Mr. Collins says, "Okay, okay, but what does it do for me?" Explain the physical improvements Mr. Collins should be able to see.

CHAPTER 31

Thyroid and Antithyroid Drugs

Critical Thinking Crossword

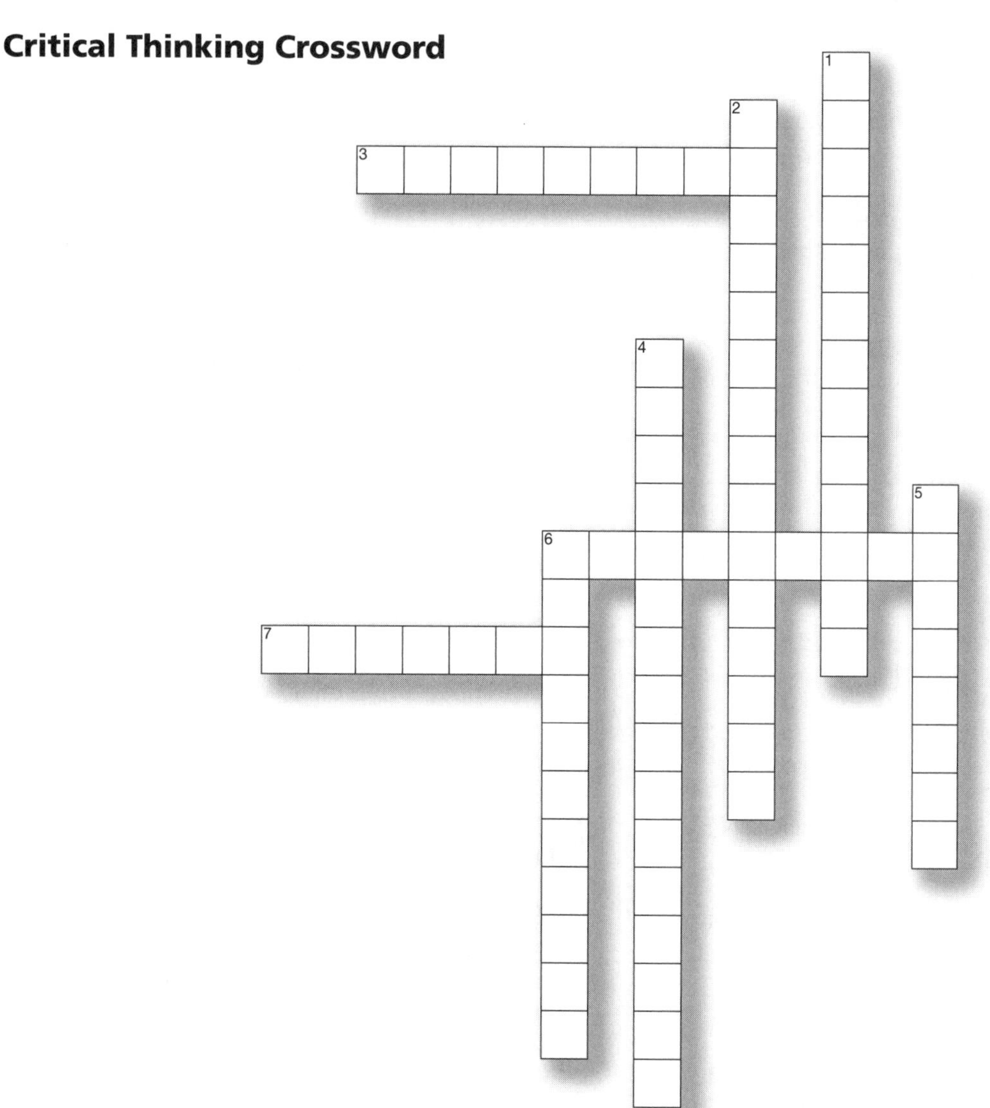

Across

3. The type of hypothyroidism that results from insufficient secretion of thyroid-stimulating hormone (TSH) from the pituitary gland
6. The principal thyroid hormone that influences the metabolic rate
7. The type of hypothyroidism that is due to the inability of the thyroid gland to perform a function

Down

1. The most commonly prescribed synthetic thyroid hormone
2. Excessive secretion of thyroid hormones
4. A drug used to treat hyperthyroidism
5. The type of hypothyroidism that stems from reduced secretion of thyrotropin-releasing hormone from the hypothalamus
6. Another name for TSH

Chapter Review and NCLEX® Examination Preparation

Select the best answer for each question.

1. A patient who is beginning therapy with levothyroxine (Synthroid) asks the nurse when the medication will start working. What is the nurse's best answer?
   a. Immediately
   b. Within a few days
   c. Within a few weeks
   d. Within a few months

2. A patient wants to switch brands of levothyroxine (Synthroid). What is the nurse's best response?
   a. "If you do this, you should reduce the dosage of your current brand before starting the new one."
   b. "Levothyroxine has been standardized, so there is only one brand."
   c. "It shouldn't matter if you switch brands; they are all very much the same."
   d. "You should check with your physician before switching brands."

3. Patient teaching for a patient taking antithyroid medication should include the need to avoid which foods?
   a. Soy products and seafood
   b. Bananas and oranges
   c. Dairy products
   d. Processed meats and cheese

4. Which information should be included in the nurse's teaching of patients taking thyroid medications? *(Select all that apply.)*
   a. Keeping a log or journal of individual responses and a graph of pulse rate, weight, and mood would be helpful.
   b. The medication should be discontinued if the adverse effects become too strong.
   c. The medication should be taken at the same time every day.
   d. Nervousness, irritability, and insomnia may be a result of a dosage that is too high.
   e. Thyroid replacement drugs should be taken after meals.

5. A patient is scheduled for a radioactive isotope study. Upon review of his medications, the scheduling nurse notes that he takes levothyroxine (Levothroid) daily. Which statement is correct regarding the use of this medication before a radioactive isotope study?
   a. The patient should continue to take the medication as ordered.
   b. The patient should skip the medication on the morning of the test.
   c. The patient should stop the medication about 4 weeks before the test.
   d. The patient should reduce the dosage 1 week before the test.

6. Levothyroxine, 88 mcg PO is ordered. What is 88 mcg expressed as mg? ________________

Critical Thinking and Application

Answer the following questions on a separate sheet of paper.

7. Mrs. W., age 43, comes into the clinic complaining of hair loss, lethargy, and constipation. "I just can't eat anything," she says. As the nurse takes her blood pressure, he notices that her skin feels thickened. She also seems to have a lump in her neck. Which of the disorders discussed in this chapter is Mrs. W. most likely to have? Suggest several possible appropriate medications. Which of those is generally preferred? Why?

8. Ms. H. has had Graves' disease for 3 years. Today she reports symptoms of diarrhea, muscle weakness, fatigue, and palpitations. Also, she says that despite the diarrhea, she often has an increased appetite. She is also having trouble sleeping and wonders whether she is undergoing menopause because she suffers flushing, heat intolerance, and altered menstrual flow. As the nurse asks her questions about these symptoms, it is noted that she seems irritable. This is understandable given her multiple symptoms; however, the nurse has known Ms. H. since she began treatment for Graves' disease, and she has never acted this way before, no matter how bad she felt. What will the nurse suspect is happening with Ms. H.?

9. After undergoing a thyroidectomy as treatment for a thyroid tumor that turned out to be benign, Rebecca is given a prescription for levothyroxine (Levothroid). "I thought I would be cured after this surgery!" she exclaimed. "Why do I have to take a pill every day?" What will the nurse explain to Rebecca?

10. The nurse is examining changes in a medication administration record after new orders were written. One new medication order reads, "levothyroxine, 200 mg, once a day." The nurse suspects an error. What is wrong with this order?

Case Study

Read the scenario and answer the following questions on a separate sheet of paper.

Goldie, a 38-year-old teacher, has come to the clinic complaining of having "no energy or appetite" and yet her weight has increased by 15 pounds in the last month. You note that her hair is thin and her skin is dull. Laboratory work reveals an elevated level of TSH.

1. What do Goldie's symptoms suggest? What medication do you expect to be ordered for her?

2. Explain the concept of "euthyroid" as it would relate to Goldie's condition.

3. One month after therapy has begun, Goldie calls the office to complain that she "can't sleep at all" since she started taking the medication. She says she tries to take it at the same time every morning but often forgets and takes it at dinnertime. What teaching, if any, does she need to help her with this problem?

CHAPTER 32

Antidiabetic Drugs

Chapter Review and NCLEX® Examination Preparation

Select the best answer for each question.

1. When administering insulin, the nurse must keep in mind that which is the most immediate and serious adverse effect of insulin therapy?
   a. Hyperglycemia
   b. Hypoglycemia
   c. Bradycardia
   d. Orthostatic hypotension

2. A dose of long-acting insulin has been ordered for bedtime for a diabetic patient. The nurse expects to give which type of insulin?
   a. Regular
   b. Lispro
   c. NPH
   d. Glargine

3. A patient is to be placed on an insulin drip to control his high blood glucose levels. The nurse knows that which is the only type of insulin that can be given intravenously?
   a. Regular
   b. Lispro
   c. NPH
   d. Glargine

4. While monitoring a patient who is receiving insulin therapy, the nurse observes for which signs of hypoglycemia?
   a. Decreased pulse and respiratory rates and flushed skin
   b. Increased pulse rate and a fruity, acetone breath odor
   c. Irritability, sweating, and confusion
   d. Increased urine output and edema

5. When giving oral acarbose (Precose), the nurse should administer it at what time?
   a. With the first bite of a meal
   b. 15 minutes before a meal
   c. 30 minutes before a meal
   d. 1 hour after eating

6. A patient taking rosiglitazone (Avandia) tells the nurse, "There's my insulin pill!" Which information will the nurse provide to the patient regarding the mechanism of action of rosiglitazone?
   a. "It stimulates the beta cells of the pancreas to produce insulin."
   b. "It decreases insulin resistance."
   c. "It inhibits hepatic glucose production."
   d. "It decreases intestinal absorption of glucose."

7. The nurse is reviewing the history of a patient who will be taking the amylin mimetic drug pramlintide (Symlin). Which condition is a contraindication to the use of this drug?
   a. Hypertension
   b. Coronary artery disease
   c. Hypothyroidism
   d. Gastroparesis

8. The sliding-scale insulin order reads: "Do bedside glucose testing before meals. For glucose results over 150 mg/dL, give regular (Humulin R) insulin, 1 unit for every 20 mg/dL over 150 mg/dL." If the blood glucose level is 238 mg/dL, the patient will receive ______ unit(s) of insulin.

Critical Thinking and Application

Answer the following questions on a separate sheet of paper.

9. What is the mechanism of action of each drug?
   a. pramlintide (Symlin)
   b. exenatide (Byetta)
   c. metformin (Glucophage)

10. Alice occasionally experiences hypoglycemia as a result of her diabetes drug therapy.
    a. What signs and symptoms of hypoglycemia should Alice be taught about?
    b. The nurse knows that one of the early signs of hypoglycemia is irritability. Why is this true?
    c. If Alice experiences hypoglycemia at home, what are the treatment options?

11. The nurse's co-worker is in the medication room preparing a dose of Novolin-R to administer to a patient.
    a. Before he administers the medication, how will the nurse's co-worker verify the order?
    b. When the nurse enters the room, she notices that the insulin is cloudy. When the nurse tells her co-worker to discard it, he says, "Insulin is supposed to look this way." Who is right, the nurse or her co-worker?
    c. The nurse examines the vial. A date on the label indicates that it has been on the shelf in this room for 2 months. Is this a problem?

12. Mrs. F., a 48-year-old homemaker, is 5 feet tall and weighs 180 pounds. During a routine physical, laboratory studies indicate an elevated blood glucose level. The nurse's assessment of Mrs. F. reveals that she is a smoker with mild hypertension. The physician suspects type 2 diabetes.
    a. What initial treatment is indicated for Mrs. F.? Explain your answer.
    b. At a follow-up visit 3 months later, Mrs. F.'s blood glucose level is still elevated. She has quit smoking, however, and has been walking for exercise. What treatment is indicated now?

13. Dennis is a 40-year-old taxicab dispatcher who takes glipizide (Glucotrol). He comes to the emergency department late one Sunday evening complaining that he feels weak, he vomited earlier, he has a headache, and his face "feels hot." You note that Dennis has profound flushing and is sweating.
    a. What do Dennis's signs and symptoms indicate?
    b. What may have caused this? How can you tell?

14. The patient is taking insulin every morning with sliding-scale coverage. The specified dosages are: NPH insulin, 20 units, every morning before breakfast, and regular insulin, sliding-scale coverage, before meals and at bedtime, as follows:
    - Blood glucose level lower than 200 mg/dL: no additional coverage
    - Blood glucose level 200 to 249 mg/dL: 2 units regular (Humulin R) insulin
    - Blood glucose level 250 to 299 mg/dL: 4 units regular (Humulin R) insulin
    - Blood glucose level 300 to 349 mg/dL: 6 units Regular (Humulin R) insulin
    - Blood glucose level higher than 350 mg/dL: call for orders

    How much insulin will the patient receive in the following circumstances?
    a. Before breakfast, if her blood glucose level is 275 mg/dL
    b. Before lunch, if her blood glucose level is 199 mg/dL
    c. Before dinner, if her blood glucose level is 328 mg/dL

15. A patient who has been taking metformin (Glucophage) for type 2 diabetes mellitus needs to have a radiology exam with contrast dye. What is the nurse's best action regarding the metformin?

Case Study

Read the scenario and answer the following questions on a separate sheet of paper.

The physician is planning to prescribe glipizide (Glucotrol) for Mr. D., a 50-year-old financial advisor with a history of renal failure. In particular, Mr. D. requires treatment for the short-term elevation in blood glucose level that occurs after he eats.

1. Why would glipizide be a good choice for Mr. D.?

2. When should he take this drug? Explain.

3. A few weeks later, Mr. D. comes down with the flu. He is vomiting and has been unable to eat all day. What should he do, and why?

CHAPTER 33

Adrenal Drugs

Chapter Review and NCLEX® Examination Preparation

Select the best answer for each question.

1. A 50-year-old man has been taking prednisone (Deltasone) following a severe reaction to poison ivy. He notices that the dosage of the medication decreases. During a follow-up office visit, he asks the nurse why he must continue the medication and why he cannot just stop taking it now that the skin rash is better. What is the nurse's best response?
   a. "Sudden discontinuation of this medication may result in adrenal insufficiency."
   b. "You would experience withdrawal symptoms if the drug were discontinued abruptly."
   c. "Cushing's syndrome may develop as a reaction to a sudden drop of serum cortisone levels."
   d. "You can stop taking the medication if his rash is better."

2. Which medication is the preferred oral glucocorticoid for antiinflammatory or immunosuppressant purposes?
   a. fludrocortisone (Florinef)
   b. dexamethasone
   c. prednisone (Deltasone)
   d. hydrocortisone (Solu-Cortef)

3. When monitoring a patient who is taking corticosteroids, the nurse observes for which adverse effects? *(Select all that apply.)*
   a. Fragile skin
   b. Increased glucose levels
   c. Nervousness
   d. Hypotension
   e. Weight loss
   f. Drowsiness

4. A patient has Cushing's syndrome. The nurse expects which drug to be used to inhibit the function of the adrenal cortex in the treatment of this syndrome?
   a. dexamethasone
   b. aminoglutethimide (Cytadren)
   c. hydrocortisone (Solu-Cortef)
   d. fludrocortisone (Florinef)

5. A patient who has been taking corticosteroids has developed a "moon face" and facial redness, and has many bruises on her arms. Which is the most appropriate nursing diagnosis?
   a. Risk for infection
   b. Imbalanced nutrition: Less than body requirements
   c. Deficient fluid volume
   d. Disturbed body image

6. Because corticosteroids may cause sodium retention, the nurse should closely monitor patients with which condition when administering corticosteroids?
   a. Diabetes mellitus
   b. Seizure disorders
   c. Heart failure
   d. Hyperthyroidism

7. The order reads "dexamethasone, 1.5 mg, twice a day." The medication is available in 3-mg tablets. How many tablets will the nurse give? ___________

Critical Thinking and Application

Answer the following questions on a separate sheet of paper.

8. Ms. R., a 30-year-old hospital receptionist, is receiving glucocorticoid therapy after a kidney transplant. The nurse is reviewing her drug regimen with her when she says that she frequently uses aspirin or ibuprofen to treat problems like headaches or menstrual cramps. She also mentions that she enjoys walking for exercise and likes to visit sick children on the hospital's pediatric ward when she has time. What issues will the nurse discuss with Ms. R.?

9. Peter, a 21-year-old mechanic, has developed a severe skin rash after a camping trip. The physician is planning to prescribe prednisone (Deltasone). The nursing assessment reveals that Peter has type 1 diabetes.
   a. Does that finding affect Peter's treatment? Explain your answer.
   b. To help minimize gastrointestinal effects, what advice will the nurse have for someone taking an oral form of a systemic adrenal drug?

10. The nurse is watching a student nurse prepare to apply a topical glucocorticoid to a patient's skin rash. After donning gloves, she places some of the medication on her finger. Should the nurse intervene, or is the student nurse doing fine so far? What other consideration is involved in determining the technique for applying a topical drug?

11. Nina has been prescribed a steroid drug delivered via inhaler. What special instructions will the nurse give her?

Case Study

Read the scenario and answer the following questions on a separate sheet of paper.

Julie is in the urgent care center because of an exacerbation of asthma. She is usually able to control it with inhaled bronchodilators, but the physician decides to give her a short course of prednisone (Deltasone) in a dose that started high and then tapered down over a week's time.

1. Why is the dose tapered instead of just discontinued after a week?

2. What are potential effects of long-term therapy?

3. Is this drug a glucocorticoid or mineralocorticoid? Explain the difference.

4. What time of day will she take this drug? Explain.

CHAPTER 34

Women's Health Drugs

Chapter Review and NCLEX® Examination Preparation

Select the best answer for each question.

1. When reviewing the health history of a patient who wants to begin taking oral contraceptives, the nurse recalls that which conditions are contraindications to this drug therapy? *(Select all that apply.)*
   a. Multiple sclerosis
   b. Pregnancy
   c. Thrombophlebitic disorders
   d. Hypothyroidism
   e. Abnormal vaginal bleeding

2. When the nurse is teaching patients about postmenopausal estrogen replacement therapy, which statement is correct?
   a. "The smallest dose that is effective will be prescribed."
   b. "Oral forms should be taken on an empty stomach for best absorption."
   c. "Estrogen therapy should be long-term to prevent menopausal symptoms."
   d. "If estrogen is taken, supplemental calcium will not be needed."

3. When combination oral contraceptives are given to provide postcoital emergency contraception, the nurse should remember which fact?
   a. They are not effective if the woman is already pregnant.
   b. They should be taken within 12 hours of unprotected intercourse.
   c. They are given in one dose.
   d. They are intended to terminate pregnancy.

4. When reviewing an order for dinoprostone cervical gel (Prepidil), the nurse recalls that this drug is used for which purpose?
   a. To induce abortion during the third trimester
   b. To improve cervical inducibility ("ripening") near term for labor induction
   c. To soften the cervix in women who are experiencing infertility problems
   d. To reduce postpartum uterine atony and hemorrhage

5. A pregnant woman is experiencing contractions. The nurse remembers that drugs such as terbutaline are used to prevent contractions during which timeframe?
   a. Before the 20th week of gestation
   b. Between the 20th and 37th weeks
   c. After the 37th week
   d. At any time during the pregnancy if delivery is not desired

6. What patient teaching is appropriate for a patient taking alendronate (Fosamax)? *(Select all that apply.)*
   a. Take on an empty stomach.
   b. Take at night just before going to bed.
   c. Take with an 8-oz glass of water.
   d. Take with a sip of water.
   e. Take first thing in the morning upon arising.
   f. Do not lie down for at least 30 minutes after taking.

7. The patient is to receive medroxyprogesterone (Depo-Provera), 500 mg, weekly on Mondays for four weeks. The medication is available in vials of 400 mg/mL. How many mL will the nurse administer with each injection? ________________

Critical Thinking and Application

Answer the following questions on a separate sheet of paper.

8. Isabelle is a 48-year-old woman exhibiting symptoms of menopause. Assessment of Isabelle reveals a history of depression and mild arthritis.
   a. What will the nurse need to ask Isabelle and why?
   b. The physician decides to prescribe estrogen therapy. At this time, what does the nurse know about the dose and the length of time it will be administered?

9. Ms. K. is a 25-year-old paralegal with diabetes. She is at the physician's office today because her menstrual periods have ceased. The physician has decided to prescribe a hormonal drug.
   a. Which drug will the physician likely prescribe?
   b. What adjustments to Ms. K.'s existing drug regimen might need to be made?

10. Jacklyn receives a prescription for norethindrone and ethinyl estradiol (Ortho-Novum) for birth control purposes. At a follow-up visit 4 months later, she tells the nurse, "I'm really messing up. I take the pills for 3 weeks, but when I'm off them for a week, sometimes I don't remember to start again!"
    a. What might the nurse suggest to help Jacklyn?
    b. Jacklyn then expresses concern that her menstrual bleeding, now that she is taking birth control pills, is "nothing compared with what it used to be." She asks the nurse whether she is okay. What will the nurse tell Jacklyn?

11. Ms. J., a sales associate in a bookstore, is being treated for fertility problems. She is currently on a drug regimen that includes human chorionic gonadotropin and clomiphene (Clomid). Why is she taking two fertility drugs?

12. Mrs. I. has been taking estrogen therapy for several weeks. During a routine checkup, she sheepishly tells the nurse that she has not been able to quit smoking yet. She also mentions that she is going to Aruba for a vacation the next month. What patient teaching does Mrs. I. require?

13. Mrs. S., age 33, comes in for her yearly gynecologic examination, and the physician recommends alendronate (Fosamax), 5 mg daily. Mrs. S. experienced early menopause last year and asks the nurse, "Why did the doctor wait until now to start me on estrogen? I didn't need it before."
    a. What will the nurse explain about the purpose of this medication?
    b. What risk factors might Mrs. S. have to support therapy with alendronate?

14. Mr. G. is receiving 400 mg of megestrol (Megace). This drug is a progestin, a female hormone. Why is a male patient receiving this medication?

Case Study

Read the scenario and answer the following questions on a separate sheet of paper.

Ms. O., a 34-year-old computer programmer, is having mild contractions. She is in the 30th week of gestation, and the physician determines that she is experiencing premature labor.

1. What drug is the physician likely to prescribe, and how does it work?

2. In what position do you place Ms. O. before starting the intravenous infusion. Why?

3. Ms. O.'s contractions stop, and she is sent home on maintenance ritodrine therapy. At a follow-up visit, her blood glucose and electrolyte levels are checked. Why?

4. During her 39th week of gestation, her contractions return. Will she receive this same therapy?

CHAPTER 35

Men's Health Drugs

Chapter Review and NCLEX® Examination Preparation

Select the best answer for each question.

1. A 19-year-old college football player asks his friend's mother, who is a nurse, about taking steroids to help him "beef up" his muscles. Which statement is true?
   a. There should be no problems as long as he does not exceed the recommended dosage.
   b. Long-term use may cause a life-threatening liver condition.
   c. He would need to be careful to watch for excessive weight loss.
   d. These drugs also tend to increase the male's sperm count.

2. In which situations would androgens be prescribed for a woman? *(Select all that apply.)*
   a. Development of secondary sex characteristics
   b. Fibrocystic breast disease
   c. Ovarian cancer
   d. Treatment of endometriosis
   e. Postmenopausal osteoporosis prevention
   f. Metastatic breast cancer

3. A patient will be receiving testosterone therapy for male hypogonadism and has a new prescription for transdermal testosterone (Testoderm). The nurse needs to include which teaching about the use of this medication?
   a. The patch should be applied only to the scrotum.
   b. The patch should not be applied to the scrotum.
   c. If the adverse effects become bothersome, the patient should stop using the patch.
   d. The patch should be applied to a different area of the upper body each day.

4. Before a patient begins therapy with finasteride (Proscar), the nurse should make sure that which laboratory test has been performed?
   a. Blood glucose level
   b. Complete blood count
   c. Urinalysis
   d. Prostate-specific antigen (PSA) level

5. A patient is taking finasteride (Proscar) for the treatment of benign prostatic hyperplasia. His wife, who is 3 months pregnant, is worried about the adverse effects that may occur with this drug. Which statement by the nurse is the most important at this time?
   a. "Gastric upset may be reduced if he takes this drug on an empty stomach."
   b. "He should notice therapeutic effects of increased libido and erection within 1 month."
   c. "This medication should not even be handled by pregnant women because it may harm the fetus."
   d. "He may experience transient hair loss while taking this medication."

6. A male patient wants to know if there are any drugs that can be used for baldness. The nurse knows that which drug, in low dosages, is used for androgenetic alopecia in men?
   a. finasteride (Propecia)
   b. vardenafil (Levitra)
   c. danazol (Danocrine)
   d. oxandrolone (Oxandrin)

7. A patient is to receive testosterone cypionate (Depo-Testosterone) 300 mg every 2 weeks as an intramuscular injection. The medication is available in two strengths: 100 mg/mL and 200 mg/mL.
   a. Which is the most appropriate strength? ________________
   b. How many mL will the nurse administer per injection? ________________

Critical Thinking and Application

Answer the following questions on a separate sheet of paper.

8. Mr. M. is being treated for hypogonadism. He has been taking intramuscular injections of testosterone cypionate (Depo-Testosterone) but has complained about the pain caused by the injections. Today he will be switched to an oral dosage form. He expects to get "testosterone pills." However, the nurse remembers the poor performance of the drug when given via that route, and she tells him that it will probably not be testosterone itself.
   a. Mr. M. is skeptical of switching drugs and asks for more information. Explain specifically why oral testosterone does not work well.
   b. What does the nurse predict Mr. M. will receive instead?
   c. Discuss potential contraindications that might apply to this patient.

9. Mr. M. is prescribed methyltestosterone buccally. He reports that he gets "tired" of waiting for the buccal tablet to dissolve and asks whether he can swallow or chew it, at least after it is mostly dissolved.
   a. If Mr. M. lets most of the tablet dissolve on its own, is it acceptable to compromise, for the sake of patient compliance, by letting him chew or swallow the rest?
   b. "And while we're on the subject," Mr. M. says, "I'm going on a fishing trip next week. I'd like not to have to bother with the pills. Can we work something out so that I stop temporarily and pick back up with the treatment as soon as I get back?" What do you say?

10. Mr. O. has been prescribed finasteride (Proscar) for his benign prostatic hyperplasia. He asks, "How does it work?" The nurse explains that it will cause his prostate to decrease in size and alleviate discomfort. He is concerned about taking this new drug. What are the most important things for the nurse to include in his patient teaching plan?

11. Compare the application methods for the following forms of testosterone: Testoderm patch, Androderm patch, and AndroGel.

Case Study

Read the scenario and answer the following questions on a separate sheet of paper.

Mr. E., age 72, has asked the physician for "help with a private matter." He tells the physician that he would like to try Viagra, "that drug that helps with a certain problem."

1. What assessment findings may contraindicate the use of sildenafil (Viagra) by Mr. E.?

2. If he is a candidate for therapy with Viagra, what patient teaching should he receive?

3. What concerns would there be about his liver function? About his vision?

4. When should he take this medication?

CHAPTER 36

Antihistamines, Decongestants, Antitussives, and Expectorants

Chapter Review and NCLEX® Examination Preparation

Select the best answer for each question.

1. The nurse who is providing patient teaching about antihistamine use will include which information? *(Select all that apply.)*
   a. Antihistamines are best tolerated when taken with meals.
   b. The patient can chew gum if he or she experiences dry mouth.
   c. Drowsiness is a frequent side effect of antihistamines.
   d. Over-the-counter medications are generally safe to use with antihistamines.
   e. The patient should avoid drinking alcoholic beverages while on these drugs.

2. A patient asks the nurse for advice about one of the newer antihistamines that does not cause drowsiness. Which of these drugs is appropriate?
   a. loratadine (Claritin)
   b. diphenhydramine (Benadryl)
   c. dimenhydrinate (Dramamine)
   d. meclizine (Antivert)

3. Which drugs are considered first-line drugs for the treatment of nasal congestion? *(Select all that apply.)*
   a. Antihistamines such as diphenhydramine
   b. Decongestants such as naphazoline
   c. Antitussives such as dextromethorphan
   d. Expectorants such as guaifenesin
   e. Inhaled corticosteroids such as beclomethasone

4. When giving an antitussive, the nurse remembers that they are used primarily for what reason?
   a. To relieve nasal congestion
   b. To thin secretions to ease removal of excessive secretions
   c. To stop the cough reflex when the cough is nonproductive
   d. To suppress productive and nonproductive coughs

5. The nurse is administering an expectorant and will provide which teaching?
   a. Avoid fluids for 30 to 35 minutes after the dose.
   b. Drink extra fluids, unless contraindicated, to aid in expectoration of sputum.
   c. Avoid driving or operating heavy machinery while taking this medication.
   d. Expect secretions to become thicker.

6. A patient has been self-medicating with diphenhydramine (Benadryl) to help her sleep. She calls the clinic nurse to ask, "Why do I feel so tired during the day after I take this pill? I get a good night's sleep!" Which statement by the nurse is correct?
   a. "You are probably getting too much sleep."
   b. "You are taking too much of the drug."
   c. "This drug is not really meant to help people sleep."
   d. "This drug often causes a 'hangover effect' during the day after taking it."

7. A patient is to receive guaifenesin, 300 mg, via his nasogastric tube. The available medication is syrup, 100 mg/5mL. How many mL will the nurse administer? 15mL

Critical Thinking and Application

Answer the following questions on a separate sheet of paper.

8. Why are histamine-1 (H_1) blockers most beneficial when given early in a histamine-mediated reaction?

9. Do the traditional antihistamines have any advantages over the newer, nonsedating antihistamines? Explain your answer.

10. Mrs. L. was seen in the office several days ago with a common cold. She has been on decongestant therapy with naphazoline nasal spray (Privine) since that time. Today she calls to say, "I thought I was getting over this, but suddenly my nose is more stuffed up than ever." Does Mrs. L. possibly need a stronger dosage of the decongestant? Explain your answer.

11. Keith has been using a topical nasal decongestant for the past few days. He calls the physician's office to report that he is feeling nervous and dizzy and that his heart seems to be racing. What might be the cause of Keith's symptoms?

12. How does benzonatate (Tessalon Perles) differ from other antitussive drugs in its mechanism of action? In its drug interaction profile?

13. One day the nurse encounters her neighbor Irene as she is returning home from work. Irene is on her way to the drugstore, she tells the nurse, because she has been experiencing a nonproductive cough and wants to get a cough medicine "to loosen things up." The nurse recalls that Irene mentioned a few months ago that she has problems with her thyroid. Will the nurse wish Irene good luck and continue on her way? Explain your answer.

14. Lisa is a 5-year-old patient who has bronchitis accompanied by a nonproductive cough. The physician has prescribed Robitussin DM for the cough. Lisa's father tells the nurse that his 11-year-old son was prescribed Robitussin A-C several months earlier for a severe cough. He asks whether his son's cough medicine would help Lisa because "there's plenty left in the bottle." What will the nurse tell him?

15. Britney gave birth recently and is breastfeeding her baby. She calls the pediatrician's office because she wants to take an over-the-counter antihistamine for her allergies. "It's okay now that I've given birth, right?" What is the nurse's best answer?

Case Study

Read the scenario and answer the following questions on a separate sheet of paper.

James, a 35-year-old electrician, is seen in the emergency department with a rash on his arms and hands that appeared after he was working in his yard. You suspect that the physician will prescribe topical diphenhydramine (Benadryl), but during the nursing assessment, James tells you that he has diabetes.

1. How does James's diabetes affect his possible treatment with diphenhydramine?

2. If James does receive a topical diphenhydramine preparation, what other drug might be found in combination with it?

The topical medication did not help his rash, and James has been switched to oral diphenhydramine. He tells you that he expects to return to work tomorrow and hopes this medication "does the trick."

3. What cautions, if any, should James be aware of while taking this medication?

4. Are there any concerns with drug interactions?

CHAPTER 37

Bronchodilators and Other Respiratory Drugs

Chapter Review and NCLEX® Examination Preparation

Select the best answer for each of the following.

1. The nurse is teaching a group of patients about the use of bronchodilators. It is important to remind them that using bronchodilators too frequently may cause which adverse effects? *(Select all that apply.)*
   a. Blurred vision
   b. Increased heart rate
   c. Decreased heart rate
   d. Nausea
   e. Nervousness
   f. Tremors

2. For patients taking a leukotriene antagonist, the nurse should include which information in the patient teaching?
   a. If a dose is missed, the patient may take a double dose to maintain blood levels.
   b. The patient should gargle or rinse the mouth after using the inhaler.
   c. The medication should be taken at the first sign of bronchospasm.
   d. Improvement should be seen within a week of use.

3. Which drug acts by blocking leukotrienes, thus reducing inflammation in the lungs?
   a. albuterol (Proventil)
   b. cromolyn (Intal)
   c. theophylline (Elixophyllin)
   d. montelukast (Singulair)

4. A patient in status asthmaticus has not yet responded to epinephrine. The nurse will expect which drug to be used next?
   a. albuterol (Proventil)
   b. aminophylline
   c. cromolyn (Intal)
   d. montelukast (Singulair)

5. When a patient is taking parenteral xanthine derivatives such as aminophylline, the nurse should monitor for which adverse effect?
   a. Decreased respirations
   b. Hypotension
   c. Tachycardia
   d. Hypoglycemia

6. A patient who is taking a beta-adrenergic agonist for bronchodilation may also take which type of inhaled drug for its antiinflammatory effects?
   a. Corticosteroid
   b. Anticholinergic
   c. Xanthine derivative
   d. Antileukotriene

7. A patient has a new prescription for a Combivent (ipatropium bromide/albuterol sulfate) metered-dose inhaler. The patient is to take two puffs, four times a day. The inhaler contains 200 "puffs." In how many days should the patient replace the inhaler?

   ____

Critical Thinking and Application

Answer the following questions on a separate sheet of paper.

8. Describe briefly how idiopathic asthma differs from allergic asthma.

9. Tom, a 70-year-old retiree who smoked for 40 years, has been diagnosed with chronic obstructive pulmonary disease (COPD); the treatment regimen prescribed includes theophylline (Theo-Dur). After a few weeks, Tom tells the nurse that he is experiencing nausea and "bad heartburn at night." The laboratory studies show the level of theophylline in his blood to be 30 mcg/mL. What might be wrong with Tom, and how can it be corrected?

10. Sylvia has come to the clinic today complaining of nausea, palpitations, and anxiety. She says that her heart feels "as if it's going to fly out of my chest."

Physical examination confirms an increased heart rate. Sylvia's records indicate that she has asthma for which she uses an albuterol inhaler. What will the nurse suspect might be wrong with Sylvia, and what will the nurse advise her to do?

11. Mrs. V., a 65-year-old office manager, has arthritis, glaucoma, and emphysema. The physician is planning prophylactic treatment for her emphysema.
    a. What three types of drugs might be considered for treatment of COPD?
    b. What factor must the physician keep in mind when determining the best drug for Mrs. V.?

12. Several months ago, the physician prescribed an orally administered corticosteroid for Mr. Z., who has chronic bronchial asthma.
    a. What are the disadvantages of administering the corticosteroids orally? Is there a better alternative route?
    b. Today the physician adds beclomethasone dipropionate (Beclovent) to Mr. Z.'s drug regimen and also reduces the dosage of the oral corticosteroid. Is that safe?

13. Sam is a 10-year-old girl who is to be treated with theophylline (Elixophyllin) for her asthma. Sam's mother asks whether she can crush the tablets to make them easier for Sam to swallow. Is that advisable?

14. Alice has been treated for asthma for several months and has the following inhalers: albuterol (Proventil) and fluticasone (Flovent). Which one should she choose if she experiences an asthma attack? Explain your answer.

15. Justin calls the nurse at the office because he experiences "palpitations and a racing heart" every morning after breakfast. He is taking theophylline (Theo-Dur) as part of his treatment for asthma. Upon questioning, he states that he has been drinking an extra cup of coffee in the morning "to get going" because his coughing has kept him from sleeping well. What could be his problem?

Case Study

Read the scenario and answer the following questions on a separate sheet of paper.

Jennie has been treated for adult-onset asthma for 3 years. Today she has started taking montelukast (Singulair), one 10-mg tablet daily.

1. How does this medication differ from traditional antiasthma drugs?

2. Jennie says, "I hope this medicine works better than the other one I took when I had an asthma attack." What should be your reply?

3. Jennie takes ibuprofen (Advil) on occasion for arthritic pain. What should you advise about taking this medication with montelukast?

4. After 3 months, Jennie stops taking the montelukast. She says, "My symptoms are better, and I don't want to take medicine unless I need it." Is this appropriate?

CHAPTER 38

Antibiotics Part 1

Critical Thinking Crossword

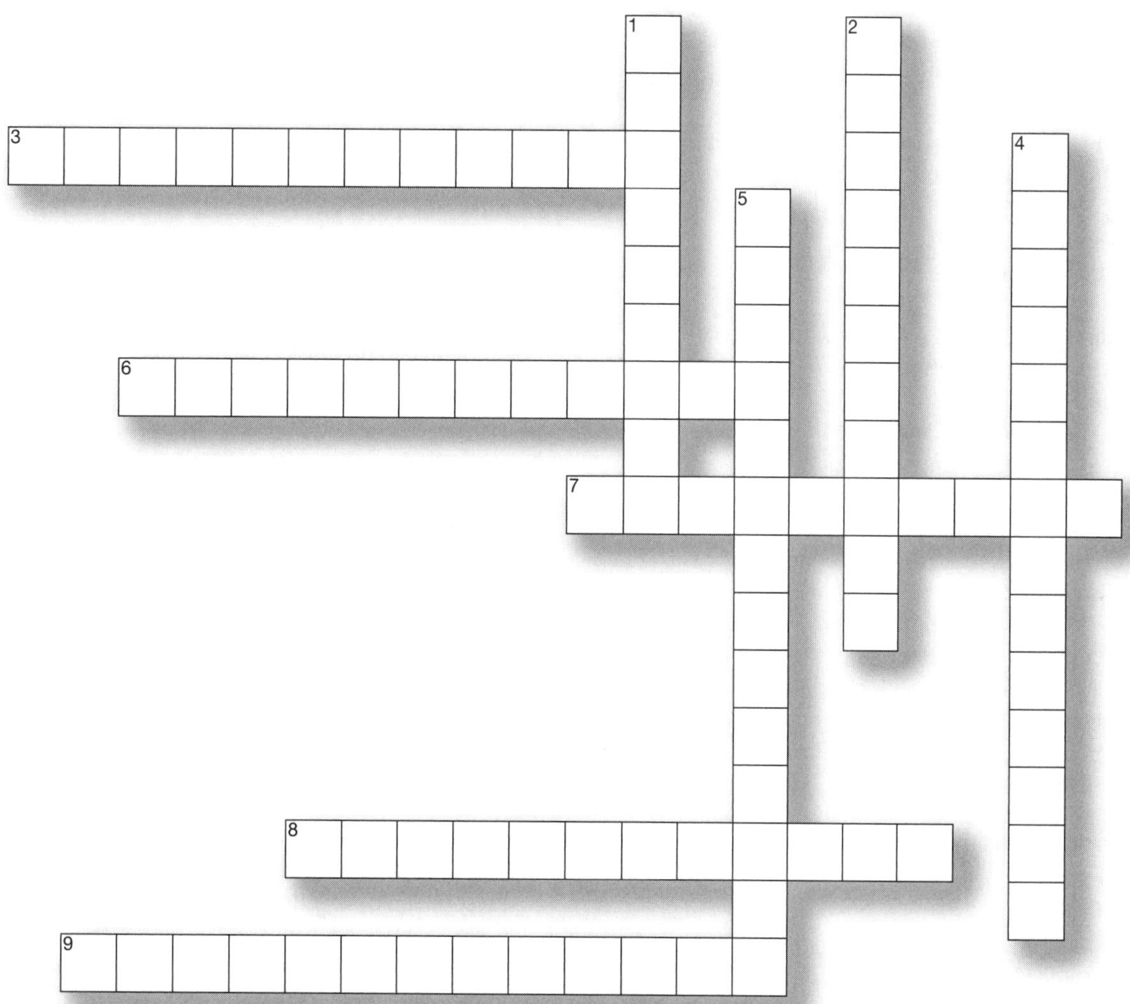

Across

3. Antibiotics taken before exposure to an infectious organism in an effort to prevent the development of infection
6. The classification for the drug doxycycline
7. An antibiotic derived from a fungus or mold often seen on bread or fruit
8. Antibiotics that kill bacteria
9. The classification for the drug cefazolin

Down

1. The classification for the drug erythromycin
2. The classification for the drug sulfisoxazole
4. Antibiotics that inhibit the growth of bacteria
5. An infection that occurs during antimicrobial treatment for another infection and involves overgrowth of a nonsusceptible organism

Chapter Review and NCLEX® Examination Preparation

Select the best answer for each question.

1. The nurse is reviewing the drugs ordered for a patient. A drug interaction occurs between penicillins and which drugs? *(Select all that apply.)*
   a. Alcohol
   b. Oral contraceptives
   c. Digoxin
   d. Nonsteroidal antiinflammatory drugs
   e. Warfarin
   f. Anticonvulsants

2. Which intervention is important for the nurse to perform before beginning antibiotic therapy?
   a. Obtain a specimen for culture and sensitivity.
   b. Give with an antacid to reduce gastrointestinal (GI) upset.
   c. Monitor for adverse effects.
   d. Restrict oral fluids.

3. The nurse will instruct a patient who is receiving a tetracycline antibiotic to take it using which guideline?
   a. It should be taken with milk.
   b. It should be taken with 8 oz of water.
   c. It should be taken 30 minutes before iron preparations are taken.
   d. An antacid should also be taken to decrease GI discomfort.

4. A patient is to receive antibiotic therapy with a cephalosporin. When assessing the patient's drug history, the nurse recognizes that an allergy to which drug class may be a possible contraindication to cephalosporin therapy?
   a. Cardiac glycosides
   b. Thiazide diuretics
   c. Penicillins
   d. Macrolides

5. When asked about drug allergies, a patient says, "I can't take sulfa drugs because I'm allergic to them." Which question should the nurse ask next?
   a. "Do you have any other drug allergies?"
   b. "Who prescribed that drug for you?"
   c. "How long ago did this happen?"
   d. "What happened when you took the sulfa drug?"

6. Which statement accurately describes the action of antiseptics?
   a. They are used to kill organisms on nonliving objects.
   b. They are used to kill organisms on living tissue.
   c. They are used to sterilize equipment.
   d. They are used to inhibit the growth of organisms on living tissue.

7. During a class on health care–associated infections, the nurse shares several facts about these infections. Which statements about health care–associated infections are true? *(Select all that apply.)*
   a. They are contracted in the home or community.
   b. They are contracted in a hospital or institution.
   c. They are more difficult to treat.
   d. The organisms that cause these infections are more virulent.
   e. The infection is incubating at the time of admission.

8. A patient is to receive 2 million units of penicillin G potassium per day, every 6 hours in IV piggyback doses. The medication is available in vials of 1 million units/50 mL, and each dose needs to be mixed in 50 mL of D_5W. How many mL will the nurse draw up for each IV piggyback dose? ________________

Critical Thinking and Application

Answer the following questions on a separate sheet of paper.

9. Mr. R., a 50-year-old banker, is scheduled for colorectal surgery tomorrow. The surgeon is planning to administer a prophylactic antibiotic. What drug is frequently used for this purpose, and why?

10. Sean is a 19-year-old college freshman who has been diagnosed with gonorrhea. The physician has prescribed doxycycline therapy. During the nursing assessment, Sean discusses his diet, which includes "lots of meat, milk, and veggies." Sean also tells the nurse that he jogs frequently and is a member of the tennis team.
    a. In addition to instruction about sexually transmitted diseases, what patient teaching does Sean require?
    b. A few days later, Sean calls and complains of an upset stomach and diarrhea. What does the nurse suspect might be wrong with Sean?

11. Sandra, a 59-year-old homemaker, has bronchitis and has been taking an antibiotic for 1 week. She calls the nurse and complains of severe itching and a whitish discharge in her vaginal area. What has happened, and what caused it?

Case Study

Read the scenario and answer the following questions on a separate sheet of paper.

A 78-year-old patient, admitted to the hospital with a stroke 2 days earlier, has developed a urinary tract infection. His Foley catheter is draining urine that is cloudy and dark yellowish orange with a strong odor. Strands of pus are also visible in the urine. He is receiving an intravenous heparin infusion and has a history of type 2 diabetes. The physician orders co-trimoxazole (Bactrim).

1. What should be assessed before giving this medication?
2. Are there any potential drug interactions?
3. Why was this particular antibiotic chosen?
4. Is this antibiotic bactericidal or bacteriostatic? Explain.

CHAPTER 39

Antibiotics Part 2

Chapter Review and NCLEX® Examination Preparation

Select the best answer for each question.

1. When patients are receiving aminoglycosides, the nurse must monitor for tinnitus and dizziness, which may indicate which problem?
   a. Cardiotoxicity
   b. Hepatotoxicity
   c. Ototoxicity
   d. Nephrotoxicity

2. A patient is being prepared for colon surgery and will be receiving neomycin (Neo-Fradin) tablets during the day before surgery. He asks the nurse why he needs to take this medicine before he even has surgery. What is the nurse's best response?
   a. "This medicine helps to clear out your bowels before surgery."
   b. "It helps to reduce the number of bacteria in your intestines before surgery."
   c. "It is given to sterilize your bowel before surgery."
   d. "It is given to prevent an infection after surgery."

3. A patient has been admitted to the unit with a stage IV pressure ulcer. After 2 days, the wound culture results come back positive for methicillin-resistant *Staphylococcus aureus* (MRSA). The nurse knows that the drug of choice for the treatment of MRSA infection is which drug?
   a. vancomycin (Vancocin)
   b. gentamicin (Garamycin)
   c. ciprofloxacin (Cipro)
   d. colistimethate (Coly-Mycin)

4. A patient who is receiving vancomycin (Vancocin) therapy should notify the nurse immediately if which effects are noted? *(Select all that apply.)*
   a. Ringing in the ears
   b. Dizziness
   c. Hearing loss
   d. Fullness in the ears
   e. Nausea

5. During an infusion of colistimethate (colistin), the nurse will stop the infusion if the patient complains of which adverse effects? *(Select all that apply.)*
   a. Numbness
   b. Vertigo
   c. Upset stomach
   d. Insomnia
   e. Dizziness

6. A patient will be taking oral neomycin (Neo-Fradin) before having bowel surgery. The order reads, "Give 1 g per hour for 4 doses PO." The patient cannot swallow pills, so an oral solution has been ordered. The solution is 125 mg/5mL. How many mL will the nurse give for each 1-g dose? ____________

Critical Thinking and Application

Answer the following questions on a separate sheet of paper.

7. Angie has a severe infection and is receiving an aminoglycoside once a day. She says, "They tell me I have a terrible infection. Why am I not getting the antibiotic more than once a day? I don't understand!" What will the nurse tell her?

8. Explain the concept of "trough" levels during aminoglycoside therapy and the way in which renal function is monitored.

9. Greg has been taking amiodarone (Cordarone) for a heart rhythm problem. He has developed an infection from an open wound, and the sensitivity report indicates that levofloxacin (Levaquin) is the best choice to fight this infection. Are there any concerns?

10. Nitrofurantoin (Macrodantin) has been ordered for a patient who has a severe urinary tract infection caused by *Escherichia coli*. Explain why this drug is used for this type of infection.

Case Study

Read the scenario and answer the following questions on a separate sheet of paper.

Virgil has been admitted to your unit and placed on aminoglycoside therapy as part of treatment for a urinary tract infection with *Pseudomonas*. He is 65 years old, awake and alert, but anxious about his problem and wants to "hurry up and get better."

1. For which two serious toxicities will you monitor, what are their symptoms, and how can they be prevented?

2. The physician adds penicillin to Virgil's drug regimen. Explain the reason for this.

3. Virgil's "trough" aminoglycoside level is 3.0 mcg/mL, and his serum creatinine level is increased from 2 days earlier. Are these results a concern? What should you do? Explain.

CHAPTER 40

Antiviral Drugs

Chapter Review and NCLEX® Examination Preparation

Select the best answer for each question.

1. The nurse is administering acyclovir (Zovirax) and recalls that it is considered the drug of choice for treatment of which viral infection?
   a. Cytomegalovirus (CMV)
   b. Human immunodeficiency virus (HIV)
   c. Respiratory syncytial virus (RSV)
   d. Varicella-zoster virus (VZV)

2. When administering ganciclovir (Cytovene), the nurse keeps in mind that the main dose-limiting toxicity for this drug is which condition?
   a. Renal failure
   b. Gastrointestinal disturbances
   c. Peripheral neuropathy
   d. Bone marrow suppression

3. When reviewing the health history of a patient who is to receive foscarnet (Foscavir), the nurse knows that which condition would be a contraindication to its use?
   a. Renal failure
   b. CMV retinitis
   c. Asthma
   d. Immunosuppression

4. When reviewing the use of amantadine (Symmetrel), the nurse expects that the drug would be used most appropriately in which patient?
   a. A 29-year-old man who tests positive for HIV
   b. A 22-year-old woman who is in her eighth month of pregnancy and tests positive for HIV
   c. A heart transplant patient who is to receive prophylaxis for influenza A
   d. Older adult patients who require prophylaxis for influenza B

5. A patient calls the clinic nurse to ask for oseltamivir (Tamiflu) "because I was exposed to the flu over the weekend at a family reunion." The nurse knows that Tamiflu is indicated for which condition? *(Select all that apply.)*
   a. Prevention of infection after exposure to influenza virus types A and B
   b. Reduction of the duration of influenza by several days in adults
   c. Treatment of topical herpes simplex virus infections
   d. Reduction of the severity of shingles symptoms
   e. Treatment of lower respiratory tract infections caused by respiratory syncytial virus

6. The order reads, "Give acyclovir, 0.25 g IVPB now." The medication comes in a vial that contains 1000 mg. The label reads, "Add 20 mL of diluent for a solution that contains 50 mg/mL." The medication will be added to 100 mL D_5W for IV piggyback infusion. How many mL of reconstituted medication will the nurse add to the 100-mL bag for infusion?

   ____

Critical Thinking and Application

Answer the following questions on a separate sheet of paper.

7. Why are so few antiviral drugs available? Why are viruses so difficult to kill?

8. Amy is 12 weeks into her pregnancy when she discovers that she is HIV-positive. Amy is very upset and says, "I won't live long enough to have this baby. We're both going to die." Is it possible to treat Amy and/or the fetus? Explain your answer.

9. Bailey, a 53-year-old teacher with osteoporosis, has shingles.
   a. What drug will the nurse expect the physician to prescribe?
   b. What instructions will the nurse give Bailey regarding any dietary considerations?
   c. Several months later, Bailey calls the office to say that her symptoms have returned. What action will the nurse expect to be taken now?

10. Brenda is a 2-year-old who has bronchopneumonia caused by RSV.
    a. What antiviral drug is used to treat RSV?
    b. Brenda's mother wonders whether the treatment will be completed before Brenda's birthday, which is just 2 weeks away. What will the nurse tell her?

11. A 25-year-old man has acquired immunodeficiency syndrome (AIDS). He was treated with zidovudine (Retrovir) for several months, but now the physician has switched him to didanosine powder (Videx). What frequently is the reason that patients are switched from zidovudine to another anti-HIV drug?

12. The nurse overhears a co-worker explaining to a student nurse the procedure for administering acyclovir intravenously. After the acyclovir is diluted in sterile water, the co-worker says, "We'll administer this over at least an hour." Should the nurse intervene? Explain your answer.

13. Stacy has had flu symptoms for 4 days and feels miserable. She calls the nurse practitioner in the clinic to ask for "that medicine, Tamiflu, that is supposed to make the flu symptoms better." Should Stacy receive this medication at this time? Explain.

14. Matt has had an organ transplant. What antiviral drug may be used, even though he does not have a viral infection at this time?

Case Study

Read the scenario and answer the following questions on a separate sheet of paper.

Mr. C., a 30-year-old stockbroker, has been diagnosed with genital herpes simplex type 2 (HSV-2) infection. The physician has prescribed topical acyclovir (Zovirax).

1. What patient teaching do you provide to Mr. C. regarding administration of this drug?

2. Mr. C. asks you how long it will take for the acyclovir to cure his herpes. What is your reply?

3. What else should you discuss with Mr. C., who is married?

4. HSV-2 is closely related to which other viruses?

CHAPTER 41

Antitubercular Drugs

Chapter Review and NCLEX® Examination Preparation

Select the best answer for each question.

1. A patient will be receiving long-term isoniazid (INH) therapy. What laboratory tests are most important for the nurse to monitor during therapy?
   a. Liver enzyme levels
   b. Hematocrit and hemoglobin level
   c. Creatinine level
   d. Platelet count

2. The nurse should include which information in the teaching plan for a patient who is taking isoniazid (INH)?
   a. Urine and saliva may be reddish-orange.
   b. Pyridoxine (vitamin B_6) may be needed to prevent neurotoxicity.
   c. Injection sites should be rotated daily.
   d. The medication should be taken with an antacid to reduce gastric distress.

3. Patients who are in the initial period of treatment for tuberculosis need to be taught to perform which procedures? *(Select all that apply.)*
   a. Wash their hands and cover their mouths when coughing or sneezing to reduce the spread of tuberculosis.
   b. Throw away dirty tissues with care.
   c. Be sure to get adequate rest, nutrition, and relaxation.
   d. Skip medication doses occasionally if gastric distress occurs.
   e. Medication therapy will be discontinued when symptoms of tuberculosis are gone.

4. A patient with newly diagnosed tuberculosis asks the nurse for how long he will need to take "all this medicine." The nurse replies that drug therapy for active tuberculosis may need to last how long?
   a. 6 months
   b. 12 months
   c. 24 months
   d. A lifetime

5. The nurse is explaining antitubercular therapy to a patient. The patient asks, "Why do I have to take so many different medications?" What is the nurse's best response?
   a. "It helps to prevent drug-resistance."
   b. "It makes sure that the disease is cured."
   c. "These medications will reduce symptoms immediately."
   d. "You will have fewer side effects."

6. The patient is to receive isoniazid (INH) 0.3 g daily. The medication is available as 100-mg tablets. How many tablets will the nurse administer per dose?

   ____

Critical Thinking and Application

Answer the following questions on a separate sheet of paper.

7. Diane, a 33-year-old proofreader, has been prescribed prophylactic isoniazid (INH) treatment.
   a. What laboratory studies should be performed before the start of therapy? Why?
   b. After Diane has taken isoniazid for 2 months, the physician significantly reduces her dosage of the drug. Why might that be?

8. Ms. I. is undergoing antitubercular therapy that includes streptomycin.
   a. How is streptomycin administered?
   b. For what adverse effects will the nurse monitor?
   c. Ms. I. takes an oral contraceptive. Is that a concern given Ms. I.'s antitubercular therapy? Explain your answer.

9. Why would an eye examination be performed before instituting antitubercular therapy?

10. Mr. F., a 42-year-old marketing executive, is on antitubercular therapy. During his first follow-up visit, he is evasive when the nurse asks him about his compliance with his therapy regimen. He does tell the nurse that he has been very busy lately, entertaining various clients "at everything from cocktail parties to big sit-down dinners."
    a. What issues will the nurse discuss with Mr. F.?
    b. Several weeks later, Mr. F. returns for another follow-up visit. On examination, the nurse sees no apparent signs of the tuberculosis. How can Mr. F.'s therapeutic response be confirmed?

11. Frannie is a homeless 68-year-old woman who lives in a shelter some of the time. She was diagnosed at the community health clinic with tuberculosis and antitubercular therapy has been instituted.
    a. What patient education issues are of particular concern in Frannie's case?
    b. Frannie is staying at the shelter and seems to be handling her medication regimen well, but one day she comes by the clinic to tell the nurse that she is afraid the medication may be bad for her. "Whenever I go to the bathroom, everything is reddish-orange," she says. What do you suspect is going on and what do you tell Frannie?

Case Study

Read the scenario and answer the following questions on a separate sheet of paper.

George, a 73-year-old retired plant foreman, has been diagnosed with tuberculosis. Nursing assessment reveals a history of gout and diabetes. He also has a history of heavy drinking.

1. What considerations will the physician keep in mind when deciding on a first-line drug for George?

2. George tells you that he has been told that he has a "liver problem." His medical record mentions that he is a slow acetylator. How does this affect his therapy?

3. How will his history of "heavy drinking" affect his therapy?

4. You instruct George about taking vitamin B_6 along with the isoniazid (INH) therapy. When he asks you why this is necessary, what will you tell him?

CHAPTER 42

Antifungal Drugs

Chapter Review and NCLEX® Examination Preparation

Match each definition with the corresponding term.

1. _____ Single-celled fungi that reproduce by budding
2. _____ One of the major groups of antifungal drugs; includes amphotericin B and nystatin
3. _____ A very large, diverse group of eukaryotic, thallus-forming microorganisms that requires an external carbon source
4. _____ One of the major groups of antifungal drugs; includes ketoconazole and miconazole
5. _____ A term for yeast infection of the mouth
6. _____ One of the older antifungal drugs that acts by preventing susceptible fungi from reproducing
7. _____ The oldest antifungal drug
8. _____ An antifungal drug commonly used to treat candidal diaper rash
9. _____ An infection caused by fungi
10. _____ Multicellular fungi characterized by long, branching filaments called *hyphae*, which entwine to form a mycelium

a. Thrush
b. Molds
c. griseofulvin
d. Mycosis
e. Polyenes
f. Fungi
g. Azoles
h. amphotericin B
i. nystatin
j. yeast

Select the best answer for each question.

11. An infant has thrush. The nurse expects to administer which drug for the treatment of thrush?
    a. amphotericin B (Fungizone)
    b. fluconazole (Diflucan)
    c. nystatin (Mycostatin)
    d. miconazole (Monistat)

12. During an infusion of amphotericin B, the nurse monitors for which adverse effects? *(Select all that apply.)*
    a. Abdominal pain
    b. Fever
    c. Malaise
    d. Diarrhea
    e. Chills
    f. Rash

13. A patient calls the gynecologic clinic because she has begun to menstruate while taking medication for a vaginal infection. She asks the nurse, "What should I do about taking this vaginal medicine right now?" Which is the nurse's best response?
    a. "You should stop the medication until the menstrual flow has stopped."
    b. "Just take the medication at night only."
    c. "You should stop the medication for 3 days, then start it again."
    d. "It's okay to continue to take the medication."

14. A patient will be receiving a one-dose treatment for vaginal candidiasis. The nurse expects to administer which drug?
    a. ketoconazole (Nizoral)
    b. fluconazole (Diflucan)
    c. griseofulvin
    d. terbinafine (Lamisil)

15. The nurse is administering an antifungal drug to a patient who has a severe systemic fungal infection. Which drug is most appropriate for this patient?
    a. amphotericin B (Fungizone)
    b. fluconazole (Diflucan)
    c. griseofulvin
    d. flucytosine

16. The order reads: Give amphotericin B (Fungizone), 20 mg in 300 mL D_5W over 6 hours. The nurse will set the infusion pump to what rate? ____________

Critical Thinking and Application

Answer the following questions on a separate sheet of paper.

17. Why are there so few oral and parenteral drugs to treat mycotic infections?

18. Mr. K. has been diagnosed with cryptococcal meningitis, and the physician has prescribed fluconazole (Diflucan).
    a. Why did the physician choose this drug rather than one of the other azole antifungals?
    b. The results of Mr. K.'s cerebrospinal fluid culture eventually come back negative. When he hears the good news, he says, "Great! I'm tired of taking this medicine." What will be the nurse's response?

19. The physician is planning intravenous amphotericin B (Fungizone) therapy for James.
    a. What guidelines will the nurse follow in diluting the drug?
    b. What adverse effects will the nurse expect James to experience?
    c. Should the nurse stop the infusion if those effects occur? Explain your answer.

20. Lewis has a severe fungal infection for which the physician has prescribed an antifungal medication. During the nursing assessment, Lewis tells the nurse that he hopes the infection will clear up soon because he is going on a cruise in a week and he plans to "party every night!" What patient teaching issues will the nurse discuss with Lewis?

21. Chrissie has thrush and has a prescription for nystatin oral troches. After a few days, she calls the physician to report that her mouth is not better. "I've been chewing them slowly every time I take one. I don't understand why it's not working!" she says. What is the nurse's response?

22. David has been diagnosed with a severe fungal infection and the physician has prescribed a lipid formulation of amphotericin B (Fungizone). Why was this formulation ordered and what are the advantages and disadvantages?

Case Study

Read the scenario and answer the following questions on a separate sheet of paper.

Sally, a 68-year-old hospital volunteer, has been diagnosed as having pneumonia with invasive aspergillosis. She has been treated for 2 weeks without showing much improvement and the physician is considering starting voriconazole (Vfend) therapy. Sally is also receiving a medication for treatment of a cardiac dysrhythmia.

1. What is the reason for starting voriconazole therapy now rather than earlier?

2. What consideration may arise depending on the cardiac medication she is taking?

3. What should be monitored while she is taking voriconazole?

CHAPTER 43

Antimalarial, Antiprotozoal, and Anthelmintic Drugs

Chapter Review and NCLEX® Examination Preparation

Select the best answer for each question.

1. Before beginning antiprotozoal therapy, the nurse should assess for which possible contraindications?
   a. Underlying renal, cardiac, thyroid, or liver disease and pregnancy
   b. Porphyria and glucose-6-phosphate dehydrogenase (G6PD) efficiency
   c. Glaucoma, cataracts, anemia, and petechiae
   d. Constipation, gastritis, and lactose intolerance

2. The nurse should warn the patient taking thiabendazole (Mintezol) about which possible adverse effect?
   a. Reddish-orange urine
   b. Urine with an asparagus-like odor
   c. A metallic taste in the mouth
   d. Severe halitosis

3. A patient is taking quinine therapy for a mild case of malaria. The physician has decided to add a sulfonamide or tetracycline drug along with the quinine. When the nurse gives the patient the prescription for this new medication, the patient is upset about having to take "another pill." What is the nurse's best explanation for the second drug?
   a. "The antibiotic treats bacterial infections that accompany malaria."
   b. "The antibiotic reduces the severe adverse effects of quinine."
   c. "The antibiotic will help the quinine to work more effectively against the malaria."
   d. "The antibiotic therapy is also needed to kill the parasite that causes malaria."

4. Which drug is used mainly for the management of *Pneumocystis jirovecii* (formerly *Pneumocystis carinii*) pneumonia? *(Select all that apply.)*
   a. metronidazole (Flagyl)
   b. pentamidine (NebuPent)
   c. primaquine
   d. pyrantel (Antiminth)
   e. atovaquone (Mepron)

5. The nurse is reviewing anthelmintic therapy. Which statement is true regarding anthelmintic therapy?
   a. The medication can be stopped once symptoms disappear.
   b. Anthelmintics are more effective in their parenteral forms.
   c. Anthelmintics are broad in their actions and can be substituted easily for one another if a given medication is not well-tolerated.
   d. Specific anthelmintic drugs target specific organisms.

6. Several people have contracted a protozoal infection after a group trip to another country. The nurse is aware that which patient is at the highest risk of dying from a protozoal infection?
   a. A teenager with no health problems
   b. An adult with diabetes mellitus
   c. An adult who had a kidney transplant a year ago
   d. An adult with a history of myocardial infarction

7. A patient with *Pneumocystis jirovecii* pneumonia will be receiving pentamidine (NebuPent) intravenously. The order reads, "Give 4 mg/kg/day once daily." The medication comes in a vial of 300 mg and is to be reconstituted with 5 mL of sterile water, with a resulting concentration of 60 mg/mL. The dose will then be added to a 100-mL bag of D_5W for the infusion. What is the dose for this patient and how many mL of medication will the nurse add to the infusion bag? The patient weighs 154 pounds.

   ____

Critical Thinking and Application

Answer the following questions on a separate sheet of paper.

8. Professor H. has just returned from a research sabbatical in Africa where she did not adequately protect herself from mosquito exposure; thus, she has contracted malaria. What kind of parasite causes malaria? Which drug is recommended if the parasite is in the exoerythrocytic phase of development? What exactly is the exoerythrocytic phase?

9. Professor H.'s physician would like to prescribe the drug the nurse identified in the answer to question 8. The nurse should assess this patient for which kind of contraindications?

10. Professor H.'s husband, who accompanied her on her trip, has even more recently begun to develop signs of malaria. He is given chloroquine (Aralen), a 4-aminoquinoline derivative. Unlike his wife, however, Mr. H. sees no diminishing of his symptoms. His strain of malaria appears to be chloroquine-resistant. What alternative(s) will the nurse suggest for Mr. H.?

11. The medical clinic has a full waiting room this morning. Patient A is being seen for an intestinal disorder that he acquired after swimming in a local lake. Patient B has acquired immunodeficiency syndrome (AIDS) and is showing early signs of pneumonia. Patient C is being treated and evaluated on a regular basis for a sexually transmitted disease. Here's your challenge: All three patients have something in common in terms of the causes of their disorders. Describe what that could be. Second, based on that commonality, predict what disorder, of those discussed in this chapter, each patient may have. (Hint: One patient has giardiasis.) Third, select the drugs you feel the physician is likely to prescribe for each patient.

Case Study

Read the scenario and answer the following questions on a separate sheet of paper.

Sandra, age 15, has been diagnosed with an infestation of intestinal roundworms, specifically ascariasis, after a visit to another country. You are preparing to medicate her with pyrantel.

1. How is this infestation diagnosed?

2. What are the contraindications to therapy with pyrantel?

3. The recommended dosage for pyrantel is 11 mg/kg, up to a maximum of 1 g, in a one-time dose. If Sandra weighs 57 kg, what dose should she receive?

4. What are expected adverse effects of this medication?

CHAPTER 44

Antiinflammatory and Antigout Drugs

Chapter Review and NCLEX® Examination Preparation

Select the best answer for each question.

1. When teaching a patient about the common adverse effects of therapy with nonsteroidal antiinflammatory drugs (NSAIDs), the nurse should mention which possible adverse effect?
   a. Dizziness
   b. Heartburn
   c. Palpitations
   d. Diarrhea

2. A 13-year-old patient has the flu, and her mother is concerned about her fever of 103° F (39.4° C). Which medication should the nurse suggest the mother use to treat the teen's fever?
   a. aspirin
   b. acetaminophen (Tylenol)
   c. indomethacin (Indocin)
   d. naproxen (Aleve)

3. A patient is receiving treatment with allopurinol (Zyloprim) for an acute flare-up of gout. Which statements should be included when the nurse provides patient teaching? *(Select all that apply.)*
   a. "Be sure to avoid alcohol and caffeine."
   b. "Take the medication with meals to prevent stomach problems."
   c. "You need to take this medication on an empty stomach to improve absorption."
   d. "You need to increase fluid intake to up to 3 liters per day."
   e. "Call your physician immediately if you note any skin rashes or abnormalities."

4. When reviewing the health history of a patient who is to receive NSAID therapy, the nurse keeps in mind that contraindications for the use of these drugs include which conditions?
   a. Pericarditis
   b. Osteoarthritis
   c. Bleeding disorders
   d. Juvenile rheumatoid arthritis

5. A patient is receiving gold injections as treatment for arthritis. The nurse should tell the patient which information?
   a. "Injections will be given via the intravenous route."
   b. "The medication is more effective if fluids are restricted."
   c. "Relief from symptoms can be expected in a few days."
   d. "Relief from symptoms may take 3 to 4 months."

6. A college student is in the urgent care center after experiencing a severe ankle sprain during a basketball game. The nurse expects that which pain reliever will be ordered for this patient?
   a. ketorolac (Toradol)
   b. aspirin
   c. indomethacin (Indocin)
   d. meloxicam (Mobic)

7. A newborn infant has a high fever, and the order for acetaminophen reads, "Give acetaminophen 30 mg PO every 6 to 8 hours PRN temperature over 101° F." The infant weighs 6 pounds. The dosage range for acetaminophen for neonates is 10 to 15 mg/kg/dose.
   a. Is the ordered 30-mg dose within the safe range for this newborn? ______________
   b. If so, what is the amount of medication the nurse will give for this dose? ______________

Critical Thinking and Application

Answer the following questions on a separate sheet of paper.

8. Ms. B. is brought into the emergency department exhibiting the following symptoms: tinnitus, hearing loss, dimming vision, and dizziness. She is also very thirsty and sweating profusely, and has had severe nausea and vomiting. On examination the nurse discovers that she has an increased heart rate and is experiencing some confusion. At first she appears drowsy and then begins to hyperventilate. The nurse

suspects salicylism, but her colleague says, "No, this is acute salicylate intoxication." If he is correct, how was he able to tell? What causes each?

9. Ms. B. turns out to have acute toxicity stemming from a salicylate overdose. Describe an appropriate treatment plan.

10. Mr. C. comes to the emergency department with symptoms that are similar to Ms. B.'s but not as extensive. He is experiencing drowsiness, confusion, and disorientation, and had a seizure while en route to the hospital. What is wrong? What would the nurse expect if the situation were allowed to progress?

11. How will Mr. C.'s treatment differ from Ms. B.'s?

12. Mr. H. has come to the clinic complaining of a severe flare-up of his gout. He tells the nurse that he does not take his medicine on a regular basis because it "kills" his stomach. He also says that he hates to take medicine but hates the gout more. He has a prescription for allopurinol (Zyloprim) and a follow-up appointment for next week. What patient teaching does Mr. H. need?

13. Eileen has had arthritic joint pain for months and her current pain management regimen has been less than successful. During a checkup today, she tells the nurse that she has heard of a new drug, Toradol, which "works wonders." She wants to try it for "a couple of months" to see if it can help her. What will the nurse tell her?

14. What could happen if Eileen takes the ketorolac (Toradol) on a long-term basis?

15. Your neighbor calls you over to "check out this aspirin bottle" that she found in her medicine cabinet. It has a strong vinegary odor. She wants to know if she can still take it for her headaches. What will you tell her?

Case Study

Read the scenario and answer the following questions on a separate sheet of paper.

Sadie has been taking indomethacin (Indocin) as part of therapy for osteoarthritis but lately has noticed that it has been less effective. Her physician has decided to try celecoxib (Celebrex). Sadie has a history of hepatitis (15 years earlier).

1. What advantages might there be to treatment with celecoxib rather than indomethacin?

2. What potential adverse effects should you warn Sadie about before she takes this medication? What should she report?

3. What allergies are important to assess before Sadie takes this medication?

4. She asks you if she can drink her usual glass of wine each evening while taking this medication. What will you tell her?

CHAPTER 45

Immunosuppressant Drugs

Chapter Review and NCLEX® Examination Preparation

Select the best answer for each question.

1. When monitoring patients on immunosuppressant therapy, the nurse must keep in mind that the major risk factor for patients taking these drugs is which condition?
   a. Severe hypotension with potential renal failure
   b. Increased susceptibility to opportunistic infections
   c. Decreased platelet aggregation
   d. Increased bleeding tendencies

2. A patient is experiencing rejection of a transplanted organ. The nurse expects which drug to be given to manage this?
   a. azathioprine (Imuran)
   b. cyclosporine (Sandimmune)
   c. muromonab-CD3 (Orthoclone OKT3)
   d. tacrolimus (Prograf)

3. A patient who is taking cyclosporine (Sandimmune) calls the office to say that he has heard that some food or beverages can increase the effectiveness of this drug. The nurse recognizes that he is talking about which of the following?
   a. Dairy products
   b. Orange juice
   c. Grapefruit juice
   d. Red wines

4. When teaching patients who are taking oral doses of immunosuppressants, how will the nurse instruct the patient to take the medication?
   a. With food to minimize gastrointestinal upset
   b. On an empty stomach to increase absorption rate
   c. Only when adverse effects are tolerable
   d. With antacids

5. The nurse providing teaching for patients taking immunosuppressants will include which information? *(Select all that apply.)*
   a. The mouth and tongue should be inspected carefully for white patches.
   b. Allergic reactions to these drugs are rare.
   c. Patients should avoid crowds to minimize the risk of infection.
   d. Patients should report any fever, sore throat, chills, or joint pain.
   e. Patients should take oral forms with food to avoid gastrointestinal upset.

6. Which drug is the only immunosuppressant currently indicated for the treatment of multiple sclerosis?
   a. glatiramer acetate (Copaxone)
   b. azathioprine (Imuran)
   c. basiliximab (Simulect)
   d. daclizumab (Zenapax)

7. A patient is about to undergo transplant surgery and will be receiving a preoperative dose of cyclosporine (Sandimmune) 8 hours before the surgery. The ordered dose is "cyclosporine, 6 mg/kg/dose, IV, give 8 hours preoperatively." The patient weighs 275 pounds. The medication is available as 50 mg/mL.
   a. How many mg is the dose for this patient?
   ____
   b. How many mL will the nurse administer for this dose? ______________

Critical Thinking and Application

Answer the following questions on a separate sheet of paper.

8. Mrs. F. is about to undergo kidney transplant surgery. The physician plans for her to start taking daclizumab (Zenapax).
   a. Mrs. F. asks the nurse why. How will the nurse answer?
   b. Describe the laboratory studies to be performed and documented. How often should they be performed? What purpose do they serve?
   c. Three days before her surgery, an oral antifungal drug is added to Mrs. F.'s regimen. "Why do I have to take this, too?" she asks. How will the nurse answer?

9. A patient on cyclosporine (Neoral) therapy is convinced that the cyclosporine is upsetting his stomach. What can be done to alleviate this problem?

10. A hospitalized patient has asked the nurse to mix the doses of cyclosporine in his cup with milk before he drinks it. What will the nurse do?

11. Tess has had a renal transplant. She is being given muromonab-CD3 (Orthoclone OKT3) intravenously, 5 mg/day in a single bolus. On the second day, she begins to exhibit chest pain, dyspnea, and wheezing. Her leukocyte count is 4000/mm^3. What is happening?

12. John has relapsing-remitting multiple sclerosis and is in the hospital because of an acute exacerbation. The physician talks to him about a "different type" of therapy with an immunosuppressant drug. What drug will be used, and how can it help John?

Case Study

Read the scenario and answer the following questions on a separate sheet of paper.

Mr. K. had renal transplant surgery 6 months ago and so far has had no problems with organ rejection. He is taking cyclosporine (Sandimmune) in a maintenance dose. He wants to go back to work and is in for a checkup before approval is given for a return to his job.

1. He asks if he will have to continue the cyclosporine. What is your response?

2. He complains of difficulty swallowing, and as you examine his mouth, you look for signs of oral candidiasis. What findings would indicate that he has this condition?

3. After 2 weeks at work, Mr. K. calls to report that he has the flu. He has a sore throat, chills, and achy joints, and he is very tired. What is your advice?

4. When you receive his most recent white blood cell count, you note that the results are 2900/mm^3. Is this a concern, and what action, if any, will be taken?

CHAPTER 46

Immunizing Drugs and Biochemical Terrorism

Chapter Review and NCLEX® Examination Preparation

1. Complete the following chart by filling in all missing information.

Drug	Active or Passive?	Purpose
a.	b.	Herpes zoster prevention (over age 60)
Hib	c.	d.
e.	Active	Hepatitis B prophylaxis
f.	g.	Postpartum antibody suppression
BCG vaccine	h.	i.
DTaP	j.	k.
Tetanus immunoglobulin	l.	m.
Td	n.	o.

Select the best answer for each question.

2. The immunity that is passed from a mother to her nursing infant through antibodies in breast milk is known as which type of immunity?
   a. Artificially acquired passive immunity
   b. Naturally acquired passive immunity
   c. Active immunity
   d. Genetic immunity

3. Which of the following contain substances that trigger the formation of antibodies against specific pathogens?
   a. Antivenins
   b. Serums
   c. Toxoids
   d. Vaccines

4. When reviewing various immunizing drugs, the nurse recalls that some products provide long-lasting immunity against a particular pathogen. Which is an example of this?
   a. Poliovirus vaccine, live oral
   b. Tetanus immune globulin
   c. Rh_o(D) immune globulin
   d. Black widow spider antivenin

5. The nurse is preparing to give a second dose of DTaP vaccine to a 6-month-old infant. The infant's mother tells the nurse that the last time he received this vaccination, the injection site on his leg became warm, slightly swollen, and red. Which is the nurse's best action?
   a. Explain that these effects can be expected and give the medication.
   b. Give half the prescribed dose this week and the other half next week if tolerated well.
   c. Skip the dose and notify the physician.
   d. Wait 6 months and then administer the dose.

6. A nurse has been stuck by a used needle while starting an intravenous line. Which preparation is used as prophylaxis against disease after exposure to blood and body fluids?
   a. Hib vaccine
   b. Rh_0(D) immune globulin
   c. Hepatitis B immune globulin
   d. Hepatitis antitoxin

7. The nurse is providing patient teaching to a 24-year-old woman regarding the human papillomavirus virus (HPV) vaccine. Which statement by the woman indicates that more teaching is needed? *(Select all that apply.)*
   a. "This vaccine only takes one injection."
   b. "I need to have this vaccine before I turn 26."
   c. "It is safe to take this vaccine if I am pregnant."
   d. "This vaccination prevents the virus that commonly causes cervical cancer."
   e. "My 12-year-old sister should take this vaccine, too."

8. A newborn will be receiving her first dose of hepatitis B vaccine (inactivated). The dose is 5 mcg IM at birth, then again at 1 month and 6 months. Five mcg is equivalent to how many mg? _______________

Critical Thinking and Application

Answer the following questions on a separate sheet of paper.

9. Jim, a cabinetmaker, is cut by a woodworking tool and comes to the clinic for stitches. When the nurse asks him about his tetanus vaccination history, he says, "I have no idea when my last tetanus shot was—I thought once I had all the shots for school that I was set for life! Surely I don't need any more." What will the nurse explain to Jim?

10. Mrs. T., an 82-year-old widow, is in the office for a follow-up appointment to evaluate her emphysema. The physician recommends that she have an influenza virus vaccine. As the nurse prepares the injection, Mrs. T. says, "I had a flu shot last year—why do I need another one this year?" What is the nurse's explanation to her?

11. Mr. S. brings his toddler, Carl, in for a 12-month well-child checkup. Before the nurse gives the measles-mumps-rubella (MMR) vaccine injection, what adverse effects will she tell Mr. S. to watch for in Carl's response to the immunization? What can be done to relieve these adverse effects?

12. There have been news reports about anthrax threats. Your neighbor is worried and asks you which type of anthrax is the most deadly. What does he mean by "which type," and what is the answer to his question?

13. Paul has received several immunizations in preparation for an overseas trip. He expected to feel some soreness at the injection sites, but the next morning he wakes up with swelling of the face and tongue, difficulty breathing, shortness of breath, nausea and vomiting, and a fever of 102° F (38.9° C). What is happening, and what should he do?

Case Study

Read the scenario and answer the following questions on a separate sheet of paper.

You are volunteering at a local animal shelter and helping to care for a sick dog that has just been admitted. During the examination, the dog nipped both you and the veterinarian. A little later, the veterinarian tells you that she fears that the dog has rabies and that both of you have been exposed. The veterinarian tells you that she has received a vaccine for rabies but that you will need to be vaccinated immediately.

1. Is rabies a virus or a bacteria?

2. Did the vaccine the veterinarian received previously give her active or passive immunization? Explain.

3. Will the vaccine you receive give you active or passive immunization? Explain why this particular type of vaccine is preferred in your situation.

4. How will your vaccine(s) be given?

CHAPTER 47

Antineoplastic Drugs Part 1: Cancer Overview and Cell Cycle–Specific Drugs

Critical Thinking Crossword

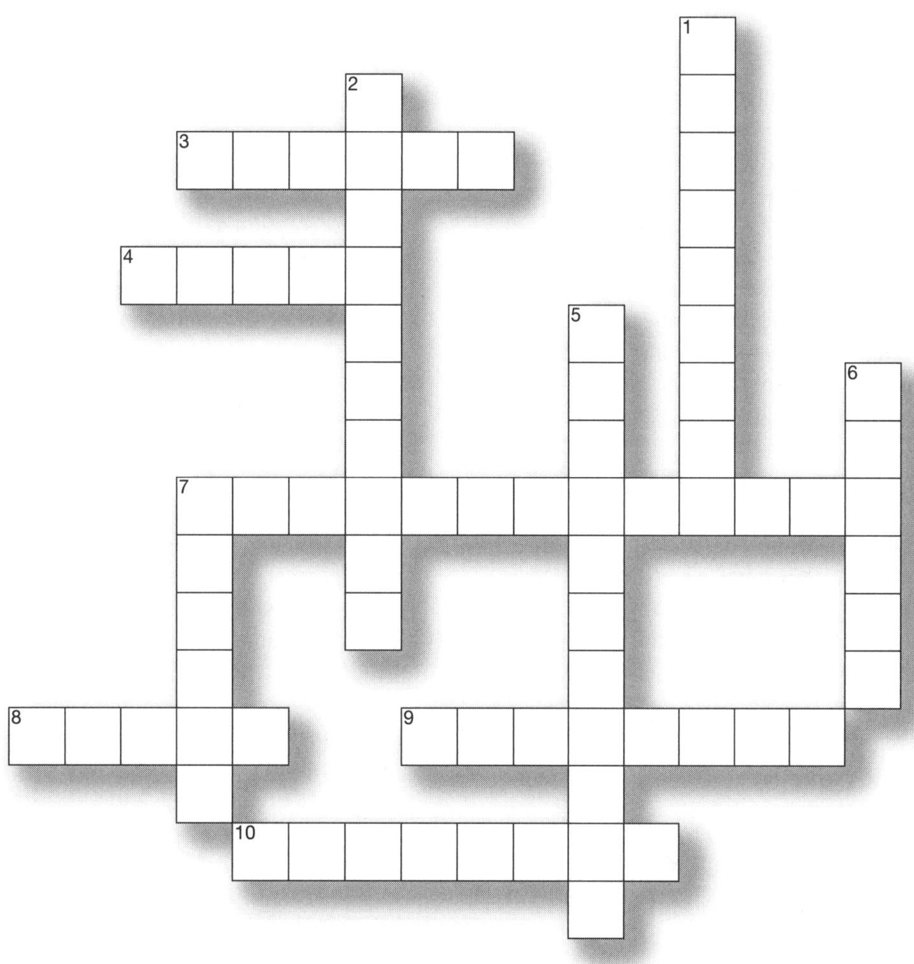

Across

3. Mr. H. is told that his cancer has metastasized. His physician explains to him that this means it has __________ to other areas of his body.
4. Your patient is receiving methotrexate. Your instructor asks for a full description of its mechanism of action, so you explain that it will inhibit dihydrofolic reductase from converting __________ acid to a reduced folate and thus ultimately prevent the synthesis of DNA and cell reproduction. The result, you explain, is that the cell will die.
7. Mr. B. has just undergone a series of chemotherapeutic treatments when it is discovered that the antineoplastic drug has leaked into surrounding tissues; in other words, __________ of the drug has occurred.
8. Mr. C. is very interested in his chemotherapy process. As you are discussing a drug's action, he hears you use the term __________, and he asks you what it means. You explain that this is the point at which the lowest neutrophil count occurs after administration of a chemotherapy agent that causes bone marrow suppression.

9. Ms. F. has been given her first chemotherapy treatment. However, it soon becomes apparent that the adverse effects she is experiencing prevent her from being given dosages that will be high enough to be effective. These are dose-__________ adverse effects.
10. Ms. H. has a hematologic malignancy. Her bone marrow is being rapidly replaced with leukemic blasts; she also has abnormal numbers (and forms) of immature white blood cells in her circulation, and even her lymph nodes, spleen, and liver are being infiltrated. Ms. H.'s type of cancer is known as _________.

Down

1. Ms. P. had a biopsy performed on the same day that Ms. L. (6 Down) did. When her biopsy specimen is analyzed, however, the results are the opposite of Ms. L.'s; that is, her lump is considered __________.
2. Mr. K. has been treated with methotrexate for its folate-antagonistic properties. Now, however, he seems to be experiencing a toxicity reaction. The treatment he will receive will be ________ rescue.
5. Mr. G. is receiving chemotherapy with a drug that is considered cytotoxic during any phase of the cellular growth cycle. This drug is known as cell-cycle ________.
6. Ms. L. recently underwent biopsy of a lump near her breast. Several days later, her physician calls and tells her that the lump is noncancerous and therefore is not an immediate threat to life. She is relieved to hear, then, that it is __________.
7. Mr. Y.'s physician is not surprised to find that methotrexate is killing the cells of Mr. Y.'s stomach, which results in nausea and vomiting; the methotrexate therapy is displaying a strong __________ potential in this patient.

Chapter Review and NCLEX® Examination Preparation

Select the best answer for each question.

1. When administering antineoplastic drugs, the nurse needs to keep in mind that the general adverse effects of these drugs include: *(Select all that apply.)*
   a. bone marrow suppression.
   b. infertility.
   c. diarrhea.
   d. urinary retention.
   e. nausea and vomiting.
   f. stomatitis.

2. A patient will be receiving chemotherapy with paclitaxel (Taxol). What will the nurse expect to do along with administering this drug?
   a. Administer platelet infusions.
   b. Provide acetaminophen (Tylenol) as needed.
   c. Keep the patient on "nothing-by-mouth" status because of expected nausea and vomiting.
   d. Premedicate with a steroid, H_2 receptor antagonist, and antihistamine.

3. As the nurse is preparing to give the patient chemotherapy, the patient asks the nurse why more than one drug is used. The nurse will explain that combinations of chemotherapeutic drugs are used to:
   a. prevent drug resistance.
   b. reduce the incidence of adverse effects.
   c. decrease the cost of treatment.
   d. reduce treatment time.

4. If extravasation of an antineoplastic drug occurs, what will the nurse do first?
   a. Remove the intravenous catheter immediately.
   b. Stop the drug infusion without removing the intravenous catheter.
   c. Aspirate residual drug or blood from the tube if possible.
   d. Administer the appropriate antidote.

5. During chemotherapy, the nurse will monitor the patient for which symptoms of stomatitis?
   a. Indigestion and heartburn
   b. Severe vomiting and anorexia
   c. Ulcerations of the mouth
   d. Diarrhea and perianal irritation

6. A patient is receiving leucovorin as part of his chemotherapy regimen. The nurse expects that the patient is receiving which antineoplastic drug?
   a. cladribine (Leustatin)
   b. fluorouracil (Adrucil)
   c. vincristine (Oncovin)
   d. methotrexate (Trexall)

7. A patient will be receiving chemotherapy with IV cladribine (Leustatin). The order reads, "Give 0.09 mg/kg each day for 7 days." The medication is to be added to 500 mL of normal saline and is available in a 1-mg/mL solution. The patient weighs 200 pounds.
   a. How many mg is each daily dose? __________
   b. How many mL of medication will be added to each infusion? __________

Case Study

Read the scenario and answer the following questions on a separate sheet of paper.

Allen, a 40-year-old physician, has been diagnosed with acute lymphocytic leukemia and will be receiving chemotherapy with methotrexate (Trexall). He is scheduled to receive his first treatment today.

1. What is methotrexate's classification, and how does it work?

2. What laboratory test results should be checked before he receives this medication?

3. Allen tells you that he often has problems with ankle pain from an old injury and takes ibuprofen (Motrin) for relief. Is this a concern?

4. What other medications may be given along with the methotrexate chemotherapy and why?

CHAPTER 48

Antineoplastic Drugs Part 2: Cell Cycle–Nonspecific and Miscellaneous Drugs

Chapter Review and NCLEX® Examination Preparation

Select the best answer for each question.

1. While hanging a new infusion bag of a chemotherapy drug, the nurse accidentally spills a small amount of solution on the floor. What is the nurse's best action?
   a. Let it dry, then mop the floor.
   b. Wipe the area with a paper towel.
   c. Use a spill kit to clean the area.
   d. Ask the housekeeping department to wipe the floor.

2. The nurse is reviewing the medication list for a patient who will be receiving mitotane (Lysodren) treatments. A drug from which class would cause the most concern if administered along with the mitotane?
   a. Benzodiazepine
   b. Thyroid replacement hormone
   c. Insulin
   d. Beta-blocker

3. A patient receiving chemotherapy for a testicular tumor complains of hearing a "loud ringing sound" in his ears. The nurse expects what to happen next?
   a. The therapy will continue as ordered.
   b. The therapy will be stopped until the patient's hearing is evaluated.
   c. The therapy will be withheld for a day, then resumed.
   d. The therapy will be stopped until renal studies are performed.

4. When teaching a patient who is receiving outpatient chemotherapy about potential problems, the nurse needs to mention signs and symptoms of an oncologic emergency, which include which of the following? *(Select all that apply.)*
   a. Swollen tongue
   b. Alopecia
   c. Blood in the urine
   d. Nausea and vomiting
   e. Temperature of 100° F (37.8° C) or higher
   f. Chills

5. The nurse monitors very closely for signs of liver toxicity when which antineoplastic drug is given?
   a. doxorubicin (Adriamycin)
   b. cisplatin (Platinol)
   c. bevacizumab (Avastin)
   d. mitotane (Lysodren)

6. A patient who has cancer is to receive a course of chemotherapy with doxorubicin (Adriamycin). Which coexisting condition will require very close monitoring while the patient is taking this drug?
   a. Hypertension
   b. Diabetes mellitus
   c. Gout
   d. Cardiomyopathy

7. A patient will be receiving cisplatin chemotherapy. The order reads, "Give 100 mg/m^2 in 1000 mL D_5W over 22 hours." The nurse will program the infusion pump to deliver the infusion at what rate?

   ____

Critical Thinking and Application

Answer the following questions on a separate sheet of paper.

8. Describe the concept of cytoprotection and provide some examples of how this may be accomplished during chemotherapy.

9. Mrs. S. has been receiving bleomycin to treat a lung tumor, and lately she has been experiencing

increased difficulty breathing. She tells the nurse, "I guess this cancer is getting worse. The medicine is not working." Will the nurse agree or is there another possible concern?

10. During a busy evening shift, a physician tells the nurse that he wants to start Mrs. N.'s chemotherapy immediately. The physician asks the nurse to mix the drug as soon as possible and start the infusion. Should the nurse do this? Explain your answer.

11. Mr. G., who had been receiving an infusion of mechlorethamine (Mustargen), has an infiltrated intravenous site. He wants the nurse to pull out the intravenous line immediately because "it hurts so much." What will the nurse do? How will this extravasation be treated?

Case Study

Read the scenario and answer the following questions on a separate sheet of paper.

Dottie, age 63, has been diagnosed with mid-stage ovarian cancer and will be receiving chemotherapy with cisplatin (Platinol) after surgery. She is understandably anxious about the therapy but says she wants to "beat the cancer."

1. Cisplatin is associated with three main toxicities. Describe each one.

2. Before she receives the therapy, what will be assessed?

3. During therapy, Dottie complains of an "odd tingling" in her toes. Is this a concern? Explain.

4. Dottie tells you that she'd rather "drink nothing" when she is feeling nauseated. Is this a concern? Explain what you need to teach her about fluids.

CHAPTER 49

Biologic Response–Modifying and Antirheumatoid Drugs

Chapter Review and NCLEX® Examination Preparation

Match each definition with its corresponding term. (Note: Not all terms will be used.)

1. _____ A type of cytokine that promotes resistance to viral infection in uninfected cells
2. _____ Cytokines that regulate the growth, differentiation, and function of bone marrow stem cells
3. _____ Cytokines that are produced by sensitized T lymphocytes upon contact with antigen particles
4. _____ An immunoglobulin that binds to antigens to form a special complex
5. _____ A substance that is foreign to the human body
6. _____ The primary functional cells of the cell-mediated immune system
7. _____ The specific cells of the humoral immune system

a. Colony-stimulating factors
b. Antibody
c. B lymphocytes (B cells)
d. T lymphocytes (T cells)
e. Interferons
f. Lymphokine-activated killer cells
g. Lymphokines
h. Antigen
i. Memory cells

Select the best answer for each question.

8. When giving interferon drugs, the nurse knows that what is the best time to administer them?
   a. In the morning, before the patient rises
   b. At mealtimes
   c. Between meals
   d. At bedtime

9. A patient with a critically low hemoglobin level and hematocrit is to receive a drug that will stimulate the production of red blood cells. The nurse expects that the patient will receive which drug?
   a. filgrastim (Neupogen)
   b. epoetin alfa (Epogen)
   c. sargramostim (Leukine)
   d. oprelvekin (Neumega)

10. While teaching a patient about the possible adverse effects of the interferons, the nurse should mention which effects? *(Select all that apply.)*
    a. Myalgia
    b. Fever
    c. Diarrhea
    d. Fatigue
    e. Chills
    f. Dizziness

11. A patient is starting therapy with adalimumab (Humira) after a course of therapy with methotrexate failed to improve the patient's condition. The nurse recognizes that this patient is being treated for which condition?
    a. Advanced-stage cancer
    b. Multiple sclerosis
    c. Severe rheumatoid arthritis
    d. Systemic lupus erythematosus

12. A patient is to receive 400 mcg of filgrastim (Neupogen) subcut daily for 1 week. The vial contains 480 mcg/1.6 mL. How many mL will the nurse draw up into the syringe for the dose?

    ____

Critical Thinking and Application

Answer the following questions on a separate sheet of paper.

13. Sonja is to receive interferon therapy as part of the treatment for cancer. Sonja is very athletic and participates in sports activities on a regular basis. The

physician explains that there is a dose-limiting adverse effect of this type of drug that may have a huge effect on her daily activities. What is this adverse effect and how will it concern Sonja?

14. Trevor is receiving chemotherapy as part of his treatment for Hodgkin's disease. As he begins therapy, he tells the nurse, "I've seen those commercials about the drugs that increase your white blood cell count. Can't I start taking one of them now to keep my counts from getting so low?" What are the drugs he is referring to and what is your answer?

15. Brittany has a history of thrombocytopenia, and the results of today's laboratory work have indicated a critically low platelet count. She has received 2 units of platelets, but the physician has decided to give her a medication to improve her platelet counts. What drug will be given, how will it be given, and what concerns are there while her platelet count is so low?

16. Dusten will be receiving treatments with methotrexate (Trexall) for severe rheumatoid arthritis. The nurse is reviewing the medication administration record (MAR) and sees the following transcribed order, "methotrexate, 7.5 mg per day PO." What will be the nurse's next action?

Case Study

Read the scenario and answer the following questions on a separate sheet of paper.

Connie, a 58-year-old cashier, is in the hospital because of extreme weakness. She has received hemodialysis three times a week for chronic renal failure for the last 2 years. The laboratory results revealed a critically low hematocrit and hemoglobin level, and the physician has ordered a transfusion of 2 units of packed red blood cells. However, Connie states that she cannot accept the blood transfusion because of her religious beliefs. As a result, there are orders to begin therapy with epoetin alfa (Epogen).

1. How does epoetin work?

2. What laboratory test results should be monitored while she is taking this medication and why?

3. Connie is concerned about the source of this drug. What can you tell her about this?

4. She is going to be taking this drug at home. What is the route by which it will be given?

5. When Connie realizes that she will be giving herself injections up to three times a week, she complains, "Isn't there something else I can take? I don't want that many shots!" Is there an alternative?

CHAPTER 50

Acid-Controlling Drugs

Chapter Review and NCLEX® Examination Preparation

Match each definition with its corresponding term. (Note: Not all terms will be used; some definitions may have more than one answer.)

1. _____ Drugs known as *H_2 blockers* that reduce acid secretion in the stomach
2. _____ Drugs that block all acid secretion in the stomach
3. _____ A cytoprotective drug
4. _____ The cells responsible for producing and secreting hydrochloric acid in the stomach
5. _____ A type of antacid that can cause diarrhea
6. _____ Antacids that have constipating effects
7. _____ The cause of many peptic ulcers
8. _____ Drugs used to relieve the painful symptoms associated with gas
9. _____ A type of antacid that may contribute to the development of kidney stones
10. _____ A drug that can result in systemic alkalosis

a. Aluminum-containing antacids
b. Calcium-containing antacids
c. Magnesium-containing antacids
d. Antiflatulents
e. Proton pump inhibitors
f. *Helicobacter pylori*
g. Sodium bicarbonate
h. Histamine type 2 receptor antagonists
i. Sucralfate
j. Chief cells
k. Parietal cells

Select the best answer for each question.

11. A patient with renal failure wants to take an antacid for "sour stomach." The nurse needs to consider that some antacids may be dangerous when taken by patients with renal failure and should recommend which type of antacid?
    a. Activated charcoal
    b. Aluminum-containing antacids
    c. Calcium-containing antacids
    d. Magnesium-containing antacids

12. A patient with peptic ulcer disease will be starting medication therapy. He tells the nurse that he smokes and wonders if that will affect his treatment. Which is the nurse's best response?
    a. "Smoking has no effect on these medications."
    b. "The actions of antacids are less potent when you smoke."
    c. "Smoking has been shown to decrease the effectiveness of H_2 blockers."
    d. "Smoking has been shown to increase the adverse effects of H_2 blockers."

13. Which drug class would be used as first-line therapy for gastroesophageal reflux disease (GERD) that has not responded to customary medical treatment?
    a. H_2 blockers
    b. Antacids
    c. Mucosal protectants
    d. Proton pump inhibitors

14. The nurse is administering a proton pump inhibitor during morning medication rounds. Which statements about proton pump inhibitors are true? *(Select all that apply.)*
    a. They should be taken 1 hour before antacids.
    b. They should be taken 30 to 60 minutes before meals.
    c. They should be taken with meals.
    d. They are part of the treatment of patients with *H. pylori* infections.
    e. There are very few adverse effects with these drugs.

15. A pregnant woman asks the nurse about taking an antacid for indigestion. What is the nurse's best response?
    a. "You won't be allowed to take an antacid while you are pregnant."
    b. "Let's check with your obstetrician to see what is recommended."
    c. "Go ahead and use an aluminum-based antacid."
    d. "Sodium bicarbonate would be the safest choice."

16. The patient is to receive pantoprazole (Protonix) 40 mg, mixed in 100 mL of D_5W over 30 minutes, IV. The nurse will set the infusion pump to what rate?

    ____

Critical Thinking and Application

Answer the following questions on a separate sheet of paper.

17. Your neighbor, Mr. M., comes over to get advice on antacids. He says he has taken Maalox "for years" for indigestion, but it is no longer helping. He asks, "Can you recommend another antacid or one of those expensive, fancy pills that the pharmacy sells? Or should I just take baking soda?" What is your response?

18. Mrs. K. is advised to take omeprazole (Prilosec) to treat her severe case of GERD; nothing else has worked. Develop a patient teaching plan that will instruct Mrs. K. in how this medication should be taken.

19. Mr. A. has called to ask which antacid he should take. He has been to the store and is confused by the great variety on the shelves. He says he needs something for "occasional heartburn" when he eats something too spicy. He has a history of heart failure and is taking antihypertensive drugs. What type of antacid should he take and what other instructions will he need?

20. Mr. S. is taking enteric-coated aspirin for mild arthritis symptoms. He tells the nurse that he plans to take the aspirin with his favorite antacid, Maalox, because he does not want any stomach problems. What will the nurse tell him?

21. Frank has been diagnosed with a peptic ulcer caused by *H. pylori* infection. He has been told that he will be started on Regimen 1 drug therapy for this disease. What does this mean?

Case Study

Read the scenario and answer the following questions on a separate sheet of paper.

Edna, age 78, has been self-treating with antacids for "heartburn" for 6 months. After an upper gastrointestinal tract endoscopy, she has been diagnosed with GERD. The decision has been made to start treatment with cimetidine (Tagamet). Edna has been generally healthy except for a history of asthma. She says that she does not smoke but that she enjoys going to a Bingo session every Saturday for a few hours where there is smoking, beer, and pizza.

1. When Edna sees the prescription for cimetidine, she asks, "Why do I need a prescription? I can buy this over the counter!" What will you say in reply?

2. How will the cimetidine help her GERD?

3. What cautions, if any, are associated with the use of cimetidine?

4. Will staying in a smoke-filled room affect her therapy? Explain.

CHAPTER 51

Bowel Disorder Drugs

Critical Thinking Crossword

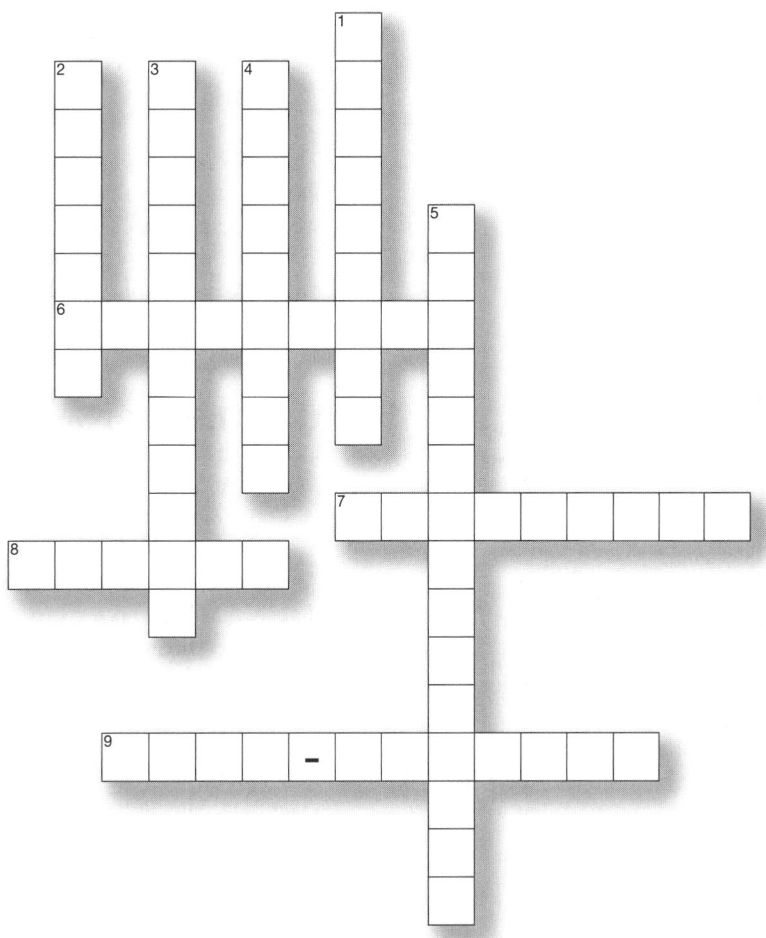

Across

6. A laxative that softens the stool
7. Another word for intestinal floral modifier
8. Laxatives that increase osmotic pressure in the small intestine, increasing water content and resulting in distention
9. Laxatives that absorb water into the intestine, increasing bulk and distending the bowel (two words)

Down

1. Acts by coating the walls of the gastrointestinal tract, binding to causative bacteria or toxin to allow elimination via the stool
2. These laxatives also act to decrease bowel motility
3. A laxative that increases fecal water content in the large intestine, resulting in distention, increased peristalsis, and evacuation
4. A laxative that stimulates the nerves that supply the intestine, which results in increased peristalsis
5. Acts by decreasing peristalsis and muscular tone of the intestine, thus slowing the movement of substances through the gastrointestinal tract

Chapter Review and NCLEX® Examination Preparation

Select the best answer for each question.

1. The nurse is reviewing the use of bismuth subsalicylate (Pepto-Bismol). For which patient would be this medication the most appropriate choice?
   a. A 7-year-old child who has chickenpox
   b. A 23-year-old woman who has severe abdominal pain
   c. A 45-year-old man who is complaining of constipation
   d. A 58-year-old man who developed diarrhea after traveling out of the country

2. The nurse should teach a patient who is self-treating with bismuth subsalicylate (Pepto-Bismol) to avoid which drug because of the possibility of toxicity?
   a. aspirin
   b. acetaminophen (Tylenol)
   c. calcium supplements
   d. vitamin tablets

3. A patient asks for a medication that will provide rapid relief of constipation. After ruling out possible contraindications, the nurse should suggest which drug?
   a. psyllium (Metamucil)
   b. methylcellulose (Citrucel)
   c. docusate sodium (Colace)
   d. magnesium hydroxide (Milk of Magnesia)

4. A patient has been given PEG-3350 in a solution of polyethylene glycol (GoLYTELY) as preparation for a colonoscopy. He started having diarrhea after about 45 minutes. Two hours later, he tells the nurse that "the diarrhea has not stopped yet." What will the nurse do?
   a. Give the patient an antidiarrheal drug, such as loperamide (Lomotil).
   b. Give the patient another dose of the GoLYTELY to finish cleansing his bowel.
   c. Remind the patient that it may take up to 4 hours to completely evacuate the bowel.
   d. Report this to the physician immediately.

5. A 79-year-old woman visits the clinic today and tells the nurse that her "bowels just aren't right." She wants advice on the best laxative to take so that she can have a bowel movement every day. Which is an appropriate response by the nurse? *(Select all that apply.)*
   a. "A normal bowel pattern does not necessarily mean that you will have a bowel movement every day."
   b. "Try taking Metamucil with sips of water."
   c. "You can try taking Milk of Magnesia every other day—it's a mild laxative."
   d. "Increasing fluids and fiber in your diet are better alternatives than laxative use."
   e. "Mineral oil would be safe for long-term use if needed."

6. The order reads: "Give lactulose (Chronulac) 5 g, PO daily after breakfast." The patient is a child who weighs 55 pounds. The medication is available as a syrup in a unit-dose package that contains 10 g/15 mL. How many mL will the nurse administer per dose? ____________________

Critical Thinking and Application

Answer the following questions on a separate sheet of paper.

7. Anna has called the health clinic in a panic. She says that she has been taking Pepto-Bismol for diarrhea and noticed this morning that her tongue "is a funny color." She asks, "Have I overdosed on this stuff? What should I do?" What will the nurse tell Anna?

8. Mrs. B. is a 65-year-old retiree with osteoporosis and glaucoma. She has recently developed diarrhea and the physician is considering antidiarrheal therapy. Mrs. B. tells the nurse that her husband recently "had a bout of diarrhea" for which he took Donnatal. Mrs. B. wonders whether Donnatal would help in her case. What will the nurse tell her?

9. Hillary has come to the physician's office complaining of constipation. During the nurse's assessment, Hillary mentions that she recently started graduate school and has not had time lately to keep up her usual exercise regimen and that her diet "is a disaster." She says that, on some days, all she has time to do is grab a milkshake or cheese and crackers at the student center. She also tells the nurse that she has been taking antacids for "heartburn." What might be causing Hillary's constipation?

10. Ira, a 45-year-old accountant, has chronic constipation.
    a. What are the advantages of bulk-forming laxatives in treating Ira's problem?
    b. The physician prescribes psyllium. What instructions will the nurse give Ira regarding its administration?

11. Drake is a 5-year-old boy with constipation. The physician has ordered treatment with glycerin suppositories.
    a. Why is glycerin a good choice for Drake?
    b. For what adverse effects will the nurse monitor?

12. Five-year-old Kyle has diarrhea for which the physician has ordered an antidiarrheal drug.
    a. How will the dosage likely be determined?
    b. The next day Kyle's mother calls to tell the nurse that Kyle seems to be no better and that his abdomen "looks bloated" and is painful. What will the nurse do?

Case Study

Read the scenario and answer the following questions on a separate sheet of paper.

Charles, a 54-year-old accountant, recently completed a 2-week course of antibiotic therapy for pneumonia. He still has a slight cough and is now experiencing severe diarrhea.

1. What is the probable cause of his diarrhea?

2. What antidiarrheal drug is indicated for Charles?

3. How does this drug work?

4. Is this drug considered a drug or a dietary supplement? Explain.

CHAPTER 52

Antiemetic and Antinausea Drugs

Chapter Review and NCLEX® Examination Preparation

Select the best answer for each question.

1. The nurse is giving medication to reduce nausea. Which drugs are known to cause drying of secretions and drowsiness when given?
   a. Antihistamines
   b. Antidopaminergic drugs
   c. Serotonin blockers
   d. Tetrahydrocannabinoids

2. A nurse is reviewing chemotherapy with a newly hired nurse on the oncology unit. Which class of antinausea drugs has proven to be very effective in preventing chemotherapy-induced nausea and vomiting? *(Select all that apply.)*
   a. Antihistamines
   b. Antidopaminergic drugs
   c. Serotonin blockers
   d. Anticholinergics
   e. Tetrahydrocannabinoids

3. When reviewing the drugs used for nausea and vomiting, the nurse recalls that which drug is a synthetic derivative of the major active substance in marijuana?
   a. ondansetron (Zofran)
   b. metoclopramide (Reglan)
   c. prochlorperazine (Compazine)
   d. dronabinol (Marinol)

4. A patient is undergoing chemotherapy. When giving antiemetics, the nurse will remember that these drugs are most effective against nausea given when?
   a. Before meals
   b. At bedtime
   c. Before the chemotherapy begins
   d. Just after the chemotherapy begins

5. When giving dronabinol (Marinol) to a patient with acquired immunodeficiency syndrome (AIDS), the nurse knows that this drug may also have what effect in addition to reducing nausea?
   a. Euphoria
   b. Enhanced appetite
   c. Reduced pain
   d. Enhanced sleep

6. A patient calls in to the clinic to ask for something for his upset stomach. He admits to "eating a lot of food that's bad for me" the night before and wants something to help him to feel better. The nurse expects which drug will be most appropriate for this patient?
   a. metoclopramide (Reglan)
   b. prochlorperazine (Compazine)
   c. aprepitant (Emend)
   d. phosphorated carbohydrate solution (Emetrol)

7. A patient is about to receive his first chemotherapy treatment with a drug that is known to cause severe nausea and vomiting. One of the premedication orders reads, "Give ondansetron (Zofran) PO 24 mg one-half hour before chemotherapy begins." The medication is ordered in a syrup that contains 4 mg/5mL because the patient does not like to take pills. How many mL of medication will the nurse administer for this dose? ____________

Critical Thinking and Application

Answer the following questions on a separate sheet of paper.

8. Petra has gastroesophageal reflux disease, and the physician has ordered oral metoclopramide (Reglan).
   a. What instructions will the nurse give Petra regarding administration of the medication?
   b. A few days later, Petra calls to say that she thinks the medication is "too strong." She also mentions that her evening routine includes "a couple of glasses of wine." What will the nurse tell Petra?

9. Nellie has been prescribed prochlorperazine (Compazine) via an intramuscular injection. She is on "nothing-by-mouth" status and has no intravenous access at this time. The nurse is preparing the injection when Nellie says, "I hate shots. Can't I just take it by mouth?" What alternatives are there for this drug, and what will the nurse do?

10. Chuck, age 33, is in a later stage of AIDS. He has lost much weight and has no appetite. His physician has prescribed dronabinol (Marinol). When Chuck finds out that this medication is derived from marijuana, he becomes very upset. "Why is the doctor giving me pot?" he asks. What will the nurse explain?

Case Study

Read the scenario and answer the following questions on a separate sheet of paper.

Mr. O. has been prescribed ondansetron (Zofran) during his chemotherapy, which is daily for 2 weeks.

1. For what significant drug interactions should you assess before he takes the ondansetron?

2. Mr. O. tells you that he still has nausea. He is puzzled because "I take the medicine for nausea as soon as I feel nauseated." What should you tell him?

3. One day Mr. O. complains to you that he gets a headache every time the ondansetron is administered. What should you do?

CHAPTER 53

Vitamins and Minerals

Chapter Review and NCLEX® Examination Preparation

Match each definition with the corresponding term.

1. _____ Specialized protein that catalyzes chemical reactions in organic matter
2. _____ A deficiency of cyanocobalamin
3. _____ A nonprotein substance that combines with a protein molecule to form an active enzyme
4. _____ A condition caused by a vitamin D deficiency that is characterized by soft, pliable bones
5. _____ An inorganic substance ingested and attached to enzymes or other organic molecules
6. _____ An organic compound essential in small quantities for normal physiologic and metabolic functioning of the body
7. _____ A condition resulting from an ascorbic acid deficiency that is characterized by weakness and anemia
8. _____ An essential organic compound that can be dissolved and stored in the liver and fatty tissues
9. _____ Biologically active chemicals that make up vitamin E compounds
10. _____ A disease of the peripheral nerves caused by an inability to assimilate thiamine
11. _____ An essential organic compound that can be dissolved in water but is not stored in the body for long periods of time
12. _____ A disease resulting from a niacin deficiency or a metabolic defect that interferes with the conversion of tryptophan to niacin

a. Beriberi
b. Coenzyme
c. Enzyme
d. Fat-soluble vitamin
e. Mineral
f. Pellagra
g. Pernicious anemia
h. Rickets
i. Scurvy
j. Tocopherols
k. Vitamin
l. Water-soluble vitamin

Select the best answer for each question.

13. When giving vitamins, the nurse needs to remember that certain vitamins can be toxic if consumed in excess amounts. These include which vitamins? *(Select all that apply.)*
    a. Vitamin A
    b. Vitamin C
    c. Niacin
    d. Vitamin D
    e. Vitamin K
    f. Folic acid

14. A patient believes that taking megadoses of vitamin C is healthy. What should the nurse tell the patient about megadoses of vitamin C?
    a. They are usually nontoxic because vitamin C is water-soluble.
    b. They can produce nausea, vomiting, headache, and abdominal cramps.
    c. Megadoses of vitamin C can lead to scurvylike symptoms.
    d. They may cause dangerous heart dysrhythmias.

15. A patient has ingested an excessive amount of water-soluble vitamins. The nurse expects what to happen?
    a. The body will store them in muscle and fat tissue until needed.
    b. They are stored in the liver until needed.
    c. They circulate in the blood, bound to proteins, until needed.
    d. Excess amounts are excreted in the urine.

16. When reviewing the diet of a patient who has a calcium deficiency, the nurse recalls that efficient absorption of calcium in the diet requires adequate amounts of which substance?
    a. Magnesium
    b. Intrinsic factor
    c. Coenzymes
    d. Vitamin D

17. The order reads, "Give vitamin K (AquaMEPHYTON) 2 mg subcutaneously now." The patient is a child, age 5. The medication is available in an ampule, 1 mg/0.5 mL. How many mL will the nurse draw up for the injection? ____________

Critical Thinking and Application

Answer the following questions on a separate sheet of paper.

18. Mrs. S. has developed vitamin D deficiency as a result of long-term use of lubricant laxatives. She is advised to take supplements for her vitamin D deficiency. However, the physician also advises her to get vitamin D through more natural sources, both dietary and endogenous. "What did he mean by 'endogenous'?" she asks the nurse. How will the nurse explain to Mrs. S. what is meant by an endogenous source? Make a list of foods rich in vitamin D as well.

19. Ms. E. has recently undergone an ileal resection, which is understandably affecting her digestive functions. She is experiencing some signs of malabsorption. When routine laboratory tests are performed, the nurse discovers that she is mildly anemic.
    a. What type of anemia does the nurse expect?
    b. What about her condition is contributing to this deficiency?
    c. Create a hand-held patient education card for Ms. E., concentrating on diet. Be sure to include a list of foods that contain the vitamin or vitamins of which she is most likely to suffer a deficiency.

20. Mr. G. is hospitalized with severe hypocalcemia. Your colleague Jeffrey recommends immediately beginning a rapid infusion of intravenous calcium. The physician's order requires infusion of 1% procaine. Refute or defend the rationales of both Jeffrey and Mr. G.'s physician. In either case, what should you watch out for when giving intravenous calcium? Back up your response with your own data.

Case Study

Read the scenario and answer the following questions on a separate sheet of paper.

After Mr. W. is treated for colitis with a broad-spectrum antibiotic, he begins to show signs of vitamin K deficiency.

1. How did this happen? How will he receive supplements?

2. What function does vitamin K serve in the human body?

3. Despite the infrequent occurrence of this deficiency, what other patient populations can sometimes be at risk for it?

4. What dietary supplements can you recommend?

CHAPTER 54

Nutritional Supplements

Critical Thinking Crossword

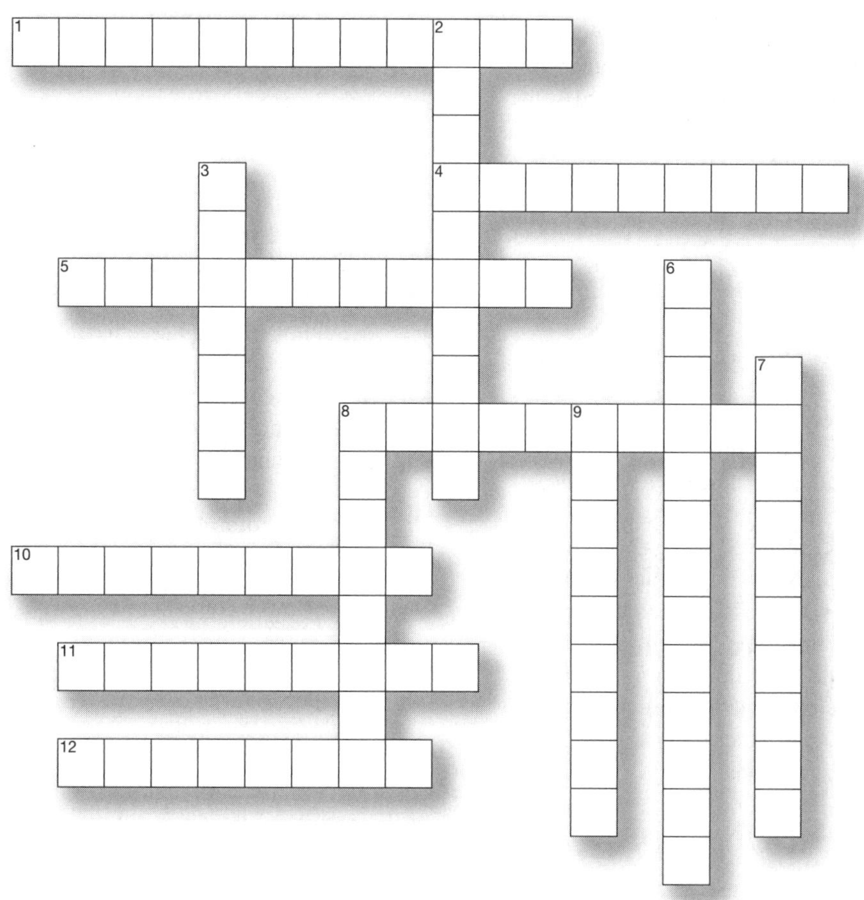

Across

1. Mr. G. is receiving __________ when it is determined that he is going to need nutritional supplementation as well. When you see that he is taking this drug, however, you ask if the feeding can wait until his other drug therapy has run its course. You are concerned that the nutritional supplement will inactivate this drug because of high gastric acid content or prolonged emptying time.
4. Ms. C. needs amino acids in nutritional supplements. The main use, or primary role, of amino acids is protein synthesis, or _________.
5. Mr. H. is about to receive a __________, in which a feeding tube will be surgically inserted directly into his stomach.
8. Mrs. P. is worried about her husband, who has postsurgical nausea. She sees that his roommate is receiving total parenteral nutrition (TPN) and asks "Can't you do that for my husband, just while he's so nauseated?" TPN, you explain, is to be used only when enteral support is impossible or when the gastrointestinal tract's __________ or functional capacity is insufficient.
10. Ms. D. comes to the clinic when a cut on her hand "just won't heal up." She also says that as long as she is here, she would like to report symptoms of hair loss and scaly dermatitis. She wants a prescription for her skin problem, but the physician says, "There's something more going on here." He runs a few tests and discovers that Ms. D. also has a de-

creased platelet level and some evidence of possible fatty liver. He says he suspects that Ms. D. has essential __________ (two words) deficiency.

11. Mr. J. is having trouble getting and digesting enough dietary forms of amino acids. His physician explains that he needs nutritional supplementation through enteral nutrition to ensure that he gets enough of these amino acids, because they cannot be produced by his own body. Mr. J. is suffering from a deficiency of __________ amino acids.
12. Craig, a college sophomore, takes a great deal of interest in the supplementary nutritional product he is receiving and asks to read the label. He says, "There are some amino acids missing from this. Why aren't you giving me all of them?" You explain that some amino acids, all but eight, are manufactured in the body, using __________ sources.

Down

2. When Ms. C. (from 4 Across) asks why she needs amino acid supplemental feedings, you explain that amino acids promote growth and help with wound healing. One of the principal ways they do so is by reducing or slowing the breakdown of proteins, or __________.
3. Mr. and Mrs. R. recently appeared in a television commercial because they drink Ensure to meet a few extra nutritional needs they have experienced with aging. Their nephew recently had surgery, and while recovering, he received nasogastric delivery of a modular formulation to supplement a polymeric feeding formulation he needed. When their grandson was an infant, his parents supplemented his breastfeeding with an infant nutritional formulation. Each member of the R. clan discussed here has received some form of _________ nutrition.
6. Lauren in 8 Down is receiving __________ amino acids.
7. You are explaining to Mrs. N.'s family that the parenteral nutritional supplementation you are about to start will help her by bypassing the entire gastrointestinal system, eliminating the need for absorption, __________, and excretion.
8. Lauren, age 10, is going through a period of rapid growth. She is receiving enough essential amino acids in her diet and her body has no problems producing its normal levels of nonessential amino acids. Nevertheless, she is to receive two amino acids that are not produced in large enough quantities to support this rapid growth spurt. Lauren is to receive a supplemental source of histidine and __________.
9. Mr. K. has been receiving peripheral parenteral nutrition. One day something rather rare occurs: his vein becomes inflamed. You notify the physician. "Left untreated," she tells you, "this could have become really severe. He could even have lost his arm eventually if you hadn't caught this so quickly." Mr. K., of course, has __________.

Chapter Review and NCLEX® Examination Preparation

Select the best answer for each question.

1. The nurse is assessing a patient who is receiving a peripheral TPN infusion. The maximum concentration of dextrose in peripheral TPN infusions should be which percentage?
   a. 10%
   b. 20%
   c. 50%
   d. 100%

2. A patient has a need for a nutritional supplement that contains complex nutrients derived from proteins, carbohydrates, and fat. However, this patient is intolerant to milk. The nurse knows that which product would be most suitable for this patient?
   a. Casec
   b. Polycose
   c. Ensure
   d. Vivonex

3. When monitoring a patient who is receiving TPN through a central line, the nurse should observe for which complications? *(Select all that apply.)*
   a. Pneumothorax
   b. Aspiration
   c. Hyperglycemia
   d. Infection
   e. Air embolus

4. A patient who is just starting to take enteral nutritional supplements should be taught by the nurse to expect which most common adverse effect?
   a. Anorexia
   b. Constipation
   c. Diarrhea
   d. Flatulence

5. When reviewing a patient's need for nutritional supplementation, the nurse remembers that peripheral TPN is most appropriate for which type of patient?
   a. Patients who will receive short-term TPN (for less than 2 weeks)
   b. Patients who will receive long-term TPN (for longer than 2 weeks)
   c. Patients with severe nutritional problems
   d. Patients who wish to reduce their weight

6. Which are nursing interventions for patients receiving enteral feedings?
   a. Checking gastric residual volumes once a day
   b. Starting the infusions at the maximum rate ordered
   c. Keeping the head of the bed flat
   d. Giving tube feeding formulas that are at room temperature
7. A patient is receiving a PEG tube feeding of Glucerna at 70 mL/hour via a feeding pump. What will be the PEG tube intake over a 24-hour period?

Critical Thinking and Application

Answer the following questions on a separate sheet of paper.

8. Ms. S. has one of the newer tubes for nasogastric feeding.
   a. What are the advantages and disadvantages of these newer tubes?
   b. What symptoms would she develop if she were lactose intolerant?
   c. Her tube feeding rate is 50 mL/hr. After 24 hours, you note that the residual amount is 120 mL. What will the nurse do?

9. Mr. R., who is on TPN therapy, has a weak pulse, hypertension, tachycardia, and decreased urine output. He seems somewhat confused, and the nurse notes on examining him that he exhibits pitting edema. What is wrong? Can the nurse do anything about it? What could the nurse have done differently to avoid this reaction?

Case Study

Read the scenario and answer the following questions on a separate sheet of paper.

You are caring for Mrs. T., who is receiving peripheral parenteral nutrition through an intravenous (IV) line in her right forearm. Your assessment shows that bag No. 3 is infusing at 100 mL/hr via an infusion pump, and the bag has about 300 mL remaining. The site is intact without redness or swelling.

1. Two hours later, Mrs. T. calls you because she accidentally pulled the IV line out of her arm. The remaining 300 mL of TPN has spilled on the floor. You have tried to reinsert the IV line but have not had success yet. What could occur if you cannot restart the infusion?

2. At last, the IV line has been reinserted, but you then discover that bag No. 4 has not yet been ordered from the pharmacy. What should you hang until TPN bag No. 4 is ready?

3. What else should you monitor while Mrs. T. is receiving peripheral parenteral nutrition?

CHAPTER 55

Anemia Drugs

Chapter Review and NCLEX® Examination Preparation

Select the best answer for each question.

1. Three days after beginning therapy with oral iron tablets, a patient calls the office. "I'm very worried because my bowel movements are black!" What will the nurse do?
   a. Tell the patient to stop the iron tablets.
   b. Tell the patient to take the tablets every other day instead of daily.
   c. Ask the patient to come into the office for a checkup.
   d. Explain to the patient that this is an expected effect of the medication.

2. Patients who take oral iron preparations should be warned by the nurse of the possible adverse effects, which may include which of the following?
   a. Dizziness and orthostatic hypotension
   b. Nausea, vomiting, and stomach cramps
   c. Drowsiness, lethargy, and fatigue
   d. Neuropathy and tingling in the extremities

3. The nurse is preparing to administer folic acid. What happens if folic acid is given to treat anemia without determining the underlying cause of the anemia?
   a. Erythropoiesis is inhibited.
   b. Excessive levels of folic acid may accumulate, causing toxicity.
   c. The symptoms of pernicious anemia may be masked, delaying treatment.
   d. Intestinal intrinsic factor is destroyed.

4. A patient is about to receive folic acid supplementation. The nurse knows that indications for folic acid supplementation include which of the following? *(Select all that apply.)*
   a. Megaloblastic anemia
   b. Tropical sprue
   c. Prevention of fetal neural tube defects
   d. Pernicious anemia
   e. Hemolytic anemia

5. When teaching the patient about oral iron preparations, the nurse will include which instructions? *(Select all that apply.)*
   a. Mix the liquid iron preparations with antacids to reduce gastrointestinal distress.
   b. Take the iron with meals if gastrointestinal distress occurs.
   c. Liquid forms should be taken through a straw to avoid discoloration of tooth enamel.
   d. Oral forms should be taken with juice, not milk.
   e. Iron products will turn the stools from brown to a black, tarry color.

6. The nurse is preparing to give iron sucrose (Venofer) to a 58-year-old patient, and will monitor for which common adverse effect?
   a. Hypotension
   b. Dyspnea
   c. Itching
   d. Cramps

7. A 5-year-old child who is receiving hemodialysis is to receive 8 doses of sodium ferric gluconate (Ferrlecit), 1.5 mg/kg, IV, with future dialysis sessions. The child weighs 38 pounds. How many mg is each dose? ______________

Critical Thinking and Application

Answer the following questions on a separate sheet of paper.

8. Mr. P. is prescribed intramuscular iron dextran. However, before the nurse can give him his first injection, the pharmacist suggests that she give him a smaller dose of 25 mg first. Why does the pharmacist suggest this? How should intramuscular iron dextran be administered?

9. The nurse is aware of the foods that contain iron. What other foods may either enhance the intake of iron or perhaps hinder it?

10. Mrs. S. will be taking iron for treatment of anemia, and her physician instructed her to take it with orange juice. She asks the nurse for an explanation of this. What will the nurse tell her?

11. Four-year-old David has accidentally ingested an oral iron preparation, but he is not showing any adverse effects yet. Describe the treatment plan. If the serum iron concentration is higher than 300 mcg/dL, how is the treatment plan affected?

12. What are the advantages of receiving ferric gluconate (Ferrlecit) or iron sucrose (Venofer) injections instead of iron dextran?

Case Study

Read the scenario and answer the following questions on a separate sheet of paper.

Maureen has been given ferrous fumarate (Femiron) capsules with instructions to take two capsules twice a day as part of her treatment for iron-deficiency anemia.

1. She asks you if she can take this drug with meals. What is your answer?

2. What else should you warn her to expect with this medication?

3. After a week, Maureen calls you because she does not like to swallow capsules. She says that her mother has iron tablets that are labeled ferrous sulfate. She wants to know if she can take those tablets instead. What do you tell her?

4. Because Maureen does not like the capsules, her iron preparation has been switched to an oral liquid suspension. While you are teaching her how to give herself the correct dosage, what else is important for you to tell her about liquid iron preparations?

CHAPTER 56

Dermatologic Drugs

Chapter Review and NCLEX® Examination Preparation

Select the best answer for each question.

1. Which statement accurately describes antifungal therapy for topical infections?
   a. The length of treatment required to eradicate the organism may be from several weeks to as long as a year.
   b. Antifungal therapy works best when the affected area is exposed to sunlight.
   c. Oral drugs are the preferred drugs for treating topical fungal infections.
   d. Antifungal therapy is palliative only; fungi are rarely eradicated from topical areas.

2. When instructing a patient on how to use suppositories for vaginal yeast infections, the nurse should keep in mind that suppositories will be given in which manner?
   a. Insert one every other day at bedtime for 1 week.
   b. Insert one daily at bedtime for 3 consecutive days.
   c. A one-time dose is administered in the morning.
   d. Insert every night at bedtime until symptoms stop.

3. A patient has a painful sunburn that covers a large area of her body and has asked the nurse for "something to make it feel better." The nurse keeps in mind that which formulation of topical medication will enhance the patient's comfort?
   a. Aerosol spray
   b. Gel
   c. Oil
   d. Cream

4. A patient needs a medication that has excellent emollient properties. Because she works as a swimming coach, the medication prescribed should not wash off when it comes in contact with water. If each has the same healing properties, which formulation will the nurse suggest for this patient?
   a. Aerosol spray
   b. Oil
   c. Gel
   d. Cream

5. The nurse is administering topical antiviral drugs. Which statements about these drugs are true? *(Select all that apply.)*
   a. Common adverse effects include stinging, itching, and rash.
   b. Topically applied acyclovir (Zovirax) does not cure viral skin infections but does seem to decrease the healing time and pain.
   c. Topically applied acyclovir can cure viral skin infections if applied as soon as symptoms appear.
   d. Antiviral drugs are applied topically for the treatment of both initial and recurrent herpes simplex infections.
   e. Topical antiviral drugs are used more often than systemic antiviral drugs for the treatment of viral skin conditions.

6. A 22-year-old woman is taking isotretinoin (Accutane) as part of the treatment for severe cystic acne. Which statement about isotretinoin therapy is true?
   a. This drug reduces acne by causing skin peeling.
   b. Its use is contraindicated if she is allergic to erythromycin.
   c. She will need to apply it twice a day to her face after washing her face thoroughly.
   d. She will need to use two forms of birth control while taking this medication.

7. Before using povidone-iodine (Betadine) solution to prepare skin for surgery, the nurse should ask the patient about allergies to which substance?
   a. Shellfish
   b. Penicillin
   c. Mercury
   d. Milk

8. A patient will be receiving intravenous amphotericin B (Fungizone) for a severe fungal infection that has not responded to other medications. The order reads for 75 mg in 1000 mL D_5W to infuse over 6 hours. The nurse will set the infusion pump to what rate?

   ____

Critical Thinking and Application

Answer the following questions on a separate sheet of paper.

9. Mr. M. has a topical skin infection. He is prescribed clindamycin (Cleocin T). He has never used this drug before. The nurse realizes that it is a good idea to assess him for possible sensitivity or allergies. What precautions will the nurse take?

10. The nurse is getting ready to apply topical erythromycin to a patient's skin. The affected area of the skin is not oozing or even moist, but the nurse's supervisor still requires that she wear gloves. Why?

11. Mr. L.'s two children brought "something" home from school, and within a day, he had "it" too. He tells the nurse that he has applied lindane (Kwell) to everyone's scalp, but he has come to the clinic to have his children and himself checked because he is not confident that he has "taken care of things properly." For what are Mr. L. and his children being treated? Describe for him the basic steps in using lindane. What other measures should he take?

12. Compare the implementation and precautions needed for benzoyl peroxide and tretinoin when used for acne.

13. A newly admitted patient has a stage III pressure ulcer that shows areas of exudate along with areas of healed granulation tissue. The orders for wound care include application of cadexomer iodine (Iodosorb). Explain what should be assessed before applying this medication and its purpose in wound care.

14. A patient with an infected pressure ulcer that contains an area of eschar needs to have the area surgically débrided, but instead the physician orders collagenase (Santyl) treatment of the wound. What could be the reason for this order instead of surgery and what is the purpose of this medication?

Case Study

Read the scenario and answer the following questions on a separate sheet of paper.

Judy is in the clinic today because she burned her arm last evening while frying chicken. She has a second-degree burn over a 5-inch area of her forearm. She did not apply anything to it overnight, and the wound is reddened and peeling.

1. The physician tells you that he is going to apply silver sulfadiazine (Silvadene) cream to the site. What will he need to do before applying this cream?

2. He tells Judy that the area will need to be kept covered. Why is this necessary?

3. As the physician prepares to apply the cream, you notice that he is about to reach into the medication jar with his ungloved fingers. Is this okay?

4. Are there any adverse effects associated with this medication?

CHAPTER 57

Ophthalmic Drugs

Chapter Review and NCLEX® Examination Preparation

Match each definition with the corresponding term. (Note: Not all terms will be used.)

1. _____ Adjustment of the lens of the eye to variation in distance
2. _____ Inflammation of the eyelids
3. _____ The clear, watery fluid that circulates in the anterior and posterior chambers of the eye
4. _____ An abnormal condition of the lens of the eye, characterized by loss of transparency
5. _____ Paralysis of the ciliary muscles, which prevents accommodation of the lens to variations in distance
6. _____ Excessive intraocular pressure caused by elevated levels of aqueous humor
7. _____ The mucous membrane that lines the eyelids
8. _____ Drugs that constrict the pupil
9. _____ The vascular middle layer of the eye, containing the iris, ciliary body, and choroid
10. _____ Drugs that dilate the pupil

a. Cycloplegia
b. Conjunctiva
c. Accommodation
d. Glaucoma
e. Mydriatics
f. Miotics
g. Uvea
h. Blepharitis
i. Vitreous humor
j. Aqueous humor
k. Cataract

Select the best answer for each question.

11. When reviewing the medical record of a patient with a new order for a carbonic anhydrase inhibitor, the nurse knows that which condition would be a potential problem for a patient taking this drug?
    a. Glaucoma
    b. Ocular hypertension
    c. Allergy to sulfa drugs
    d. Allergy to penicillin

12. During an ophthalmic procedure, the patient receives ophthalmic acetylcholine. The nurse is aware that which effect is the purpose of administering this drug?
    a. To produce mydriasis for ophthalmic examination
    b. To produce immediate miosis during ophthalmic surgery
    c. To cause cycloplegia to allow for measurement of intraocular pressure
    d. To provide topical anesthesia during ophthalmic surgery

13. When giving latanoprost (Xalatan) eyedrops, the nurse should advise the patient of which possible adverse effects?
    a. Temporary eye color changes, from light eye colors to brown
    b. Permanent eye color changes, from light eye colors to brown
    c. Photosensitivity
    d. Bradycardia and hypotension

14. A patient has come to the emergency department with an eye injury. After fluorescein (AK-Fluor) is applied, the physician sees an area with a green halo. This indicates which condition?
    a. A corneal defect
    b. A conjunctival lesion
    c. The presence of a hard contact lens
    d. A foreign object

15. When applying ophthalmic drugs, the nurse will follow which instructions? *(Select all that apply.)*
    a. Apply drops directly onto the cornea.
    b. Apply drops into the conjunctival sac.
    c. Apply pressure to the inner canthus for 1 minute after medication administration.
    d. Apply ointments in a thin layer.
    e. Avoid touching the eye with the tip of the medication dropper.

16. A newborn infant is about to receive medication that prevents gonorrheal eye infection. The nurse will prepare to administer which drug?
    a. dexamethasone (Maxidex) ointment
    b. gentamicin (Genoptic) solution
    c. erythromycin ointment
    d. sulfacetamide (Cetamide) solution

17. A patient has an order for an IV to infuse at 75 mL/hour. The infusion will infuse by gravity drip; the administration set delivers 15 gtt/mL. What is the gtt/min that the nurse will need to use for this infusion?

    ____

Critical Thinking and Application

Answer the following questions on a separate sheet of paper.

18. Jonathan has blue eyes; Julie has brown eyes. Why would the drug effects of the miotics on the iris be less pronounced in Julie?

19. Mrs. N., a 60-year-old librarian, has open-angle glaucoma. The physician prescribes dipivefrin (Propine).
    a. Why might the physician have chosen that drug over epinephrine?
    b. What problems will the nurse tell Mrs. N. to report?
    c. Will the nurse expect any serious reactions to the drug? Explain your answer.

20. The physician prescribes a beta-adrenergic blocker for Ned, who has ocular hypertension. Ned experiences what he calls "an allergic reaction" to the drug, and the physician changes Ned's medication to another beta-blocking drug, timolol (Timoptic). Because both of these drugs are beta-adrenergic blockers and Ned had a reaction to the first drug, why would the physician simply switch Ned to another drug in the same category?

21. The nurse is preparing to administer sulfacetamide to Tony, a patient with an eye infection.
    a. Why will the nurse cleanse Tony's eye before administering the medication?
    b. Before using the sulfacetamide, the nurse examines it and then throws the solution away and looks for another container of sulfacetamide. Why did the nurse do that?

22. Louisa has an inflammatory disorder of the eye for which the physician has prescribed a topical ophthalmic nonsteroidal antiinflammatory drug (NSAID). Why might the physician have chosen an NSAID over a corticosteroid?

23. Ms. L. has been prescribed ophthalmic corticosteroid drops for an inflammation of her eye. The next day she calls the clinic and tells the nurse, "These drops sting so much when I use them that I can't even put in my contacts." What will the nurse respond?

Case Study

Read the scenario and answer the following questions on a separate sheet of paper.

Mr. W., age 76, has developed a bacterial ocular infection and has a prescription for erythromycin ocular ointment.

1. How should this drug be administered?

2. What safety precautions should Mr. W. consider after receiving a dose of this medication?

3. After receiving the first dose, Mr. W. complains that the medication "burns and stings." What will the nurse say to Mr. W. about this?

4. Mr. W. tells the nurse, "I have some eyedrops from a few months ago when I had some allergy problems. I am sure they will help me now. Can I take them with this ointment?" What is the nurse's best response?

CHAPTER 58

Otic Drugs

Chapter Review and NCLEX® Examination Preparation

Select the best answer for each question.

1. When assessing for otitis media, the nurse remembers that common symptoms of this condition include which of the following? *(Select all that apply.)*
   a. Pain
   b. Malaise
   c. Ear drainage
   d. Hearing loss
   e. Fever

2. A patient with a middle ear infection will generally require treatment with which type of drug?
   a. Topical steroids
   b. Systemic steroids
   c. Topical antibiotics
   d. Systemic antibiotics

3. An older adult patient has a buildup of cerumen in his left ear. The nurse expects that this patient will receive which type of drug for this problem?
   a. Antifungal
   b. Wax emulsifier
   c. Steroid
   d. Local analgesic

4. Before giving eardrops, the nurse checks for contraindications to the use of otic preparations, such as which condition?
   a. Eardrum perforation
   b. Infection
   c. Presence of cerumen
   d. Mastoiditis

5. A child has a case of otitis media. The nurse knows that otitis media in children is usually preceded by:
   a. participation in a swim team.
   b. injury with a foreign object.
   c. upper respiratory tract infection.
   d. mastoiditis.

6. A child with an ear infection will be receiving amoxicillin (Amoxil) suspension PO. The order reads: "Give 125 mg (5 mL) three times a day PO." The child weighs 11 kg.
   a. How many mg of medication will this child receive in 24 hours? ____________
   b. The safe range of the medication 20 to 40 mg/kg/day. What is the safe range for this child?
   ____
   c. Is the ordered dose within the safe range?
   ____

Critical Thinking and Application

Answer the following questions on a separate sheet of paper.

7. A patient calls the physician's office complaining of severe pain in and drainage from his left ear. He also says he "had a little mishap" on his motorcycle yesterday. What will the nurse tell him?

8. Why are antiinfective drugs frequently combined with steroids?

9. André, a 30-year-old teacher, has an ear infection and has a prescription for eardrops.
   a. What will the nurse do before instilling the drops?
   b. What will the nurse warn André might happen after the drops are instilled?

10. Mrs. F., a 52-year-old office manager, has come to the clinic today complaining of a painful, "itchy" left ear. The physician diagnoses an infection of the external auditory canal and prescribes a topical antibiotic.
    a. What is the advantage of using a product containing hydrocortisone?
    b. What would be a contraindication to Mrs. F.'s use of this type of drug?

11. Why do so many otic combination products contain local anesthetic drugs?

12. Ben is a 2-year-old who attends day care, and his brother Drew is a 6-year-old kindergartner. They both require otic drugs for ear infections.
    a. What instructions will the nurse give the boys' parents regarding instillation of the drops?
    b. A few days after they are first seen, the boys' mother brings them back for a follow-up visit. Ben and Drew do not seem to be in pain and there is no redness or swelling in either child's ears. What does this mean?

13. During a home visit, the nurse observes Esther's husband preparing her eardrops. He puts a glass of water in the microwave, saying that he will soak the bottle of eardrops in hot water to warm them up.
    a. How is Esther's husband doing so far?
    b. Later, immediately after her husband instills the drops, Esther sits up and asks whether they are now doing everything right. What will the nurse tell her?

Case Study

Read the scenario and answer the following questions on a separate sheet of paper.

Mark, who is 45 years old, comes to the office complaining of a "heavy" feeling in his left ear, with slight pain and decreased hearing. When you walk into the examination room, you find Mark inserting a cotton-tipped applicator into his ear "to scratch it."

1. What do you suspect is the problem with his ears?

2. What can be done to address this problem?

3. You give Mark a container of carbamide peroxide (Debrox) drops. Before you continue, he asks you how many times a day he needs to take this medication and whether he can take it with meals. How is this medication given?

4. Why is there a combination of carbamide peroxide and glycerin in the Debrox?

Overview of Dosage Calculations

There are many important aspects to consider when doing dosage calculations, but probably the most important one is common sense. If a drug dose calculation does not seem right, then most likely it is not. The administration of drugs to patients is a shared responsibility among the patient, prescriber, pharmacist, and nurse. All those involved have a moral, ethical, and legal responsibility to ensure that the administration takes place in a safe and effective way. The nurse has a legal and a professional responsibility to ensure that his or her patients receive the right dose of the right medication at the right time and in the right manner. There are many checks and balances in the system to guarantee that this happens. The necessary basic calculations involved in the safe and accurate administration of medications to patients are described in this section.

Calculating drug doses is one small part of the overall process of pharmacologic therapy. Before you actually calculate a drug dose, you must follow many steps. The nurse should evaluate the patient and the prescribed medication for the following "rights": right patient, right drug, right dose, right time, and right route. In addition, the nurse must document correctly after the drug is given. Other principles to follow to decrease the likelihood of mistakes are to calculate doses systematically and to perform calculations consistently time after time so that the process becomes easier with each calculation. It also helps to have a peer check your calculations, especially if the dose seems unusual or the math is very difficult. Remember that common sense should prevail. If a calculation shows that you should give 25 mg of digoxin and the strongest strength is 0.25 mg, common sense should tell you that the patient should not be given 100 pills, especially since drug dosage forms are usually manufactured with the most commonly prescribed dosages in mind.

You must have basic arithmetic skills before beginning. The following basic principles may need to be reviewed:

- Basic multiplication
- Basic division
- Roman numerals
- Fractions (reducing to lowest terms, addition, subtraction, multiplication, division, mixed numbers)
- Decimals (addition, subtraction, multiplication, division)
- Ratios and percentages (changing a fraction to a percentage, changing a ratio to a percentage)
- Solving for *x* in a simple equation

RULES TO REMEMBER

- Before calculating a drug dose for a particular patient, you must first convert all units of measure to a SINGLE system, if this has not already been done. For example, do NOT attempt to guess a dosage if the drug is ordered in grains but the drug label is in milligrams. The best approach is to convert to the system used on the drug label. You may have to convert the patient's weight from pounds to kilograms if the medication is ordered to be given per kilogram of weight.
- **Rounding**. Always round your answers to the nearest dose that is measurable, after verifying that the dose is correct for that patient.
  - If a tablet is scored, you may round to the nearest half tablet.
    Example: 1.8 tablets, give 2 tablets
    1.2 tablets, give 1 tablet
  - If a tablet is unscored, call the pharmacy. It is very difficult to cut an unscored tablet accurately. Remember that enteric-coated, sustained-release, or extended-release formulations cannot be cut or crushed!
  - Recheck your calculations if the dose is more than 1 or 2 tablets.
  - To round liquids, look at the equipment you plan to use. Some syringes are marked in tenths or hundredths of a milliliter. Larger syringes are marked in 0.2-mL increments. Tuberculin syringes are marked in hundredths. For

Disclaimer: Please note that the drugs and dosages within this chapter are examples for educational purposes only; please refer to appropriate drug resources for dosage information.

liquid medications, NEVER round up to the nearest WHOLE number. If the answer is 1.8 mL, DO NOT round up to 2 mL. Rounding up in these situations may lead to overdosing. However, if you are using an electronic infusion pump, you will probably need to round to the nearest whole number.

- To round to the nearest tenth, look at the hundredths column. If it is 0.5 or more, round UP to the next tenth.
  Example: To round to the nearest tenth:
  1.78 or 1.75, round to 1.8
  1.32 or 1.34, round to 1.3
- A syringe calibrated in hundredths permits more exact measurement of small dosages. To round to the nearest hundredth, look at the thousandth column. If it is 0.005 or more, round UP to the next hundredth.
  Example: To round to the nearest hundredth:
  1.847, round to 1.85
  1.653, round to 1.65
- NOTE: Never round up liquid medications to the nearest whole number. If the answer is 1.6 mL, DO NOT round up to 2 mL! Such increases may lead to overdoses.
- PEDIATRIC DOSES are rounded to the TENTHS place, not whole numbers. Rounding to whole numbers may lead to overdoses.

■ **Leading Zeros.** Always insert a zero (0) in front of decimals when the number is less than a whole number. This draws attention to the decimal and avoids potential errors.
  Example: 0.05 is CORRECT.
  .05 is NOT correct.

■ **Trailing Zeroes.** Never place a lone zero after a decimal point. If the decimal is not noticed, a dangerous dosage error may occur.
  Example: 3 is CORRECT
  3.0 is NOT correct and may be mistaken for 30

■ **Labeling.** Always label your answers with the appropriate unit. If the problem asked for a number of tablets, write "tablets." If you are to give an injection, use "mL." Heparin and insulin, however, use "units" instead of "mg" or "mcg." Intravenous drips will either be written in terms of "mL/hr" or "gtt/mL." Problems using an intravenous infusion pump are ALWAYS asking for mL/hr. THINK about what the question is asking and then label your answer appropriately.

■ **Common Sense.** Use common sense! Drug companies typically formulate medications that are close to the usual doses and medications that can provide the ordered dose with one or two tablets. If your answer indicates that you should give 60 mL intramuscularly, CHECK IT AGAIN! Remember, you can only give 2 to 3 mL intramuscularly, depending on institution policies, so a dosage of 60 mL would be inappropriate.

INTERPRETING MEDICATION LABELS

Medication labels contain a great amount of information—much of it in small print. The drug manufacturer prints some labels; others are prepared by pharmacy technicians or pharmacists for institutional use. The most important information follows:

■ Generic name—the first letter is usually lowercase; this is the name used by all companies that produce the drug
■ Trade, brand, or proprietary name—the first letter is usually capitalized; this name is used only by the manufacturer of the drug and may be followed by the "®" symbol
■ Unit dose per milliliter, per tablet, per capsule, and so on
■ Total amount in the container
■ Route
■ Directions for preparation, if needed
■ Directions for storage
■ Expiration date

Other information, such as a specification for adult or pediatric use, may be noted on the label.

Example:

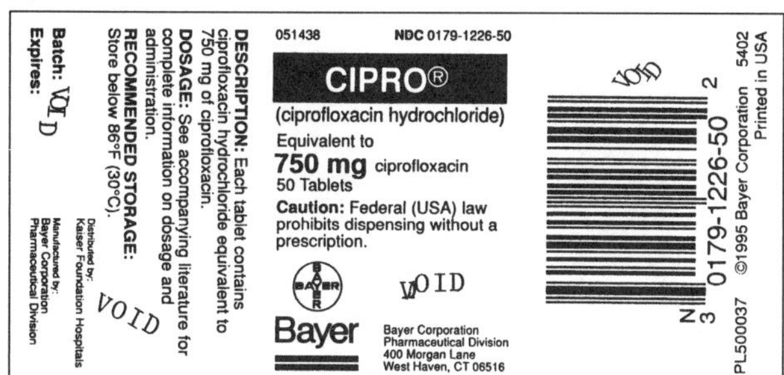

Generic name:	ciprofloxacin hydrochloride
Trade name:	Cipro
Unit dose:	750 mg per tablet
Total amount in container:	50 tablets
Route:	(It is assumed that tablets are oral route.)

For the following labels, identify the information requested:

1.

Zocor® 40 mg
(Simvastatin)
Dist. by: MERCK & CO., INC. West Point, PA 19486, USA
Store between 5-30°C (41-86°F).
60 Tablets
Lot
Exp.
NDC 0006-0749-61
6505-01-354-4546
USUAL ADULT DOSAGE: See accompanying circular.
Rx only
LIFT HERE
7975502
60 | No. 3591

Generic name: ______________________

Trade name: ______________________

Unit dose: ______________________

Total amount in container: ______________________

Route: ______________________

2.

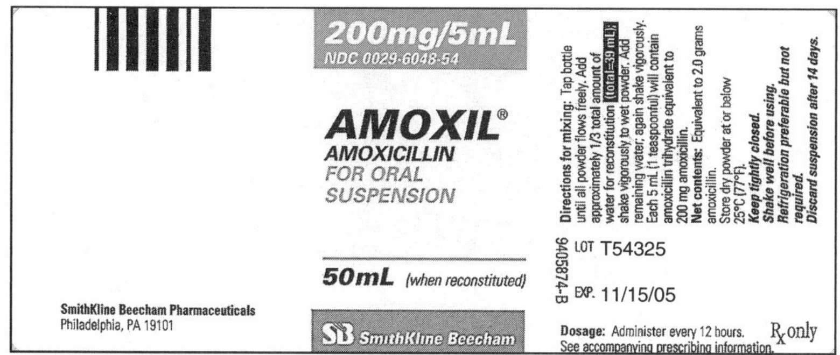

Generic name: ______________________

Trade name: ______________________

Unit dose: ______________________

Total amount in container: ______________________

Route: ______________________

3.

NDC 0009-0626-02 10 ml Vial
Depo-Provera®
Sterile Aqueous Suspension
sterile medroxyprogesterone acetate suspension, USP
400 mg per ml
For intramuscular use only
Caution: Federal law prohibits dispensing without prescription.

See package insert for complete product information.
Shake vigorously immediately before each use.
Store at controlled room temperature 15°-30° C (59°-86° F)
Each ml contains: Medroxyprogesterone acetate, 400 mg.
Also, polyethylene glycol 3350, 20.3 mg; sodium sulfate anhydrous, 11 mg; myristyl-gamma-picolinium chloride, 1.69 mg added as preservative. When necessary, pH was adjusted with sodium hydroxide and/or hydrochloric acid.
813 273 000

Upjohn
The Upjohn Company
Kalamazoo, Michigan 49001, USA

Generic name: ____________________
Trade name: ____________________
Unit dose: ____________________
Total amount in container: ____________________
Route: ____________________

4.

Single-Dose Vial For IV or IM use
Contains Benzyl Alcohol as a Preservative
See package insert for complete product information.
Per 2 mL (when mixed):
* hydrocortisone sodium succinate equiv. to hydrocortisone, 250 mg. Protect solution from light. Discard after 3 days.
814 070 205 Reconstituted ....
The Upjohn Company
Kalamazoo, MI 49001, USA

2 mL Act-O-Vial® NDC 0009-0909-08
Solu-Cortef® Sterile Powder
hydrocortisone sodium succinate for injection, USP
250 mg*

Generic name: ____________________
Trade name: ____________________
Unit dose: ____________________
Total amount in container: ____________________
Route: ____________________

SECTION I: BASIC CONVERSIONS USING RATIO AND PROPORTION

A proportion is a way of stating a relationship of equality between two ratios. The first ratio listed is EQUAL to the second ratio listed. The double colon (::) that separates the two ratios means "is the same as." The numbers at each end of the ratio equation can be called the "outside," and the two numbers in the middle of the ratio (around the "::") can be called the "inside." Ratio and proportion problems can be used to calculate ONE of the numbers in the equation if it is not known. The simple rule to use is this:

The product of the outside terms equals the product of the inside terms.

If one of the terms is not known, it is designated as *x*. The problem is then set up to solve for *x*.

Example:

The problem "1 : 100 :: 4 : *x*" actually means:
"The relationship of 1 to 100 is the same as the relationship of 4 to *x*." The *x* is unknown.

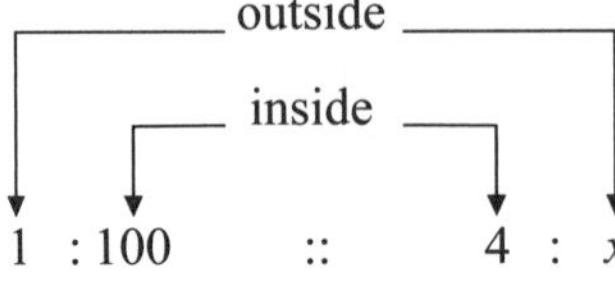

1 and *x* are the "outsides"; 100 and 4 are the "insides." To solve for *x*, multiply the "outsides" ($1 \times x$) together, multiply the "insides" (100×4) together, and form an equation:

$(1 \times x) = (100 \times 4)$
$1x = 400$
$x = 400$

Proof: You may prove your equation as follows: Insert the answer for x in the original equation, then solve.
$1 \times 400 = 400$ (outsides)
$100 \times 4 = 400$ (insides)
$400 = 400$; the answer for x is correct.

Example:
$5 : 25 :: 15 : x$
Multiply the "outsides" and the "insides" and form an equation; then solve for x.
$(5 \times x) = (25 \times 15)$
$5x = 375$
$x = 375/5$
$x = 75$

Proof:
$5 \times 75 = 375$
$25 \times 15 = 375$
$375 = 375$

Calculating ratios is one of the major foundations of drug dosage calculations. When calculating a dosage, the nurse will use the medication on hand to calculate how much of it to give for a desired dosage. The nurse uses the principle of proportion to calculate accurately how much medication to give. The following chart provides a few common equivalents used in pharmacology. These equivalents are then used in ratio and proportion problems to calculate appropriate dosages.

BASIC EQUIVALENTS

Metric Equivalents	Other Equivalents
Weight 1 mg = 1000 mcg (micrograms) 1 g = 1000 mg (milligrams) 1 kg (kilogram) = 1000 g (grams)	***Weight*** 1 gr (grain) = 60 mg 1 g (gram) = 1000 mg = gr xv (15 grains) (approximately) 1 kg = 2.2 lb
Volume 1000 mL = 1 L (liter)	***Volume*** 1 oz (ounce) = 30 mL 1 tsp (teaspoon) = 5 mL (milliliters) 1 tbsp (tablespoon) = 15 mL 2 tbsp = 30 mL

To find basic equivalents from one unit of measure to another, use the ratio and proportion approach.

Example 1: The drug dosage is 500 mg. You have scored tablets on hand that are 1 g each. How many tablets will you give?

You have *grams* on hand. You need to change the *milligrams* needed to the equivalent grams on hand.
Find the proper equivalents:
Equivalent: 1 g = 1000 mg
Next, set up the ratio and proportion equation.
On the LEFT side, put the ratio that you ***know:*** 1 g is 1000 mg
On the RIGHT side, put the ratio that you ***want to know:*** How many g (x) is 500 mg?

Know ***Want to Know***
1 g : 1000 mg :: x g : 500 mg

Solve for x: $(1 \times 500) = (1000 \times x)$; $500 = 1000x$; $x = 500/1000$; $x = 0.5$
You will give 0.5 (half) of the 1-g tablet, which equals 500 mg.

To double-check your answer, substitute your answer for the x and solve. The "outsides" should equal the "insides."
$1 \times 500 = 500$; $1000 \times 0.5 = 500$; $500 = 500$

Example 2: Cough syrup, 45 mL, is ordered. The cough syrup comes in a 2-oz bottle. How many oz do you give?
You have oz on hand. You need to give 45 mL.
Equivalent: 1 oz = 30 mL
Know: 1 oz is 30 mL; ***want to know:*** How many oz is 45 mL?

Know ***Want to Know***
1 oz : 30 mL :: x oz : 45 mL

$(1 \times 45) = (30 \times x)$; $45 = 30x$; $x = 45/30 = 1.5$ oz = 45 mL
Proof: $1 \times 45 = 45$; $30 \times 1.5 = 45$; $45 = 45$

Example 3: Mabel weighs 122 lb. How many kilograms does she weigh?

Equivalent: 1 kg = 2.2 lb

Know ***Want to Know***
1 kg : 2.2 lb :: x kg : 122 lb

$(1 \times 122) = (2.2 \times x)$; $122 = 2.2x$; $122/2.2 = x$; $x = 55.45$ lb; round off to tenths: 55.5 lb
Proof: $1 \times 122 = 122$; $2.2 \times 55.45 = 121.99$ (rounds to 122)

Example 4: You have an injectable solution that is 50-mg strength. How many mcg are in 50 mg?

Equivalent: 1 mg = 1000 mcg

Know ***Want to Know***
1 mg : 1000 mcg :: 50 mg : x mcg

$(1 \times x) = (1000 \times 50)$; $1x = 50{,}000$; $x = 50{,}000$; therefore 50 mg = 50,000 mcg
Proof: $1 \times 50{,}000 = 50{,}000$; $1000 \times 50 = 50{,}000$

Example 5: Elixir is ordered as follows: "Give 2 tsp twice a day." How many mL will you give?
Equivalent: 1 tsp = 5 mL

Know ***Want to Know***
1 tsp : 5 mL :: 2 tsp : x mL

$(1 \times x) = (5 \times 2)$; $1x = 10$; $x = 10$ mL
Proof: $1 \times 10 = 10$; $5 \times 2 = 10$; $10 = 10$
So, give 10 mL to equal 2 tsp.

Example 6: You have an injection that delivers 75 mcg. How many mg does it deliver?
Equivalent: 1 mg = 1000 mcg

Know ***Want to Know***
1 mg : 1000 mcg :: x mg : 75 mcg

$(1 \times 75) = (1000 \times x)$; $75 = 1000x$; $x = 75/1000$; $x = 0.075$
So, 75 mcg = 0.075 mg. (Don't forget the leading zero!)
Proof: $1 \times 75 = 75$; $1000 \times 0.075 = 75$; $75 = 75$

PRACTICE PROBLEMS

Calculate the following conversions.

1. 600 mg = ______________ mcg
2. 1500 mg = ______________ mcg
3. 5000 mcg = ______________ mg
4. 5 g = ______________ mg
5. 2.5 g = ______________ mg
6. 900 mg = ______________ g
7. 8 kg = ______________ g
8. 750 mL = ______________ L
9. 975 L = ______________ mL
10. 500 mL = ______________ L
11. gr xvi = ______________ mg
12. 90 mg = ______________ gr
13. 4 tsp = ______________ mL
14. 60 mL = ______________ tsp
15. 90 mL = ______________ tbsp
16. 3 oz = ______________ mL
17. 6 mL = ______________ oz
18. 90 kg = ______________ lb
19. 150 lb = ______________ kg
20. 11 kg = ______________ lb

SECTION II: CALCULATING ORAL DOSES

To calculate oral dosages of medications, use the same ratio and proportion procedures described in Section I. Label all terms, and check your answers by proving them.

The first step in doing medication dosage calculation problems is examining the order and the medication on hand. The units for both the order and the medicine on hand MUST be the same units (e.g., mg, mL). If they are not the same, then a conversion must first be done to change the ordered dose to the same units as the medication on hand.

Remember these rules:

- NEVER substitute one form of a medication for another, even if the dosage amount is the same. Parenteral forms of oral drugs are much stronger, and the resulting effects might be dangerous.
- Do not forget to place a zero in front of a decimal point (e.g., 0.75 mg). It reminds you that the number is a decimal, not a whole number.
- Are the medication ordered and the medication on hand in the same units? If not, convert the drug ordered to the units of the drug at hand.
- Place what you have on hand (what you know)—information from the label—on the LEFT side of the equation.
- Place what is ordered (what you want to know) on the RIGHT side of the equation.
- Solve the equation as described in Section I.
- ALWAYS label the units of your answer (tablets, capsules, mL, etc.).

Example 1: The prescription reads, "Give 500 mg PO." The unit dose is 250 mg/tablet. How many tablets will you give?

Ordered: 500 mg **Unit dose:** 250 mg/tablet
NOTE: Units match (mg).

Know ***Want to Know***
250 mg : 1 tablet :: 500 mg : x tablet

$(250 \times x) = (1 \times 500)$; $250x = 500$; $x = 500/250 = 2$
Answer: Give 2 tablets.
Proof: $250 \times 2 = 500$; $1 \times 500 = 500$; $500 = 500$

Example 2: The order is to give 175 mg. The tablets on hand are 350-mg scored tablets. How many tablets will you give?

Ordered: 175 mg **Unit dose:** 350 mg/tablet
NOTE: Units match (mg).

Know ***Want to Know***
350 mg : 1 tablet :: 175 mg : x tablet

$(350 \times x) = (1 \times 175)$; $350x = 175$; $x = 175/350 = 0.5$
Answer: Give 0.5 tablet (one-half of the scored tablet).
Proof: $350 \times 0.5 = 175$; $1 \times 175 = 175$; $175 = 175$

Example 3: You are asked to administer 100 mg of a drug. You have 0.05-g tablets on hand. How many tablets will you give?

Ordered: 100 mg **Unit dose:** 0.05 g/tablet
NOTE: Units do not match (mg and g).
First: Calculate: 100 mg = x g (equivalent: 1 g = 1000 mg)

Know ***Want to Know***
1 g : 1000 mg :: x g : 100 mg

$(1 \times 100) = (1000 \times x)$; $100 = 1000x$; $x = 100/1000 = 0.1$
100 mg = 0.1 g
Now that you have the ordered dose and the dose on hand in the same units, you can complete the problem.

Ordered: 0.1 g (100 mg) **Unit dose:** 0.05 g/tablet

Know ***Want to Know***
0.05 g : 1 tablet :: 0.1 g : x tablet

$(0.05 \times x) = (1 \times 0.1)$; $0.05\,x = 0.1$; $x \times 0.1/0.05 = 2$
Answer: Give 2 tablets.
Proof: $0.05 \times 2 = 0.1$; $1 \times 0.1 = 0.1$; $0.1 = 0.1$

Example 4: You are instructed to give 0.5 g of a drug. You have 250-mg tablets on hand. How many tablets will you give?

Ordered: 0.5 g **Unit dose:** 250 mg/tablet
NOTE: Units do not match (g and mg).
First: Calculate: 0.5 g = x mg (equivalent: 1 g = 1000 mg)

Know ***Want to Know***
1 g : 1000 mg :: 0.5 g : x mg

$(1 \times x) = (1000 \times 0.5)$; $1x = 500$; $x = 500$
0.5 g = 500 mg
Now that you have the ordered dose and the dose on hand in the same units, you can complete the problem.

Ordered: 500 mg (0.5 g) **Unit dose:** 250 mg/tablet

Know ***Want to Know***
250 mg : 1 tablet :: 500 mg : x tablet

$(250 \times x) = (1 \times 500)$; $250x = 500$; $x = 500/250 = 2$
Answer: Give 2 tablets.
Proof: $250 \times 2 = 500$; $1 \times 500 = 500$; $500 = 500$

Example 5: You are to administer 200 mg of guaifenesin (Robitussin) syrup. You have a bottle labeled 100 mg/5 mL. How many mL will you give?

Ordered: 200 mg **Unit dose:** 100 mg/5 mL
NOTE: Units match (mg).

Know ***Want to Know***
100 mg : 5 mL :: 200 mg : *x* mL

$(100 \times x) = (5 \times 200)$; $100x = 1000$; $x = 1000/100 = 10$
Answer: Give 10 mL.
Proof: $100 \times 10 = 1000$; $5 \times 200 = 1000$; $1000 = 1000$

PRACTICE PROBLEMS

1. Dose ordered: ascorbic acid 0.5 g PO
   Dose on hand: 500-mg tablets
   How many tablets will you give? __________

2. Dose ordered: digoxin (Lanoxin) 0.5 mg PO
   Dose on hand: 250-mcg tablets
   How many tablets will you give? __________

3. Dose ordered: sulfisoxazole (Gantrisin) 0.25 g PO
   Dose on hand: 500-mg tablets
   How many tablets will you give? __________

4. Dose ordered: diphenhydramine (Benadryl) syrup 50 mg PO
   Dose on hand: syrup 12.5 mg/5 mL
   How many milliliters will you give? _________

5. Dose ordered: 600 mg PO
   Dose on hand: gr v tablets
   How many tablets will you give? __________

6. Dose ordered: cefaclor (Ceclor) 0.1 g PO
   Dose on hand: oral suspension 125 mg/5 mL
   How many milliliters will you give? _________

7. Dose ordered: zidovudine (Retrovir) 0.3 g PO
   Dose on hand: 100-mg tablets
   How many tablets will you give? __________

8. Dose ordered: potassium chloride liquid 30 mEq PO
   Dose on hand: 20 mEq/15 mL
   How many milliliters will you give? _________

9. Dose ordered: 0.15 g PO
   Dose on hand: 50-mg capsules
   How many capsules will you give? __________

10. Dose ordered: 2 g PO
    Dose on hand: 500-mg tablets
    How many tablets will you give? __________

SECTION III: RECONSTITUTING MEDICATIONS

Many medications come in powder or crystal form and must be reconstituted by the addition of a diluent to create a liquid form. Many parenteral medications must be reconstituted before administration. Instructions for dissolving medications can be found in the literature that accompanies the medication or on the medication label. Most of the time, medications that need to be reconstituted are in delivery systems that match 50- or 100-mL IV bags, and reconstitution occurs as the nurse prepares the medication for use. However, there are still instances where you may be required to reconstitute a drug and then draw up the proper dose for parenteral use. These are examples of those instances.

For example, the instructions may read:

Add 1.2 mL normal saline to make 2 mL of reconstituted solution that yields 100 mg/mL.

This tells the user that the medication takes up 0.8 mL of space: 1.2 mL + 0.8 mL = 2 mL of medication solution. The label of the medication container will tell the user how many units, grams, milligrams, or micrograms are in each milliliter of the reconstituted drug. In this example, the dose on hand, after reconstitution, is 100 mg/mL.

Remember these rules:

- Read all instructions for reconstitution before doing anything! Be sure to ask a pharmacist if you have any questions.
- When reconstituting medications, be certain to use the exact type of diluent indicated, and add the exact amount of diluent as directed. Substitutions or inaccurate amounts of diluent can inactivate the medication or alter the concentration, thus altering the dose received by the patient.
- If the container is a multiple-dose vial, the nurse who reconstitutes the medication must put the date, time, amount of diluent used, and his or her initials on the label. Follow the facility's policy for multiple-dose vials.
- Many solutions are unstable after being reconstituted. Be sure to follow the directions on the label for proper storage of reconstituted medications. Follow the facility's policy for labeling the reconstituted solution.
- Make note of the time limit or expiration date for the reconstituted medication. Do not use the medication after it has expired.
- Ratio solutions indicate the number of grams of the medication per total milliliters of solution. For example, a medication that is designated 1:1000 has 1 g of medication per 1000 mL of solution.

In order to avoid overdosing, it is essential that the nurse choose the correct ratio solution!

- Percentage (%) solutions indicate the number of grams of the medication per 100 mL of solution. For example, a medication that is designated 10% has 10 g of drug per 100 mL of solution.
- COMPARE: "1:1000" indicates 1 g per 1000 mL
"10%" indicates 10 g per 100 mL

As you calculate parenteral dosages:

- If the amount is greater than 1 mL, round x (the amount to be given) to tenths and use a 3-mL syringe to measure it.
- Small (less than 0.5 mL, or pediatric) dosages should be rounded to hundredths and measured in a tuberculin syringe. The tuberculin syringe is calibrated in 0.01-mL increments.
- THINK! For adults, the maximum volume of an IM injection is usually 3 mL. Sometimes the dose might have to be given in two divided doses; for example, a dose of 4 mL IM would usually be divided into two 2-mL doses. However, if your calculations yield an unusual number, such as 10 mL IM, look over your calculation and repeat your math! Double-check your calculations with a peer.

Always remember to note the route ordered. IM doses and IV doses are NOT always the same amount and the drug formulations may differ. Confusing the route may have fatal results.

Example 1: You receive an order for morphine 10 mg IM. The medication vial reads: 8 mg/mL. How much morphine would you give?
Does this medication require reconstitution?
Would you use a 3-mL or a tuberculin syringe to measure this drug?

Ordered: 10 mg **Unit dose:** 8 mg/mL

Know ***Want to Know***
8 mg : 1 mL :: 10 mg : x mL

$(8 \times x) = (1 \times 10)$; $8x = 10$; $x = 10/8 = 1.25$, rounded to 1.3
Answer: 1.3 mL measured in a 3-mL syringe. This medication does not require reconstitution.
Proof: $8 \times 1.3 = 10.4$ (rounds to 10); $1 \times 10 = 10$

Example 2: The ordered dose is 500 mg IV. The medication label reads:

500 mg MEDICATION FOR INJECTION For IM or IV use Add 2.7 mL sterile water for injection. Each 1.5 mL contains 250 mg medication.

How much medication would you give?
Does this medication require reconstitution?
Would you use a 3-mL or a tuberculin syringe to measure this drug?

Ordered: 500 mg **Unit dose:** 250 mg/1.5 mL

Know ***Want to Know***
250 mg : 1.5 mL :: 500 mg : x mL

$(250 \times x) = (1.5 \times 500)$; $250x = 750$; $x = 750/250 = 3$
Answer: 3 mL measured in a 3-mL syringe. Reconstitute by adding 2.7 mL sterile water to the vial.
Proof: $250 \times 3 = 750$; $1.5 \times 500 = 750$; $750 = 750$

Example 3: You receive an order for penicillin G potassium 400,000 units IM. The medication label reads:

ONE MILLION UNITS
Penicillin G Potassium
Use sterile saline as diluent as follows:

Add	Units per mL reconstituted solution
18.2 mL	250,000
8.2 mL	500,000
3.2 mL	1,000,000

Which dilution would you choose for the ordered dose?
How much penicillin G potassium would you give?
Would you use a 3-mL or a tuberculin syringe to measure this drug?

Ordered: 400,000 units **Unit dose:** Choosing the 8.2 mL diluent amount, unit dose is 500,000/mL.

Know ***Want to Know***
500,000 units : 1 mL :: 400,000 : x mL

$(500{,}000 \times x) = (1 \times 400{,}000)$; $500{,}000x = 400{,}000$; $x = 400{,}000/500{,}000 = 0.8$
Answer: 0.8 mL measured in either a 3-mL or tuberculin syringe.
Proof: $500{,}000 \times 0.8 = 400{,}000$; $1 \times 400{,}000 = 400{,}000$; $400{,}000 = 400{,}000$

NOTE: Choose the concentration that is close to the ordered dose. Choosing the 8.2 diluent amount allows for the injection amount to be small yet easily measured. If you had chosen the 18.2 diluent amount, the injection would have been 1.6 mL; choosing the 3.2 diluent would have made the injection amount very small: 0.04 mL.

Example 4: You receive an order for epinephrine 0.6 mg subcut. The medication label reads:

1 mL ampule Epinephrine 1:1000 For subcut or IM use

What is the dose on hand?
How much epinephrine would you give?
Would you use a 3-mL or a tuberculin syringe to measure the drug?
First: Figure the dose on hand.
1:1000 = 1 g in 1000 mL = 1000 mg in 1000 mL = 1 mg in 1 mL
Then complete the problem:

Ordered: 0.6 mg **Unit dose:** 1 mg/mL

Know ***Want to Know***
1 mg : 1 mL :: 0.6 mg : x mL

$(1 \times x) = (1 \times 0.6)$; $1x = 0.6$; $x = 0.6$
Answer: 0.6 mL measured in either a 3-mL or tuberculin syringe.
Proof: $1 \times 0.6 = 0.6$; $1 \times 0.6 = 0.6$; $0.6 = 0.6$

Example 5: Magnesium sulfate 5 g IV over 3 hours is the dosage ordered. The medication label reads:

10 mL vial Magnesium sulfate 10% For IM or IV use

What is the dose on hand?
How much magnesium sulfate would you give?
First: Figure the dose on hand.
10% = 10 g in 100 mL = 0.1 g per 1 mL
Then complete the problem:

Ordered: 5 g **Unit dose:** 0.1 g/mL

Know ***Want to Know***
0.1 g : 1 mL :: 5 g : x mL

$(0.1 \times x) = (1 \times 5)$; $0.1x = 5$; $x = 5/0.1$; $x = 50$
Answer: 50 mL
Proof: $0.1 \times 50 = 5$; $1 \times 5 = 5$; $5 = 5$

PRACTICE PROBLEMS

1. Dose ordered: thiamine 200 mg IV
   On hand: 10-mL vial, 100 mg/mL
   How much will you give? __________

2. Dose ordered: gentamicin (Garamycin) 60 mg IM
   On hand: 40 mg/mL
   How much will you give? __________

3. Dose ordered: heparin 8000 units subcut
   On hand: 1-mL vial, 10,000 units/mL
   How much will you give? __________

4. Dose ordered: Medication 750 mg IV
   On hand: 1-g vial
   Instructions for reconstitution: Add 1.5 mL sterile water. Reconstituted solution will contain approximately 500 mg medication solution per mL.
   How much will you give? __________

5. Dose ordered: ampicillin 500 mg IV
   On hand: 1-g vial powder for injection
   Instructions for reconstitution: Add 66 mL sterile water. Reconstituted solution will contain 125 mg/5 mL.
   How much will you give? __________

6. Dose ordered: penicillin G potassium 300,000 units IM
   On hand: 1,000,000-units vial
   Instructions for reconstitution: Using only sterile water, add 9.6 mL to provide 100,000 units/mL, or 4.6 mL to provide 200,000 units/mL.
   Which concentration would you choose for this dose? __________
   How much will you give? __________

7. Dose ordered: epinephrine 750 mcg subcut
   On hand: 1:1000
   How much will you give? __________

8. Dose ordered: Medication 0.2 mg
   On hand: 1:5000
   How much will you give? __________

9. Dose ordered: calcium gluconate 900 mg
   On hand: calcium gluconate 10%, 100-mL vial
   How much will you give? __________

10. Dose ordered: magnesium sulfate 4 g
    On hand: magnesium sulfate 50%, 10-mL vial
    How much will you give? __________

SECTION IV: PEDIATRIC CALCULATIONS

Doses used in pediatric patients must differ from those used in adults. The most common method for calculating doses for pediatric patients is weight-based (i.e., mg/kg). In some cases, dosages may be calculated using body surface area (BSA) calculations.

Body Surface Area Calculations

The BSA is a common method used to calculate therapeutic pediatric dosages. It requires the use of a chart called a *West nomogram* (see Figure 3-1 in your text) that converts weight to square meters (m^2) of BSA. The average adult is assumed to weigh 140 lb and have a BSA of 1.73 m^2. The BSA may be used to calculate the pediatric dose of certain medications.

- For a child of normal height and weight, find the m^2 for that weight on the shaded area of the nomogram chart.
  Example: Using Figure 3-1 in your text, find the BSA for a child who weighs 40 lb and is 38 inches tall (normal height for her weight). According to the nomogram, the BSA for 40 lb is 0.74 m^2.
- For a child who is underweight or overweight, the BSA is indicated at the point where a straight line connecting the height and weight intersects the unshaded surface area (SA) column.
  Example: Using Figure 3-1, find the BSA for a child who weighs 25 lb and has a height of 30 inches (underweight). According to the nomogram, the BSA for this child is 0.51 m^2.

There are two types of BSA problems.

1. The first type involves medications for which the literature provides recommended dosages in m^2.

STEP 1: Check the order, and look up the recommended dose.
The order is for 15 mg PO.
The literature states that 40 mg/m^2 is safe for children.

STEP 2: Determine child's height and weight. Then consult the appropriate nomogram to obtain the BSA in m^2. This child weighs 22 lb and has a normal height of 70 cm. The BSA is approximately 0.46 m^2.

STEP 3: Calculate the recommended mg/m^2 dose (from the literature) using ratio and proportion. Then, for a safety check, compare it with the dose ordered.

For this calculation, what you know is the literature's recommendation (40 mg/m^2). What you want to know is the milligrams per the child's BSA (which is 0.46 m^2).

Know ***Want to Know***
40 mg : 1 m^2 :: x mg : 0.46 m^2

$(40 \times 0.46) = (1 \times x)$; $18.4 = 1x$; $x = 18.4$ (Pediatric doses are rounded to tenths place; do not round to whole numbers.)
Answer: 18.4 mg is the safe dose limit.
Decision: The order for 15 mg is safe.

Practice:
The medication ordered is 100 mg.

STEP 1: The literature recommends 50 mg/m^2 for children.

STEP 2: The child weighs 10 lb and has a normal height for his weight. The BSA is 0.27 m^2.

STEP 3: Calculate the dose for this child's BSA:

Know ***Want to Know***
50 mg : 1 m^2 :: x mg : 0.27 m^2

$(50 \times 0.27) = (1 \times x)$; $13.5 = 1x$; $x = 13.5$ (Pediatric doses are rounded to tenths place; do not round to whole numbers.)
Answer: 13.5 mg is the safe dose limit.
Decision: The order for 15 mg exceeds the safe dose limit and therefore is NOT safe. Notify the physician.

2. The second type of BSA involves situations when a recommended dose is cited in the literature for adults but not for children.

STEP 1: Determine the BSA (m^2) of the child by dividing the adult dose by 1.73 m^2 (the average adult's BSA).

STEP 2: Multiply the result by the average adult dose.

$$\frac{\text{Child's BSA } (m^2)}{\text{Average adult's BSA}} \times \text{Average adult dose of drug} = \text{Estimated child's dose}$$

Example: A 6-lb child has a BSA of 0.20 m^2, and the average adult dose of a drug is 300 mg. What would be the estimated safe dose for a child?

$$\frac{0.20 \text{ m}^2}{1.73 \text{ m}^2} \times 300 \text{ mg} = 34.68 \text{ mg}$$

Answer: 34.7 mg is the estimated safe dose for this child. (Round to tenths place for pediatric doses.)

Practice:
The average adult dose for a medication is 20 mg. The child has a BSA of 0.6 m^2. What would be the estimated safe dose for a child?

$$\frac{0.60 \text{ m}^2}{1.73 \text{ m}^2} \times 20 \text{ mg} = 6.94 \text{ mg}$$

Answer: 6.9 mg is the estimated safe dose for this child. (Round to tenths place for pediatric doses.)

Weight-Based Calculations

When calculating the proper dose according to weight, STEP 1 involves changing the weight from pounds to kilograms (if necessary).

- Be careful when converting ounces and pounds to kilograms. First, ounces must be converted to part of a pound (by dividing the ounces by 16). Remember, 16 ounces = 1 pound. Therefore 8 oz does not convert to 0.8 lb! Convert 8 ounces to pounds by dividing by 16: 8/16 = 0.5; 8 oz = 0.5 lb.
- Once you have converted ounces to pounds, then add the ounces to the pounds. For example, 10 lb 8 oz would equal 10.5 lb. You are now ready to convert pounds to kilograms.
- Remember: 1 kg = 2.2 lb. To convert 10.5 lb to kilograms, divide the pounds by 2.2.
- 1 kg : 2.2 lb :: x kg : 10.5 lb; (1 × 10.5) = (2.2 × x); 10.5 = 2.2x; x = 10.5/2.2 = 4.8 kg (rounded to tenths)
- DO NOT round pediatric weights to whole numbers!

Once you have converted the child's weight to kg, you are ready for STEP 2.

STEP 2 involves calculating the therapeutic dosage ranges for a child based on his or her weight. The nurse uses the child's weight (in kilograms) to calculate the low and high acceptable doses for that medication. This will give a range of dosage that this child could receive for this medication.

STEP 3 involves THINKING and comparing the ordered dose with the therapeutic dosage range that was calculated for that child. If the ordered dose is under or over the calculated therapeutic dosage range, then do not give the medication and notify the physician.

- **STEP 1:** Convert the child's weight from pounds to kilograms.
- **STEP 2:** Calculate therapeutic dose range (low and high).
- **STEP 3:** (1) Is the ordered dose safe (does not exceed the dosage range)?
  (2) Is the ordered dose therapeutic (falling within the recommended dosage range, not too low)?

Example 1: The ordered dose is 50 mg acetaminophen (Tylenol). The infant weighs 15 lb. The therapeutic dosage range for acetaminophen is 10 to 15 mg/kg/dose.

STEP 1: Convert pounds to kilograms by dividing 15 by 2.2.
15/2.2 = 6.82; 15 lb = 6.8 kg (Round pediatric weights to tenths, not to whole numbers.)

STEP 2: Calculate the therapeutic dosage range for this infant based on his weight.
Low dose: 10 mg/kg/dose × 6.8 kg = 68 mg/dose (note that the "kg" cancel out).
High dose: 15 mg/kg/dose × 6.8 kg = 102 mg/dose (note that the "kg" cancel out).
The therapeutic dosage range for this infant is 68 to 102 mg/dose for acetaminophen.

STEP 3: Compare the ordered dose with the therapeutic dosage range calculated in STEP 2.
Answer: The ordered dose of 50 mg is not therapeutic because it falls under the low recommended dose.

If the doctor orders 110 mg of acetaminophen for this infant, would that be a safe and therapeutic dose?
Answer: No, it would neither be safe nor therapeutic because it is higher than 102 mg.

Example 2: The ordered dose is amoxicillin (Amoxil) 275 mg q8hr PO. The patient weighs 35 lb. The therapeutic dosage range for amoxicillin is 20 to 40 mg/kg/24 hr in divided doses.

STEP 1: Convert pounds to kilograms by dividing 35 by 2.2.
35/2.2 = 15.9; 35 lb = 15.9 kg

STEP 2: Calculate the therapeutic dosage range for this child based on his weight.
Low dose: 20 mg/kg/24 hr × 15.9 kg = 318 mg/24 hr
High dose: 40 mg/kg/24 hr × 15.9 kg = 636 mg/24 hr
NOTE: These ranges are for 24 hours! The dosage is every 8 hours, so dividing 24 hours by 8 tells us that there will be 3 doses within 24 hours. To figure out the single dosage for the low and high ranges, divide each 24-hour dose by 3:
318 mg/24 hr divided by 3 doses = 106 mg/dose
636 mg/24 hr divided by 3 doses = 212 mg/dose
Answer: The safe range for a single dose of amoxicillin for this child is 106 to 212 mg/dose. (An alternate way to figure a single dose is to calculate the amount of medication the ordered dose would provide in 24 hours. In this example,

knowing there are three doses given every 8 hours in a 24-hour period, multiplying the dose ordered by 3 would yield the ordered dose for 24 hours: 275 mg × 3 doses = 825 mg/24 hr.)

STEP 3: Is the ordered dose of 275 mg therapeutic for this child?
Answer: No, the ordered dose of 275 mg exceeds the therapeutic dosage range for this patient. Consult the physician. (Note also that the calculated 24-hour dose of 825 mg/24 hr exceeds the high range of 636 mg/24 hr calculated for this child.)

Many pediatric medications come in several concentrations. It is ESSENTIAL to use the correct concentration of medication to ensure accurate dosage and prevent accidental underdosage or overdosage.

Example: Acetaminophen comes in many forms, including:
drops, 80 mg/0.8 mL
elixir, 160 mg/5 mL
liquid suspension, 160 mg/5 mL
chewable tablet, 80 mg/tablet
tablet, 325 or 500 mg/tablet
suppository, 80, 120, 325, or 650 mg

A 4-month-old infant weighs 13 lb and has a fever of 101.5° F (38.6° C). What would be the therapeutic dosage range of acetaminophen this infant could receive? The recommended range is 10 to 15 mg/kg/dose.

STEP 1: 13 lb = 5.9 kg

STEP 2: Low dose: 10 mg/kg/dose × 5.9 = 59 mg/dose
High dose: 15 mg/kg/dose × 5.9 = 88.5 mg/dose
Answer: The therapeutic dosage range for this infant is 59 to 88.5 mg/dose.
Referring to the forms of acetaminophen listed above, which form would you choose if this infant was to receive a 60-mg dose?
Answer: Choose the drops, 80 mg/0.8 mL, and administer 0.6 mL with a calibrated oral syringe or dropper. (80 mg : 0.8 mL :: 60 mg : x; x = 0.6 mL)

STEP 3: Is the ordered dose of 60 mg therapeutic for this infant?
Answer: Yes, the 60-mg dose falls within the 59 to 88.5 mg/dose range for this infant.

Why choose the drops? Remember, you are giving medication to an infant. The infant cannot take tablets; suppositories are not the first choice unless the infant cannot take oral medications, and rectal doses may be a little higher than oral doses. You should choose the medication form that is manufactured for infants and the form that will deliver the dose in an amount that is easily measured yet not too much for the infant to swallow. For example, if you chose the elixir or liquid suspension, 160 mg/5 mL, then you would need to give 2.5 mL. The 0.6 mL would be easier to administer to an infant. NOTE: Most liquid medication packages for infants and children have specific instructions for dosing and include the specific dropper to use for measuring liquids.

PRACTICE PROBLEMS

1. Your 6-year-old patient weighs 40 lb. Morphine sulfate via continuous infusion is ordered at 1 mg/hr. The therapeutic dosage range for continuous intravenous infusion is 0.025 to 2.6 mg/kg/hr.
   a. What are the low and high doses for this child? __________
   b. Is the ordered dose within a safe and therapeutic range? __________
2. A 5-year-old child weighs 33 lb. Ibuprofen is ordered at 120 mg PO q8hr. The therapeutic dosage range is 5 to 10 mg/kg/dose q6hr to q8hr, and the maximum dose is 40 mg/kg/24 hr.
   a. What are the low and high doses for this child? __________
   b. What is the maximum amount this child can receive in 24 hours? __________
   c. Is the ordered dose within a safe and therapeutic range? __________

3. A 10-year-old patient weighs 70 lb. Fortaz is ordered at 1.7 g q8hr IV. The therapeutic dosage range is 100 to 150 mg/kg/24 hr (divided q8hr IV).
   a. What are the low and high doses for this child in 24 hours? __________
   b. What are the low and high doses for this child per individual dose? __________
   c. Is the ordered dose within a safe and therapeutic range? __________

4. Your patient weighs 15 lb. The medication ordered is 150 mcg bid. The therapeutic dosage range of the medication is 0.02 to 0.05 mg/kg/day.
   a. What are the low and high doses for this child in 24 hours? __________
   b. What are the low and high doses for this child per individual dose? __________
   c. Is the ordered dose within a safe and therapeutic range? __________

5. A child weighs 34 lb. The medication ordered is 30 mg IM preoperatively. The therapeutic dosage range is 1 to 2.2 mg/kg.
   a. What are the low and high doses for this child per individual dose? __________
   b. Is the ordered dose within a safe and therapeutic range? __________

6. For a child weighing 50 lb, medication is ordered at 0.2 mg daily IV. The therapeutic dosage range is 4 to 5 mcg/kg/day.
   a. What are the low and high doses for this child per individual dose? __________
   b. Is the ordered dose within a safe and therapeutic range? __________

SECTION V: BASIC INTRAVENOUS CALCULATIONS

Intravenous (IV) fluids and medications are given over a designated period of time. For instance, the order may read:

Give 1000 mL normal saline over 8 hours IV.

For IVs that infuse with an infusion pump, the milliliters per hour is calculated (mL/hr).

For IVs that infuse by gravity, the rate at which an IV is given is measured in terms of drops per minute (gtt/min).

To calculate mL/hr and gtt/min, we need to consider what the order contains and what equipment is used. In order to calculate drops per minute we need to know the drop factor of the IV tubing. The size of the drops delivered per milliliter can vary with different types of tubing. The drop factor of a certain tubing set is printed on the packaging label.

Adding to the above order:

The drop factor for the IV tubing is 15 gtt/mL.

The order now reads:

Give 1000 mL normal saline over 8 hours IV. The drop factor is 15 gtt/mL.

STEP 1: Calculate milliliters per hour.
We know that 1000 mL is to infuse over 8 hours. We want to know how much is to infuse over 1 hour. Set up the equation:

Know ***Want to Know***
1000 mL : 8 hr :: x mL : 1 hr

$(1000 \times 1) = (8 \times x)$; $1000 = 8x$; $x = 8/1000$; $x = 125$ mL/hr
Rate: To give 1000 mL normal saline over 8 hours, give 125 mL/hr for 8 hours.
A quick way to determine the hourly rate is to divide the TOTAL VOLUME by the TOTAL TIME (if the time is in hours): 1000 mL ÷ 8 hr = 125 mL/hr.

STEP 2: Calculate the gtt/min.
To set up a gravity IV drip, further calculations are needed. To ensure the proper rate, one must count the drops per minute (gtt/min).

We know the rate is 125 mL/hr and the drop factor is 15 gtt/mL. Since we need to change from hours to minutes, another equivalent we'll need is 60 min = 1 hr.

When mL/hr is known, the formula for calculating gtt/min is as follows:

$$\frac{\text{drop factor (gtt/mL)}}{\text{time (min)}} \times \text{hourly rate (mL/hr)}$$

Plugging in what we know:

$$\frac{15 \text{ gtt/mL*}}{60 \text{ min/hr}} \times 125\text{/hr} = x \text{ gtt/min}$$

*To make it easier to calculate, reduce the 15/60 fraction to 1/4 before multiplying by 125.
1/4 × 125 = 125/4 = 31.25 (round mL/hr to whole numbers)
Answer: 31 gtt/min for a gravity drip

Points to remember:

- The drop factor varies per IV tubing set manufacturer. It can range from 10 to 60 gtt/mL.
- Infusion sets that deliver 60 gtt/mL are called *microdrips*.
- **STEP 1:** To calculate mL/hr, divide the TOTAL VOLUME by the TOTAL TIME (in hours).
- **STEP 2:** To calculate gtt/min when the hourly rate is known, use the formula:

  $$\frac{\text{drop factor (gtt/mL)}}{\text{time (min)}} \times \text{hourly rate (mL/hr)}$$

- THINK! If you are using an infusion pump, you need to calculate milliliters per hour.
- THINK! Round off your answer to the nearest whole number. You cannot count a partial drop! Also, electronic infusion pumps will usually use the nearest whole number in mL. (Exceptions to this may occur in critical care or pediatric settings.)

Example 1: The order reads "200 mL to be infused for 1 hr." If the drop factor is 15 gtt/mL, how many gtt/min will be given?
Start at STEP 1 or STEP 2?
Start at STEP 1. You need to know the hourly rate in mL/hr.

STEP 1: Calculate mL/hr. Divide total volume by the total time (in hours).
200 mL over 1 hr = 200 mL/hr.

STEP 2: Calculate gtt/min using the formula:

$$\frac{\text{drop factor}}{\text{time (min)}} \times \text{hourly rate} = 15/60 \times 200 = 1/4 \times 200 = 50$$

Answer: 50 gtt/min

Example 2: The order is for 1000 mL to infuse at 150 mL/hr. The drop factor is 20 gtt/mL. How many gtt/min will be given?
Start at STEP 1 or STEP 2?
Start at STEP 2. The hourly rate, 150 mL/hr, has been given.

STEP 2: Calculate gtt/min using the formula:

$$\frac{\text{drop factor}}{\text{time (min)}} \times \text{hourly rate} = 20/60 \times 150 = 1/3 \times 150 = 50$$

Answer: 50 gtt/min

Example 3: You receive an order for 200 mL to be infused for 90 minutes. You have a microdrip set (60 gtt/mL). How many gtt/min will be given?
Start at STEP 1 or STEP 2?
Start at STEP 1. Calculate the hourly rate. Remember, 60 min = 1 hr.

STEP 1:

Know ***Want to Know***
200 mL : 90 min :: x mL : 60 min

$(200 \times 60) = (90 \times x)$; $12{,}000 = 90x$; $x = 12{,}000/90$ $x = 133.33$
Rate: 133 mL/hr (Round to nearest whole number.)

STEP 2: Calculate gtt/min using the formula:

$$\frac{\text{drop factor}}{\text{time (min)}} \times \text{hourly rate} = 60/60 \times 133 = 133$$

Answer: 133 gtt/min
Shortcut: For microdrips, when the drip factor is 60 and the time is 60 minutes, the "60s" cancel out to "1" and the result is that the ordered mL/hr = the gtt/min.

PRACTICE PROBLEMS

Calculate the following, and prove your answers.

1. Give 1000 mL lactated Ringer's solution over 6 hours. The drop factor is 15 gtt/mL.
   Start at STEP 1 or STEP 2?
   a. mL/hr: ____________
   b. gtt/min: ____________

2. Infuse 600 mL blood over 3 hours. The blood administration set has a drop factor of 10 gtt/mL.
   Start at STEP 1 or STEP 2?
   a. mL/hr: ____________
   b. gtt/min: ____________

3. Infuse 1000 mL normal saline over 12 hours, using tubing with a drop factor of 15 gtt/mL.
   Start at STEP 1 or STEP 2?
   a. mL/hr: ____________
   b. gtt/min: ____________

4. Infuse 200 mL D_5NS over 2 hours using a microdrip set.
   Start at STEP 1 or STEP 2?
   a. mL/hr: ____________
   b. gtt/min: ____________
   c. What is the drop factor? ____________

5. Infuse D_5W at 75 mL/hr. The drop factor is 10 gtt/mL.
   Start at STEP 1 or STEP 2?
   gtt/min: ____________

6. Infuse D_5W at 75 mL/hr. The drop factor is 15 gtt/mL.
   Start at STEP 1 or STEP 2?
   gtt/min: ____________

7. Infuse D_5W at 75 mL/hr. The drop factor is 20 gtt/mL.
   Start at STEP 1 or STEP 2?
   gtt/min: ____________

8. After looking at your answers for questions 5, 6, and 7, what observation can you make about the relationship between the drop factor and the resulting gtt/min?

9. Give 50 mL of an antibiotic over 30 minutes. You will be using an infusion pump.
   Start at STEP 1 or STEP 2?
   a. mL/hr: ____________
   b. gtt/min: ____________
   c. Do you need to calculate both mL/hr and gtt/min for this situation? ____________

10. Infuse 500 mL normal saline over 4 hours, using tubing with a drop factor of 60 gtt/mL.
    Start at STEP 1 or STEP 2?
    a. mL/hr: ____________
    b. gtt/min: ____________

PRACTICE QUIZ

Convert the following.

1. 750 mcg = _________ mg
2. 8 g = _________ mg
3. 250 lb = _________ kg
4. 75 kg = _________ lb
5. 3 tsp = _________ mL
6. gr x = _________ mg

Calculate the following, and prove your answers.

7. Dose ordered: indomethacin (Indocin) (oral suspension) 50 mg qid
   Dose on hand: Oral suspension 25 mg/5 mL
   How much would you give per dose? ________

8. Dose ordered: procainamide (Pronestyl) 0.5 g q4hr PO
   Dose on hand: 500-mg tablets
   How much would you give per dose? _________

9. Dose ordered: phenytoin (Dilantin) 100 mg IV now
   Dose on hand: 5-mL ampule labeled "50 mg/mL"
   How much would you give per dose? ________

10. Dose ordered: lidocaine (Xylocaine) 50 mg IV now
    Dose on hand: lidocaine 1% in 5-mL ampule
    How much would you give? ____________

11. Dose ordered: epinephrine 0.25 mg subcut now
    Dose on hand: epinephrine 1:1000 ampule
    How much would you give? ____________

12. Dose ordered: heparin 15,000 units IV bolus
    Dose on hand: heparin 10,000 units/mL (5-mL vial)
    How much would you give? ____________

13. Dose ordered: polythiazide (Renese) 1 mg PO daily
    Dose on hand: polythiazide 1-mg tablet
    Child's weight: 22 lb
    Therapeutic dosage range: 0.02 to 0.08 mg/kg once daily
    a. What is the safe and therapeutic range for this child? ____________
    b. Is the ordered dose safe and therapeutic? ____________

14. Ordered: Infuse normal saline 500 mL over 8 hours. The tubing drop factor is 15.
    a. What is the rate of the IV? ____________
    b. What is the gtt/min? ____________

15. Ordered: $D_5$1/2NS to infuse at 50 mL/hr via an infusion pump.
    a. How will this be administered—mL/hr or gtt/min? ____________
    b. What is the rate? ____________

16. Ordered: 1000 mL D_5W to infuse over 24 hours. The tubing drop factor is 60.
    a. What is the rate of the IV? ____________
    b. What is the gtt/min? ____________

17. Ordered: Medication 500 mg IV piggyback q6hr.
    Dose on hand: Medication powder for injection (See label.)

    1-g vial
    MEDICATION
    Add 5 mL sterile water for injection.
    Solution will contain 200 mg/mL.

    a. How much does this vial contain? ____________
    b. How much will you give for each dose? ____________

18. Ordered: penicillin G 200,000 units IM qid
    Dose on hand: penicillin G 5,000,000 units
    The medication label reads:

FIVE MILLION UNITS multidose vial
Penicillin G
Use sterile saline as diluent as follows:

Add	Units per mL reconstituted solution
23 mL	200,000
18 mL	250,000
8 mL	500,000
3 mL	1,000,000

   a. What concentration should you choose? ____________
   b. How much sterile saline should you add to the vial to obtain this concentration? ____________
   c. How much medication will you give? ____________
   d. How do you label the vial? ____________

19. A child weighs 31 lb
    Dose ordered: ceftriaxone sodium 600 mg IV q12hr
    Dose on hand: See label.
    Maximum safe dose: Up to 100 mg/kg/day in two divided doses

1 g ceftriaxone sodium DIRECTIONS: Add 9.6 mL sterile water for injection to equal 100 mg/mL.

    a. How much would you give for this dose? ____________
    b. What is the maximum safe dose for this child (in 24 hours)? ____________
    c. What is the maximum safe dose for this child (per dose)? ____________
    d. Is the ordered dose within a safe and therapeutic range? ____________

20. Dose ordered: digoxin (Lanoxin) 125 mcg daily
    Dose on hand: Pediatric elixir 0.05 mg/mL
    How much would you give? ____________

Answers

CHAPTER 1
The Nursing Process and Drug Therapy

Chapter Review and NCLEX® Examination Preparation/Critical Thinking and Application

1. a
2. d
3. c
4. b
5. a
6. b
7. 0.25 mg (See Overview of Dosage Calculations, Section I.)
8. 1 = d; 2 = e; 3 = b; 4 = a; 5 = c
9. S, O, O, O, S, S
10. Answers may vary slightly with each one but should include the following:
    - *Right drug*: Compare drug orders and medication labels. Consider whether the drug is appropriate for that patient. Obtain information about the patient's medical history and a thorough, updated medication history, including over-the-counter medications taken.
    - *Right dose*: Check the order and the label on the medication, and check the "rights" at least three times before administering the medication. Recheck the math calculations for dosages and contact the physician when clarification is needed. Check the dose and confirm that it is appropriate for the patient's age and size, and also check the prescribed dose against the available drug stocks and against the normal dosage range.
    - *Right time*: Assess for a conflict between the pharmacokinetic and pharmacodynamic properties of the drugs prescribed and the patient's lifestyle and likelihood of compliance.
    - *Right route*: Never assume the route of administration or change it; always check with the physician or prescriber.
    - *Right patient*: Check the patient's identity before administering a medication. Ask for the patient's name, and check the identification band or bracelet to confirm the patient's name, identification number, and allergies. The Joint Commission requires the use of two patient identifiers, such as name and birthday, Social Security Number, or medical record number.
    - *Right documentation*: Record the date and time of medication administration, name of medication, dose, route, and site of administration. Don't forget to document the patient's response to the medication.
11. a. assessment
    b. objective
    c. subjective
    d. analyze
    e. goals
    f. outcome criteria
    g. implementation
    h. evaluation

Case Study

1. See the discussion in Chapter 1 under Assessment. Important points include the following:
    - Use of prescription and over-the-counter medications
    - Use of home remedies, herbal treatments, vitamins
    - Intake of alcohol, tobacco, caffeine
    - Current or prior use of street drugs
    - Health history
    - Family history
    - Allergies
2. Answers will vary but may include the following:
    - Activity intolerance
    - Acute pain
    - Anxiety
    - Deficient knowledge
    - Fatigue
    - Ineffective breathing pattern
    - Ineffective health maintenance
    - Ineffective therapeutic regimen management
    - Noncompliance
    - Risk for aspiration
    - Risk for injury
    - Risk for falls

    Prioritization will depend on the nursing diagnoses chosen but should be developed with the patient's input.

3. The medication order is missing the route of delivery and the dose amount. You should contact the physician to clarify the incomplete order.
4. Once again, you should contact the physician and never change the medication route without an order.
5. After administering any drug, the nurse should evaluate the patient's response to the drug therapy. In this case, monitoring intake and output, monitoring vital signs, and watching for orthostatic blood pressure changes would be important.

CHAPTER 2 Pharmacologic Principles

Chapter Review and NCLEX® Examination Preparation/Critical Thinking and Application

1. 1 = c; 2 = d; 3 = a; 4 = b
2. c
3. b
4. d
5. a
6. c
7. 1600
8. b
9. h
10. i
11. e
12. f
13. a
14. d
15. c
16. Because muscles have a greater blood supply than the skin, drugs injected intramuscularly are typically absorbed faster than those injected subcutaneously. Absorption can be increased by applying heat to the injection site or by massaging the injection site, which increases the blood flow to the area and thus enhances absorption.
17. This is an example of palliative therapy—drug therapy that is not curative but is intended to make the patient as comfortable as possible.

Case Study

1. Half-life is the time it takes for one-half of the original amount of a drug in the body to be eliminated and is a measure of the rate at which drugs are excreted by the body. If the half-life is 2 hours, then in this example the drug levels would be as follows:
   4 PM = 200 mg/L
   6 PM = 100 mg/L
   8 PM = 50 mg/L
   10 PM = 25 mg/L
2. a. He has nausea and vomiting and cannot take medications by mouth. His medications will need to be given parenterally.
   b. Because of his decreased serum albumin level, lesser amount of drugs that are usually protein bound will be bound to protein, and as a result, more free drug will be circulating and the duration of drug action may be increased. In addition, his heart failure may result in decreased cardiac output and thus decreased distribution.
   c. His liver failure will result in decreased metabolism of drugs, which increases the chance for drug toxicities if the drugs accumulate.
   d. Because his liver may not be able to effectively metabolize drugs and convert them to water-soluble compounds, excretion through the kidneys may be decreased.
3. This situation illustrates prophylactic therapy to *prevent* illness or other undesirable outcome. Prophylactic intravenous antibiotic therapy may be used to prevent infection during a high-risk surgery or procedure, such as placement of the peripherally inserted central catheter.
4. Therapeutic index is the ratio between the toxic and therapeutic concentrations of a drug. A low therapeutic index means that the difference between a therapeutically active dose and a toxic dose is small. As a result, the drug has a greater likelihood of causing an adverse reaction. The nurse should monitor the patient's response carefully when a drug has a low therapeutic index.

CHAPTER 3 Life Span Considerations

Chapter Review and NCLEX® Examination Preparation/Critical Thinking and Application

1. c
2. a
3. d
4. b
5. b, c, d
6. 320 mg (See Overview of Dosage Calculations, Section IV.)
7. d
8. b
9. e
10. a
11. c
12. Keep in mind that older patients take a greater proportion of both prescription and over-the-counter (OTC) medications, and they commonly take multiple medications on a daily basis. In addition, older adults also have more chronic diseases than younger people. They may see several different specialists, each of whom may each prescribe a different set of medications. In addition, some patients self-administer OTC products to ease the discomfort of

even more ailments. This use of multiple mediations is called *polypharmacy.*

13. Drawing on the information in the box Life Span Considerations: The Elderly Patient—Pharmacokinetic Changes, a variety of physiologic changes affecting the cardiovascular, gastrointestinal, hepatic, and renal systems may be described.

Case Study

1. Children and teenagers should not take aspirin to treat chickenpox or flulike symptoms because Reye's syndrome—a rare but serious illness—has been associated with aspirin use at these ages. It is important to check for precautions when giving any medication to children.
2. If the toddler does not like or cannot take pills, have the parent ask the pharmacist for a liquid form of the medication, which may be flavored and better accepted by the child than a pill. Some pediatric medications also come in quick-dissolving oral tablets or films.
3. The most common dosage calculation method for children is the milligrams per kilogram formula. However, for OTC preparations, the manufacturer will convert kilograms to pounds to make dosing by the parents easier.
4. The 5-year-old child received 240 mg (at 160 mg/tsp, 1.5 tsp = 240 mg).
5. The parents should monitor the children's fever—the expected response is that the fever will go down. In addition, because the medication also has analgesic effects, signs of discomfort may decrease. The parents should also monitor for any adverse effects of the medication or worsening of the children's illness.

CHAPTER 4
Cultural, Legal, and Ethical Considerations

Chapter Review and NCLEX® Examination Preparation/Critical Thinking and Application

1. b
2. a
3. d
4. c
5. b
6. d
7. b, c
8. 6 mL
9. d
10. a
11. c
12. b
13. c
14. a
15. d
16. b
17. Answers will vary depending on the group identified.
    a. Barriers may include language, poverty, access, pride, and beliefs regarding medical practices.
    b. Attitudes will vary depending on the group identified.
    c. Questions may include the following topics: health beliefs and practices, past use of medicine, folk remedies, home remedies, use of over-the-counter drugs and treatments, usual responses to illness, responsiveness to medical treatments, religious practices and beliefs, and dietary habits.

Case Study

1. You should not give the drugs until it is established that the study has been reviewed by an institutional review board and that the patient has given informed consent. As a professional, the nurse has the responsibility to provide safe nursing care and it is within the nurse's realm of practice to provide information and assist the patient in facing decisions regarding health care. The nurse also has the right to refuse to participate in any treatment or aspect of a patient's care that violates personal ethical principles.
2. Principles include the following:
    - Autonomy—the patient's right to self-determination. The nurse supports this by ensuring informed consent.
    - Beneficence—the duty to do good. Will the patient be best served by this course of action?
    - Nonmaleficence—the duty to do no harm.
    - Veracity—the duty to tell the truth, especially with regard to investigational drugs and informed consent.
3. Some patients believe strongly in using home remedies instead of medications. You should assess and consider health beliefs and practices at the beginning of the therapeutic relationship.
4. The issue of confidentiality should be discussed. The researchers have a duty to respect privileged information about a patient. Measures that the researchers will use to ensure the confidentiality of participants should be discussed.

CHAPTER 5
Gene Therapy and Pharmacogenetics

Chapter Review and NCLEX® Examination Preparation/Critical Thinking and Application

1. g
2. f
3. b
4. c

5. d
6. DNA is deoxyribonucleic acid, located in the nucleus of all body cells as strands of chromosomes, collectively called *chromatin*. Protein synthesis is the primary function of DNA in the nuclei of human cells. DNA is the primary molecule in the body that serves to transfer genes from parents to offspring.
7. The goal of this scientific project was to map the entire DNA sequence (genome) of a human being. The research from this project led to an ultimate goal of developing improved prevention, treatment, and cures for disease.
8. The development of gene therapy and pharmacogenomics.
9. Recombinant DNA is DNA that has been artificially synthesized or modified in a laboratory setting. This technology is used to make recombinant forms of drugs such as hormones, vaccines, and antitoxins. An example of this technology is the alteration of the *Escherichia coli* genome so that these bacteria manufacture a recombinant form of human insulin.
10. The general goal of gene therapy is to transfer to the patient exogenous genes that will either provide a temporary substitute for, or initiate permanent changes in, the patient's own genetic functioning to treat a given disease. Although hundreds of gene therapy clinical trials have been approved by the U.S. Food and Drug Administration (FDA), no gene therapy to date has been approved for routine treatment of disease. Gene therapy techniques are being studied for the treatment of acquired illnesses such as cancer, heart disease, and diabetes.

Case Study

1. This information about Dale's cousin is significant! An unusual or other than expected reaction to a drug in family members may point to a difference in the patient's ability to metabolize certain drugs. Genetic factors may alter a patient's metabolism of a particular drug, resulting in either increased or decreased drug action.
2. The nurse will ask about the type of medication Dale's cousin received, the type of surgery, and obtain details about the reaction that occurred, as well as the treatment. The nurse will also ask if any other family members have had unusual reactions to drugs, and whether Dale himself has had any problems.
3. The family history should cover at least three generations and include the current and past health status of each family member.
4. The surgeon and anesthesiologist will work to adjust the planned drug therapy for Dale's surgery according to the genetic variation that has been identified. In addition, during surgery, the patient will be monitored closely for any unusual responses.

CHAPTER 6
Medication Errors: Preventing and Responding

Chapter Review and NCLEX® Examination Preparation/Critical Thinking and Application

1. medication error
2. idiosyncratic
3. allergic reaction
4. adverse drug reaction (ADR)
5. adverse drug event (ADE)
6. False. High-alert medications are not necessarily involved in more errors than other drugs. However, the potential for patient harm is higher with these medications.
7. False
8. To avoid medication errors: Follow the Six Rights! Carefully read all drug labels and confirm the Six Rights of medication administration. Repeat a verbal order and spell the drug name out loud. Never assume a route of administration; if an order is unclear or incomplete, clarify the order with the prescriber. Always read the label three times and check the medication order before administering the medication. See text for other possible answers.
9. Refer to Box 6-1: Examples of High Alert Medications
10. Digoxin 125 micrograms PO now
    Lasix 40 mg IV daily
    Discontinue all meds
    NPH insulin 12 units subcut every morning before breakfast
    Floxin otic 1 drop right ear bid
    Zolpidem 5 mg at bedtime if needed
11. a. One-half of a 50-mg tablet. (See Overview of Dosage Calculations Section II.)
    b. A 50-mg dose, which is a double dose.
    c. Because this medication can have an effect on the patient's blood pressure and heart rate, the nurse should immediately check and record the patient's vital signs and caution the patient about getting out of bed without help. The patient's physician should be notified, and the patient should be monitored frequently throughout the day. In addition to telling the patient about the double dose, the nurse will need to follow facility protocol for reporting a medication error, which would include completing a U.S. Pharmacopeia Medication Errors Reporting Program (USPMERP) for the national database.

Case Study

1. The nursing student should immediately inform her instructor of the error. Then together they should monitor the patient's response and follow the institution's procedure for reporting a medication error.

Reporting medication errors is a professional and ethical responsibility.

2. By checking the Six Rights before giving this medication. In this situation, she missed the right dose. In addition, if the student had understood the rationale for the medication (i.e., the low dose needed for antiplatelet therapy), then she may have avoided this error. One must be knowledgeable about medications and the rationale for their use in a particular patient before administering them.
3. According to Chapter 6, the recommendation is that the patient be told of the error both as ethical practice and because of the legal implications.
4. Yes. A medication error is defined as "any preventable adverse drug event involving inappropriate medication use by a patient or health care professional"; it may or may not cause harm to the patient.
5. The USPMERP exists to gather and disseminate safety information regarding medications. By reporting this error, the student contributes to the USPMERP database of medication errors and their causes. This service is confidential.

CHAPTER 7 Patient Education and Drug Therapy

Chapter Review and NCLEX® Examination Preparation/Critical Thinking and Application

1. b
2. d
3. Refer to the information in Chapter 25 for specific information about antihypertensive drug therapy. In addition, Table 7-1 provides information relevant to the development of teaching strategies for the 78-year-old patient.
4. Refer to Box 7-1. Ideally, a health care professional who speaks the mother's language should do the teaching. Some strategies include using pictures and illustrations, demonstrating by example, and finding an interpreter. In addition, the patient should be provided with detailed written instructions in her native language.
5. a. Answers will vary, but this nursing diagnosis should address deficient knowledge.
   b. Answers will vary, but this nursing diagnosis should address noncompliance or ineffective therapeutic regimen management.
6. Answers will vary, depending on the type of medication. Refer to the appropriate chapters for specific patient and family teaching and possible goals and expected outcomes.
7. Teaching plans will vary somewhat in format, but each should contain the following information:
   a. Some of the assessment items listed in the text in the section Assessment of Learning Needs Related to Drug Therapy.
   b. Deficient knowledge.
   c. A measurable goal with outcome criteria related to the nursing diagnosis.
   d. Specific educational strategies for providing the information needed.
   e. Specific questions designed to validate whether learning has occurred.
8. 10 mL per dose (See Overview of Dosage Calculations Section II.)

Case Study

1. Both "Deficient knowledge" and "Noncompliance" are possible answers. In this case, "Deficient knowledge" is probably the most correct, because this nursing diagnosis exists when the patient has a lack of or limited understanding about his or her medications. For example, nitroglycerin tablets should not be stored in one's pants pockets because the body heat may destroy the active compounds in the tablets. In addition, the patient was not aware of the importance of not missing doses of antihypertensive medication. Noncompliance exists when the patient does not take the medication as directed or at all, and the data collected indicate that the patient's condition has recurred or has not resolved. In this case, his blood pressure has improved from previous readings, despite what he has said about taking his medications.
2. Answers may vary. A goal for the nursing diagnosis of "Deficient knowledge" in this case may be the following: "The patient self-administers his prescribed medications on schedule without missing doses." Outcome criteria may include the following: "The patient is able to describe the schedule of medications ordered. The patient is able to state the rationale for consistent dosing of antihypertensive medications. The patient is able to state the proper storage and administration of sublingual nitroglycerin tablets. The patient is able to identify potential side effects of the prescribed medications and knows when to report them."
3. Again, answers may vary. Refer to Box 7-3. Suggestions include the following:
   - A teaching session regarding medication administration should be held with both the patient and his wife in attendance. If necessary, find out whether they have any children or neighbors nearby who may be able to assist with medications as needed.
   - Assist the patient in developing a daily time calendar for taking the medications prescribed.
   - Suggest the use of a daily or weekly pill container that can assist in reminding when doses are due. If necessary, a neighbor or the patient's son or daughter can come over periodically to fill this container.

- Discuss and provide written literature on the purposes and side effects of each medication ordered and on other important issues regarding these medications.

4. Confirm whether learning has occurred by asking the patient and his wife questions related to the teaching session. Assess their understanding of the time calendar and the concept of using pill containers. Follow-up can be accomplished via telephone as needed, and a return visit to review medications can be scheduled. In addition, the patient must keep return appointments to the office so that the therapeutic outcomes of the drug therapy (i.e., blood pressure readings) can be measured.

CHAPTER 8 Over-the-Counter Drugs and Herbal and Dietary Supplements

Critical Thinking Crossword Puzzle

Across

2. Ginger
5. Flax
7. Saw Palmetto
8. Kava

Down

1. Echinacea
2. Gingko
3. Ginseng
4. Aloe
6. Soy

Chapter Review and NCLEX® Examination Preparation/Critical Thinking and Application

1. a, b, d, f
2. d
3. d
4. b
5. c
6. 12,000 mg total per day.
7. YES, there is a concern! Acetaminophen doses should not exceed a total of 4 g per day, and hepatic toxicity may occur with excessive doses.
8. Garlic, ginger, ginkgo, ginseng, flax,and valerian
9. Older adults; children; patients with single and/or multiple acute and chronic illnesses; patients who are frail or in poor health; patients who are debilitated and nutritionally deficient; and those with suppressed immune systems. In addition, those who have a history of renal, hepatic, cardiac, or vascular disorders may have problems with over-the-counter (OTC) medications.
10. Answers will vary.

Case Study

1. The aspirin and garlic tablets may interfere with platelet and clotting functions. If the wine is taken with the kava and/or valerian, central nervous system depression may occur.
2. The Food and Drug Administration (FDA) has recently issued a warning about the use of kava and possible liver toxicity. Also, tolerance may develop in patients who use echinacea for longer than 8 weeks.
3. Because she is trying to conceive, she needs to consider the fact that the herbal drugs have not been tested or proved safe for use in pregnancy. Also, aspirin use is contraindicated in pregnancy because of its antiplatelet effects.
4. Herbal products are not required by the FDA to be proven safe or effective. They are classified as dietary supplements and are not subject to the same rules as are drugs. Therefore, the patient must receive adequate information about the herbal products, including their risks, side effects, and possible benefits.
5. Many patients believe that if a product is "natural" then it is safe. Each product should be discussed with the patient, and the patient should be instructed about possible contraindications, safe use, frequency of dosing, specifics about how to take the product, and the way to monitor for both therapeutic effects and complications or toxic effects.

CHAPTER 9 Substance Abuse

Chapter Review and NCLEX® Examination Preparation/Critical Thinking and Application

1. h
2. i
3. f
4. e
5. g
6. d
7. j
8. a
9. c
10. b
11. c
12. d
13. b, c, e
14. c
15. b
16. The nicotine transdermal system (patch) and nicotine polacrilex (gum) can be used to supply nicotine without the carcinogens in tobacco. The patches provide a stepwise reduction in delivery and work by gradually reducing the nicotine dose over time. With the gum, rapid chewing releases an immediate dose of nicotine, but this dose is about half of what the average smoker receives from one cigarette,

and the onset of action is longer than with smoking. Therefore, the reinforcement and self-reward effects of smoking are minimized. Zyban is a sustained-release form of the antidepressant bupropion and was the first nicotine-free prescription medicine used to treat nicotine dependence. Varenicline (Chantix) both activates and antagonizes the *alpha-4-beta-2* nicotinic receptors in the brain. This effect provides some stimulation to nicotine receptors, while also reducing the pleasurable effects of nicotine from smoking. This drug has demonstrated greater efficacy than bupropion.

17. Benzodiazepines are used for all three levels of ethanol withdrawal. Lower dosages are used for mild symptoms and higher dosages are needed for severe withdrawal. The oral route is preferred; however, it is often necessary to use the intravenous route for patients experiencing severe withdrawal. Patients who are experiencing severe withdrawal often require monitoring in an intensive care unit for cardiac and respiratory function, fluid and nutrition replacement, vital signs, and mental status. Restraints are indicated for a patient who is confused or agitated to protect the patient from self and to protect others (delirium tremens can be a terrifying and life-threatening state). Thiamine administration, hydration, and magnesium replacement may be indicated depending on the severity of the withdrawal state.
18. Dextromethorphan is an ingredient in several over-the-counter products, including Robitussin DM cough syrup and Mucinex DM tablets. Some adolescents have discovered that taking dextromethorphan in large amounts leads to a "high" that is accompanied by hallucinations. The hallucinations have been documented to be similar to those associated with the street drug phencyclidine (PCP). In addition, it has been found that teens who abuse dextromethorphan may also abuse other drugs such as lysergic acid diethylamide (LSD), PCP, Ecstasy, and inhalants. The hazardous short- or long-term effects that may occur with these drugs include nausea, hot flashes, reduced mental status, dizziness, seizures, loss of coordination and balance, brain damage, and death.

Case Study

1. Ethanol causes central nervous system depression.
2. Acute severe alcoholic intoxication may cause cardiovascular depression, and long-term excessive use has largely irreversible effects on the heart. Moderate amounts may either stimulate or depress respiration, but large amounts produce lethal respiratory depression.
3. First, the nurse should monitor the patient's respiratory and cardiovascular status and prevent injury from falling or aspiration from vomiting. In addition, the nurse should be alert to the patient's behavior and mental status to identify changes in his condition.

   Withdrawal from alcohol can lead to serious conditions such as delirium tremens (see question 4). Careful assessment of vital signs and mental status is imperative at this time, because early withdrawal symptoms may be an increase in blood pressure and pulse with an altered mental status.
4. Mr. C. should stay in the hospital for observation for and possible treatment of delirium tremens, which may begin with tremors and agitation and progress to hallucinations and sometimes death. See Box 9-6 for information on treatment of ethanol withdrawal.
5. Chronic excessive ingestion of ethanol is directly associated with several serious mental and neurologic disorders. Nutritional and vitamin B deficiencies can occur, which result in conditions such as Wernicke's encephalopathy, Korsakoff's psychosis, polyneuritis, and nicotinic acid deficiency encephalopathy. Seizures may also occur. In addition, long-term ingestion of ethanol may result in alcoholic hepatitis or liver cirrhosis.

CHAPTER 10
Photo Atlas of Drug Administration

Chapter Review and NCLEX® Examination Preparation/Critical Thinking and Application

1. c
2. a
3. b
4. c
5. c
6. b
7. a
8. c
9. a
10. b
11. d
12. b
13. a
14. a, b, d, e
15. 1 mL
16. a. Palpate sites for masses or tenderness and assess the amount of subcutaneous tissue.
    b. Note the integrity and size of the muscle and palpate for tenderness.
    c. Note any lesions or discoloration of the forearm.
17. See the descriptions under Figure 10-38 for each type of injection.
18. Remove the needle and ensure that the site is not bleeding. Discard the medication and syringe, draw up new medication, and repeat the procedure in a different location.

19. Rather than pouring it into a medication cup, draw small volumes of liquid medications into a calibrated oral syringe.
20. 100 divided by 4 (4 puffs/day) would equal 25 days.

Case Study

1. For the adult, the ventrogluteal site is the preferred injection site. If the woman is of average size, choose a needle that is 1 1/2 inches long and 21 to 25 gauge and insert the needle at a 90-degree angle. For the infant, the preferred site is the vastus lateralis site. The needle should be of the correct length to ensure that it reaches muscle tissue, not the subcutaneous layer.
2. For an infant or child younger than 3 years of age, the pinna of the ear should be pulled down and back before the drops are administered. The drops should be directed along the sides of the ear rather than directly onto the eardrum. The drops should be taken out of refrigeration about 30 minutes before administering them. The mother should stay with her child and ensure that the child lies on her side for 5 to 10 minutes. Gentle massage of the tragus area of the ear with her finger will help distribute the medication down the ear canal.
3. Liquid medication doses under 5 mL should be drawn up in a calibrated oral syringe.
4. Liquids are usually ordered because infants cannot swallow pills or capsules. A plastic disposable oral dosing syringe is recommended for measuring small doses of liquid medications. Position the infant so that the head is slightly elevated. Place the plastic dropper or syringe inside the infant's mouth, beside the tongue, and administer the liquid in small amounts while allowing the infant to swallow each time. Take great care to prevent aspiration. A crying infant can easily aspirate medication. Do not add the medication to a bottle of formula. The infant may refuse the feeding or may not drink all of the bottle and, as a result, would not get the entire dosage of medication.

CHAPTER 11 Analgesic Drugs

Critical Thinking Crossword

Across

3. Agonist
5. Acute
11. Superficial
13. Visceral

Down

1. Antagonist
2. Adjuvant
4. Tolerance
6. Threshold
7. Somatic
8. Chronic
9. Opioid
10. Opiate
12. Partial

Chapter Review and NCLEX® Examination Preparation

1. b
2. d
3. c
4. d
5. b, c, e
6. 3 mL (See Overview of Dosage Calculations, Section II)
7. f
8. e
9. h
10. g
11. c
12. a
13. i
14. b
15. d

Case Study

1. Superficial pain, which originates from the skin or mucous membranes.
2. A back rub. Massage to the affected area often decreases the pain. When an area is rubbed or liniment is applied, large sensory fibers from peripheral receptors carry impulses to the spinal cord. This causes impulse transmission to be inhibited and the gate to be closed. This in turn reduces recognition of the pain impulses arriving by means of the small fibers. This is the same pathway that the opioid analgesics use to alleviate pain.
3. All opioids cause some histamine release. It is thought that this histamine release is responsible for many of the unwanted side effects, such as itching.
4. The most serious side effect of opioids is central nervous system depression, which may lead to respiratory depression. Naloxone (Narcan), an opioid reversal drug, may have to be administered to reverse severe respiratory depression.
5. The use of a nonopioid analgesic with an opioid is known as *adjuvant analgesic therapy*. This allows the use of smaller doses of opioids, which accomplishes two important functions. First, it diminishes some of the side effects that are seen with higher doses of opioids, such as respiratory depression, constipation, and urinary retention. Second, it approaches the pain stimulus by another mechanism of action and has a resulting synergistic beneficial effect in reducing the pain.

CHAPTER 12
General and Local Anesthetics

Critical Thinking Crossword

Across

3. Pancuronium
6. General
7. Topical
8. Adjunctive
9. Local

Down

1. Atropine
2. Anesthetics
3. Parenteral
4. Balanced
5. Regional

Chapter Review and NCLEX® Examination Preparation/Critical Thinking and Application

1. a, c, e
2. b
3. a
4. b
5. b, c, e
6. c
7. 1 = c; 2 = a; 3 = b
8. 0.4 mL (See Overview of Dosage Calculations, Section III.)
9. Pediatric patients are more susceptible to problems such as central nervous system depression, toxicity, atelectasis, pneumonia, and cardiac abnormalities because their hepatic, cardiac, respiratory, and renal systems are not fully developed or fully functional.
10. These drugs cause paralysis but not sedation. The patient is still able to hear and feel. It is important to remain professional at all times and to take the time to reassure the patient and orient him to his surroundings, what noises mean, and what procedures are going to be done to him.
11. She will be given a combination of intravenous medications that will produce analgesia and also amnesia of the procedure, but she will still be alert enough to breathe on her own and follow verbal directions as needed. In some cases, local anesthesia will be used to enhance patient comfort. This type of sedation is called *moderate sedation*; it is associated with fewer complications and a shorter recovery time than general anesthesia.

Case Study

1. In balanced anesthesia, minimal doses of a combination of anesthetic drugs (both intravenous and inhaled) are given to achieve the desired level of anesthesia for the surgical procedure. Adjunctive drugs may also be used and commonly include sedative-hypnotics, narcotics, and neuromuscular blocking drugs (NMBDs) (depolarizing drugs such as succinylcholine and the nondepolarizing or competitive drugs such as pancuronium or d-tubocurarine). Combining several different drugs makes it possible for general anesthesia to be accomplished with smaller amounts of anesthetic gases and thereby reduces the side effects.
2. The main therapeutic use of the NMBD succinylcholine is to maintain controlled ventilation during surgical procedures. When respiratory muscles are paralyzed by NMBDs, mechanical ventilation is easier because the body's drive to control respirations is eliminated by the drug; this allows the ventilator to have total control of the respirations.
3. Multiple medical conditions (listed in Box 12-4) can predispose an individual to toxicity. These conditions increase the sensitivity of an individual to NMBDs and prolong their effects. Because the patient's temperature has decreased, hypothermia may lead to an increased sensitivity to the medication. In addition, the history of paraplegia is another condition that may predispose this patient to toxicity.
4. Anticholinesterase drugs such as neostigmine, pyridostigmine, and edrophonium are antidotes and are used to reverse muscle paralysis.
5. Local anesthesia is most commonly used in settings in which loss of consciousness, whole-body relaxation, and loss of responsiveness are either unnecessary or unwanted. A lower incidence of toxic effects is associated with the use of local anesthetics, because very little of these drugs is absorbed systemically.
6. Regardless of the type of anesthesia a patient is receiving, one of the most important nursing considerations during this time is close and frequent observation of the patient and all body systems, with specific attention to the ABCs of care (airway, breathing, and circulation) and vital signs. Resuscitative equipment, as well as any drug antidote, should be kept nearby in case of cardiorespiratory distress or arrest. Other nursing actions include monitoring all aspects of body functions, instituting safety measures, and implementing the physician's orders.

CHAPTER 13
Central Nervous System Depressants and Muscle Relaxants

Chapter Review and NCLEX® Examination Preparation/Critical Thinking and Application

1. a
2. b
3. a
4. d

5. c
6. c
7. a. 7.5 mg
   b. 3.75 mL (See Overview of Dosage Calculations, Section IV.)
8. Answers should reflect the discussion under Toxicity and Management of Overdose in the textbook. The priority of care would be to maintain the ABCs (airway, breathing, and circulation), especially respirations, because respiratory depression is likely. There is no antidote for barbiturate overdose.
9. These drugs can be taken for insomnia only if their use is limited to the short-term (less than 2 to 4 weeks). With long-term use, rebound insomnia and severe withdrawal can develop. If Jackie needs to take something to help her sleep while she is on her trip, the nonbenzodiazepine hypnotics may be an option; and, of course, you could provide patient teaching on nonpharmacologic methods to aid sleep.
10. Older patients should be started on lower dosages because they generally experience a more pronounced effect from benzodiazepines.
11. a. Ask about allergies, central nervous system (CNS) disorders, sleep disorders, diabetes, addictive disorders, personality disorders, thyroid conditions, and renal and liver function.
    b. Alcohol and CNS depressants, but also all prescribed or over-the-counter medications and herbal products used.
    c. The patient's age matters, because these drugs have increased effects in older persons and small children.
12. a. Patient teaching should include information about potential side effects and potential drug interactions. In addition, safety measures to prevent injury stemming from decreased sensorium must be emphasized.
    b. These medications are most effective when used in conjunction with rest and physical therapy.

Case Study

1. Barbiturates are considered controlled substances because of the potential for misuse and the severe effects that result if they are not used appropriately. Other hypnotic drugs are now used more frequently than barbiturates because they have fewer side effects and are safer than the older barbiturates. They also do not suppress rapid eye movement (REM) sleep to the same extent as do barbiturates.
2. Barbiturates deprive people of REM sleep (dreaming sleep), and long-term use can result in agitation and inability to deal with normal stress. In addition, when the barbiturate is stopped, the returning REM sleep may be more intense than before and lead to nightmares (a rebound effect). Barbiturates are habit-forming, they have a low therapeutic index, and severe withdrawal effects may occur when the medication is stopped. Other drugs have been shown to be safer to use for treatment of insomnia.
3. Other CNS depressants, especially alcohol, should be avoided. There may also be an additive effect when the herbal products kava or valerian are used.
4. Zaleplon is indicated for the short-term treatment of insomnia; it is not approved for long-term use. It has a very short half-life, so the patient should be taught that if sleep difficulties include early awakenings, a dose can be taken as long as it is at least 4 hours before the patient must arise. In addition, the patient should explore other nonpharmacologic options for the treatment of insomnia and try to find the cause of the sleep problems. See Box 13-1 for information on nonpharmacologic measures to promote sleep.

CHAPTER 14
Central Nervous System Stimulants and Related Drugs

Chapter Review and NCLEX® Examination Preparation/Critical Thinking and Application

1. b
2. b, c, e
3. a
4. d
5. b
6. b
7. 60 mg (See Overview of Dosage Calculation, Section IV.)
8. a. Stacey has narcolepsy.
   b. Methylphenidate, an amphetamine, or modanafil, a nonamphetamine, may be ordered.
   c. These drugs boost mental alertness, increase motor activity, and diminish the patient's sense of fatigue by stimulating the cerebral cortex and possibly the reticular activating system.
   d. Stacey should avoid other central nervous system stimulants, in particular caffeine-containing products (e.g., coffee, tea, colas, and chocolate). She should check with her physician before taking any over-the-counter drug or herbal product, and she should not consume any substance that contains alcohol. In addition, she should keep a journal to document her response to the medication.
9. Weight loss due to anorexia is associated with these drugs, and so it is important to monitor for weight gain or loss in children who are taking drugs for attention deficit hyperactivity disorder. Height and weight should be measured and recorded before therapy is initiated, and growth rate should be plotted during therapy. Nutritional status should be assessed, with attention to daily dietary intake as well as the

amount eaten before drug therapy and after therapy is initiated.
10. With orlistat, patients need to watch dietary fat intake. Restricting the intake of fat to less than 30% of total caloric intake may help decrease the occurrence of gastrointestinal side effects. Supplementation with fat-soluble vitamins may be indicated.
11. These drugs work to reduce the severity of the headaches but do not prevent headaches.

Case Study

1. Serotonin agonists work by stimulating 5-HT1 receptors in the brain; this stimulation results in constriction of dilated blood vessels in the brain and decreased release of inflammatory neuropeptides.
2. Orally administered medications may not be tolerated because of the nausea and vomiting that often accompany the headaches. Alternative formulations such as subcutaneous self-injections, sublingual forms, and nasal sprays are advantageous. They also typically have a more rapid onset of action, producing relief in some patients in 10 to 15 minutes compared with 1 to 2 hours with tablets.
3. Use of sumatriptan is contraindicated in patients with drug allergy and the presence of serious cardiovascular disease, because of the vasoconstrictive potential of these medications.
4. Foods containing tyramine should be avoided, because tyramine is known to precipitate severe headaches. Tyramine-containing foods include beer, wine, aged cheese, food additives, preservatives, artificial sweeteners, chocolate, and caffeine.
5. Keeping a journal of the occurrence of headaches, precipitating factors, and response to drug therapy is also encouraged so that the patient's progress and response to drug therapy can be followed.

CHAPTER 15
Antiepileptic Drugs

Critical Thinking Crossword

Across

2. Emergency
6. Primary
10. Hepatotoxicity
11. Seizure
12. Slowly

Down

1. Secondary
3. Convulsion
4. Benzodiazepines
5. Idiopathic
6. Phenobarbital
7. Autoinduction
8. Epilepsy
9. Phenytoin

Chapter Review and NCLEX® Examination Preparation/Critical Thinking and Application

1. d
2. a
3. b, c, d
4. c
5. b
6. c
7. a. 450 mg per day; 150 mg per dose
   b. 150 mL per dose
8. Carbamazepine undergoes autoinduction, the process by which the metabolism of a drug increases over time, which leads to lower than expected drug concentrations.
9. Jeremy's mother should be told that topiramate should be taken whole and should not be crushed, broken in half, or chewed. It does have a very bitter taste and seems to be better tolerated when taken with food. She can still give it with gelatin, as long as the dosage form remains whole.

Case Study

1. Generalized seizures, more specifically, absence seizures. These are most often seen in children.
2. She needs to be sure to measure the dose carefully with an exact graduated device or oral syringe, rather than using a household teaspoon, and to give the medication at the same time daily. She should report excessive sedation, confusion, lethargy, or decreased movement. See Patient Teaching Tips for more information.
3. She should be encouraged to keep a journal to record Mattie's signs and symptoms before, during, and after any seizure activity to measure the therapeutic effectiveness of the medication.
4. A therapeutic response to antiepileptic drugs does not mean that the patient has been cured of the seizures but only that seizure activity is decreased or absent. Further evaluation will be needed before a decision is made to stop the medication. Treatment may need to last for years or may be lifelong.

CHAPTER 16
Antiparkinsonian Drugs

Chapter Review and NCLEX® Examination Preparation/Critical Thinking and Application

1. b
2. a
3. c
4. c
5. a, c
6. b
7. 0.2 mL (Did you remember that apomorphine is ordered in milliliters?)

8. a. Dopamine must be given in this form because exogenously administered dopamine cannot pass through the blood-brain barrier; levodopa can.
   b. The addition of carbidopa avoids the high peripheral levels of dopamine and unwanted side effects induced by the very large dosages of levodopa necessary when the drug is given alone.
   c. Carbidopa does not cross the blood-brain barrier and thus prevents levodopa breakdown in the periphery. This, in turn, allows levodopa to reach and cross the blood-brain barrier. Once in the brain, the levodopa is then broken down to dopamine, which can be used directly.
9. You must ask whether Mrs. R. is lactating; if so, use of amantadine is contraindicated. In addition, pregnancy may be a contraindication to many antiparkinsonian drugs.
10. Older patients, especially men with benign prostatic hyperplasia, are at risk for urinary retention. Jane's neighbor may or may not have that condition, but his age is a major factor. Jane's age is not a concern at this time. This drug may also cause palpitations.

Case Study

1. The primary cause of Parkinson's disease is an imbalance in the two neurotransmitters dopamine and acetylcholine (ACh) in the basal ganglia of the brain. This imbalance is caused by a failure of the nerve terminals in the substantia nigra to produce dopamine, which acts in the basal ganglia to control body movements. A correct balance between dopamine and ACh is needed for the proper regulation of posture, muscle tone, and voluntary movement. The deficiency of dopamine can also lead to excessive ACh activity because of the lack of dopamine's normal balancing effect. Symptoms of Parkinson's disease do not appear until approximately 80% of the dopamine store in the substantia nigra of the basal ganglia has been depleted.
2. Drug therapy is aimed at increasing the levels of dopamine at the remaining functioning nerve terminals. It is also aimed at blocking the effects of ACh and slowing the progression of the disease.
3. Amantadine causes the release of dopamine from nerve endings that are still intact. The result is higher levels of dopamine in the central nervous system.
4. It is most effective in the early stages of Parkinson's disease, but as the disease progresses and the number of functioning nerves diminishes, amantadine's effect is also reduced. The drug is usually effective for only 6 to 12 months.
5. Patients with Parkinson's disease often experience rapid swings in response to levodopa; this fluctuating response is known as the "on-off phenomenon."

   This phenomenon is seen in patients who take levodopa for a long time. Such patients may experience periods when they have good control ("on" time) and periods when they have bad control or break-through Parkinson's disease ("off" time). Carbidopa is a peripheral decarboxylase inhibitor that does not cross the blood-brain barrier. As a result, carbidopa is able to prevent levodopa from breaking down in the periphery and allows more levodopa to reach and cross the blood-brain barrier. Levodopa-carbidopa combinations, such as Sinemet CR, may help decrease the "off" time.

CHAPTER 17
Psychotherapeutic Drugs

Chapter Review and NCLEX® Examination Preparation/Critical Thinking and Application

1. b, c, e
2. a
3. c
4. a, c, d
5. d
6. 3 tablets (See Overview of Dosage Calculations, Section II.)
7. l
8. f
9. g
10. n
11. b
12. i
13. j
14. k
15. c
16. m
17. a
18. d
19. h
20. e
21. a. If Carl is taking a benzodiazepine for his anxiety and drinking alcohol, he may be experiencing an interaction between the benzodiazepine and the alcohol, or he may have taken an overdose of the benzodiazpine.
    b. If an overdose of the benzodiazepine is suspected, Carl might be treated with gastric lavage. He might also be given flumazenil (Romazicon) to reverse the effect of the possible benzodiazepine overdose.
22. a. Mr. D. needs to be aware of the foods and drinks, including red wine, that he can no longer have because they contain tyramine.
    b. It appears that Mr. D. may have inadvertently ingested something containing tyramine, which has caused a hypertensive crisis.

23. Second-generation antidepressants offer an advantage over other antidepressants because they have fewer and less severe side effects.
24. If the antidepressant taken is a first-generation antidepressant, or tricyclic, excessive dosages could result in lethal cardiac dysrhythmias as well as seizures. These dysrhythmias are responsible for most of the deaths due to overdoses.

Case Study

1. See Table 17-2 for potential adverse effects of benzodiazepines. Most are related to their effects on the central nervous system. Patient teaching includes warning the patient to avoid driving or operating heavy equipment or machinery until he becomes accustomed to the side effects of the medication. In addition, measures should be taken to avoid orthostatic hypotension. Finally, he should avoid alcohol and other central nervous system depressants while taking this medication.
2. If he is experiencing life-altering anxiety, then he should also consider obtaining psychotherapy to assist him at this time.
3. Benzodiazepines are potentially habit-forming and addictive, with possible withdrawal symptoms such as anxiety, panic attacks, convulsions, nausea, and vomiting. The medication should not be withdrawn abruptly. Patients should always be advised to take the medication as directed and never to stop taking the medicine abruptly. Benzodiazepines should be withdrawn gradually.
4. There is a potential for benzodiazepines to cause serious life-threatening toxicities, but when taken alone in normal dosages in otherwise healthy patients, they are very safe and effective anxiolytics. When they are taken with other sedating medications or with alcohol, however, life-threatening respiratory depression or arrest can occur. An overdose of benzodiazepines may result in one or more of the following symptoms: somnolence, confusion, coma, and respiratory depression. Overdose may be treated with gastric lavage and/or administration of activated charcoal and saline laxative. The benzodiazepine-specific antidote flumazenil may be used in severe cases.
5. Buspirone has the advantages of being both nonsedating and non—habit-forming compared with the benzodiazepines.

CHAPTER 18
Adrenergic Drugs

Chapter Review and NCLEX® Examination Preparation/Critical Thinking and Application

1. d
2. d
3. a, b, d
4. a
5. c
6. 0.5 mL (See Overview of Dosage Calculations, Section III.)
7. a. The alpha-adrenergic activity of this drug causes vasoconstriction in the nasal mucosa. This produces shrinkage of the mucosa and promotes easier nasal breathing.
   b. Perhaps she administered the spray too often. Excessive use of nasal decongestants can lead to greater congestion because of a rebound phenomenon.
8. Use of the drug is contraindicated in patients who have a tumor that secretes catecholamines, such as a pheochromocytoma.
9. The action of dopamine depends on the dosage. At low dosages, it can dilate blood vessels in the brain, heart, kidneys, and mesentery, increasing blood flow to these areas. Increased renal flow may help remove excess fluid volume. At higher infusion rates, dopamine can improve contractility and cardiac output.
10. The toxic effects of adrenergic drugs are mainly an extension of their common adverse effects, such as seizures, hypotension or hypertension, dysrhythmias, and other effects, but the two most life-threatening toxic effects involve the central nervous system and cardiovascular system. Seizures can be managed effectively with diazepam. An extreme elevation in blood pressure poses the risk of hemorrhage in the brain and elsewhere in the body. To lower the blood pressure quickly, a rapid-acting beta-adrenergic blocking drug can be used to reverse the adrenergic effects. Most of the adrenergic drugs have very short half-lives; therefore, their effects are relatively short-lived. Stopping the drug should quickly cause the toxic symptoms to subside. The treatment of overdoses often focuses on treating the symptoms and supporting the patient's respiratory and cardiac functions.
11. a. He is probably having an anaphylactic reaction to the antibiotic.
    b. First, the nurse must stop the medication! Then she will have someone else notify the physician while she stays with the patient to monitor and support the ABCs (airway, breathing, and circulation).
    c. Epinephrine is the drug of choice for anaphylactic reactions.

Case Study

1. Before giving this medication, the nurse should assess for hypersensitivity to albuterol and assess breath sounds and vital signs (blood pressure, pulse rate, respiratory rate) to obtain a baseline for comparative purposes. Because this medication may

cause tachycardia and cardiac dysrhythmias, the patient's pulse rate and rhythm should be monitored during the treatment. Afterward, the nurse should assess the patient's vital signs and breath sounds again, and assess for therapeutic response to the medication.

2. The onset of inhaled albuterol is almost immediate; it would take more time for orally administered albuterol to be absorbed and to become effective. Therefore, the inhaled form will take effect faster than the oral form.
3. These are expected side effects of the albuterol and will soon wear off.
4. Salmeterol is indicated for asthma and prevention of bronchospasms in patients who may need long-term maintenance therapy for their asthma. Patients should be taught that salmeterol is not to be used for relief of acute symptoms, and education about its dosing is important. Dosing of salmeterol is usually at 2 puffs twice daily 12 hours apart for maintenance. For prevention of exercise-induced asthma, the recommendation is 2 puffs 1/2 to 1 hour before exercise and no additional dosing for 12 hours. If Maureen is still taking the inhaled steroid, then the bronchodilator should be taken first, and she should wait approximately 5 minutes before using the steroid inhaler. All equipment should be rinsed, and the patient should be encouraged to perform mouth care after the use of any inhaled forms of medication.

Chapter 19 Adrenergic-Blocking Drugs

Chapter Review and NCLEX® Examination Preparation/Critical Thinking and Application

1. a, b, d
2. a
3. c
4. b
5. d
6. 83 mL per hour (See Overview of Dosage Calculations, Section V.)
7. Extravasation can cause vasoconstriction and ultimately tissue death (necrosis). If the vasoconstriction is not reversed quickly, the whole limb can be lost. Phentolamine, an alpha-blocker, can reverse this potent vasoconstriction and restore blood flow to the ischemic, vasoconstricted area. When phentolamine is injected subcutaneously in a circular fashion around the extravasation site, it causes alpha-adrenergic receptor blockade and vasodilation. This in turn increases blood flow to the ischemic tissue and thus prevents permanent damage.
8. Some beta-blockers are considered cardioprotective because they inhibit stimulation by the circulating catecholamines released during muscle damage, such as that caused by a myocardial infarction. When a beta-blocker occupies their receptors, the circulating catecholamines cannot bind to their receptors. Thus, the beta-blockers "protect" the heart from being stimulated by these catecholamines, which would only further increase the heart rate and the contractile force, and thereby increase myocardial oxygen demand.
9. She should take her apical pulse for 1 full minute and monitor her blood pressure because cardiac depression can occur with these drugs. If her systolic blood pressure decreases to lower than 100 mm Hg or her pulse decreases to fewer than 60 beats/min, she should contact her physician. She should also report any weight gain, especially of more than 2 pounds in a week, as well as any weakness, shortness of breath, or edema.
10. A common problem with the alpha-blockers such as tamsulosin is that when patients first start taking these drugs, they may experience lightheadedness and orthostatic hypotension. Patients should quickly develop a tolerance to this effect. He should be taught to take care when standing up to prevent falling if he gets lightheaded; taking the first dose at bedtime may help. In addition, other adverse effects of blurred vision, dizziness, and drowsiness may lead to injuries if he should fall. Special care must be taken for safety until he knows how he responds to the medication.

Case Study

1. Nonselective beta-blockers (which block both $beta_1$ and $beta_2$ receptors) may precipitate bradycardia and hypotension; their use is contraindicated in asthma. Therefore, if the patient has heart disease as well as respiratory disease, a $beta_1$-blocker, or "cardioselective" drug, would be very beneficial because it would not produce constriction or increased airway resistance as would $beta_2$-blockers.
2. When a beta-blocker is given, it occupies receptors and prevents circulating catecholamines (which are released when a myocardial infarction occurs) from binding to these receptors. The beta-blocker thus prevents stimulation of the heart by these catecholamines, which would further increase heart rate, contractile force, and myocardial oxygen demand. In addition, cardioselective $beta_1$-blockers such as atenolol block the $beta_1$-adrenergic receptors on the surface of the heart. This reduces myocardial stimulation, which in turn reduces heart rate, slows conduction through the atrioventricular node, prolongs sinoatrial node recovery, and decreases myocardial oxygen demand by decreasing myocardial contractile force (contractility).

3. Table 19-4 lists beta-blocker–induced adverse effects. Patient teaching should include instructions to monitor the apical pulse for 1 full minute and monitor blood pressure because of the cardiac depression that can occur, and to notify the physician if systolic blood pressure decreases to lower than 100 mm Hg or pulse decreases to fewer than 60 beats/min. Patients should also report any weight gain, especially a gain of 2 pounds or more in a 24-hour period or 5 pounds or more in a week, as well as any weakness, shortness of breath, and edema. The patient should also be taught about orthostatic changes and cautioned to rise slowly when getting up to avoid syncope. For other teaching points, see Patient Teaching Tips in the text.
4. Make sure that patients are weaned off these medications slowly, if this is indicated, because of the possible rebound hypertension or chest pain that rapid withdrawal can precipitate.

CHAPTER 20 Cholinergic Drugs

Chapter Review and NCLEX® Examination Preparation/Critical Thinking and Application

1. h
2. g
3. f
4. b
5. j
6. e
7. i
8. a
9. c
10. b
11. b
12. d
13. c
14. b, c, d, f
15. a
16. 17 gtt/min (16.7 rounds to 17) (See Overview of Dosage Calculations, Section V.)
17. SLUDGE stands for Salivation, Lacrimation, Urinary incontinence, Diarrhea, Gastrointestinal cramps, and Emesis.
18. a. Bethanechol is the drug of choice.
    b. None. Bethanechol use is contraindicated in patients with a genitourinary obstruction. The drug should be discontinued immediately.
19. a. Cholinergic crisis
    b. Ensure that atropine, the antidote, is readily available.
20. a. She should experience less eyelid drooping (ptosis), less double vision (diplopia), less difficulty swallowing and chewing, and/or less weakness.
    b. She should report any increased muscle weakness, abdominal cramps, diarrhea, or difficulty breathing.

Case Study

1. There are no "cures" for Alzheimer's disease, but there are several drugs available for management of symptoms. Their use can sometimes yield enough improvement in a patient's mental status to make a noticeable improvement in the quality of life for patients as well as caregivers and family members. However, individual response to these medications does vary from patient to patient. Available drugs include donepezil (Aricept), tacrine (Cognex), galantamine (Razadyne, Reminyl), rivastigmine (Exelon), and memantine (Namenda).
2. Rivastigmine is also approved for treating dementia that is associated with Parkinson's disease.
3. Direct-acting cholinergic agonists bind to cholinergic receptors and activate them. Indirect-acting cholinergic agonists act by making more acetylcholine (ACh) available at the receptor site. As a result, ACh binds to and stimulates the receptor. They do this by inhibiting the action of cholinesterase, the enzyme responsible for breaking down ACh.
4. Adverse effects of rivastigmine include dizziness, headache, nausea and vomiting, diarrhea, and anorexia (loss of appetite). Administering this drug with meals helps decrease the gastrointestinal side effects, although absorption may also be decreased. Patients who become dizzy with the therapy should be assisted with ambulation. Doses should be titrated carefully to help minimize adverse effects.

CHAPTER 21 Cholinergic-Blocking Drugs

Chapter Review and NCLEX® Examination Preparation/Critical Thinking and Application

1. a, c, f
2. a, c, d
3. b
4. c
5. b
6. 0.6 mL
7. Atropine sulfate is used preoperatively to reduce salivation and excessive secretions in the respiratory and gastrointestinal tracts. Glycopyrrolate (Robinul) is also used for this purpose.
8. a. Initially, Mr. M. should be treated with hospitalization and close, continuous monitoring (including continuous electrocardiographic monitoring). The stomach should be emptied with gastric lavage. Fluid therapy and other standard measures used to treat shock should be

instituted as needed. Activated charcoal may be effective in removing the drug that has already been absorbed.
   b. In the case of hallucinations, physostigmine has proven helpful, although its use as an antidote for cholinergic blocker overdose is controversial because it has the potential to produce severe adverse effects such as seizures and cardiac asystole, and it should therefore be reserved for the treatment of patients who show extreme delirium or agitation or who could inflict injury upon themselves.
9. Antihistamines can have additive effects with cholinergic blockers, resulting in increased effects.
10. a. In the treatment of symptomatic bradycardia, higher dosages of atropine result in an increase in heart rate because of the cholinergic-blocking effects on the heart's conduction system. Atropine blocks the inhibitory vagal (cholinergic) effects on the pacemaker cells of the sinoatrial and atrioventricular nodes, which will hopefully lead to an increased heart rate due to unopposed sympathetic stimulation.
    b. Atropine has a therapeutic effect in cases of exposure to organophosphate insecticides because of its anticholinesterase effects.

Case Study

1. Tolterodine should not be used in patients with narrow-angle glaucoma or urinary retention. Mrs. W.'s "eye problems" should be evaluated further.
2. Tolterodine appears to be associated with a much lower incidence of dry mouth. This may be due to tolterodine's specificity for the bladder as opposed to the salivary glands.
3. When these cholinergic-blocking drugs are used to treat urinary incontinence, the inability to sweat or perspire should be managed with an increase in fluids and avoidance of extreme heat. Mrs. W. needs to avoid overheating when working outside.
4. Although this drug may be associated with a lower incidence of dry mouth, it may still cause this unpleasant side effect because it is a cholinergic-blocking drug. Dry mouth may be managed best by drinking adequate fluids, chewing gum, performing frequent mouth care, sucking on sugar-free hard candy, and using saliva substitute products.

CHAPTER 22
Heart Failure Drugs

Chapter Review and NCLEX® Examination Preparation/Critical Thinking and Application

1. c
2. d
3. a
4. b
5. a, b, c, d, f
6. 0.25 mg
7. Vomiting, headache, fatigue, and dysrhythmia are adverse effects of cardiac glycosides. The presence of a serum potassium level of more than 5 mEq/L, along with these symptoms, means that administration of digoxin immune Fab is indicated for the treatment of severe digoxin toxicity.
8. Because of digoxin's fairly long duration of action and half-life, the physician has prescribed a loading, or "digitalizing," dose for Mr. D. to bring the serum levels of the drug up to a therapeutic level more quickly. The usual loading dose is 1 to 1.5 mg/day, whereas the usual maintenance dose is 0.125 to 0.5 mg/day.
9. At this time, nesiritide is generally used in the intensive care setting as a final effort to treat severe, life-threatening heart failure, often in combination with several other cardiostimulatory medications. It is recommended that its use should be strictly limited to treatment of patients with acutely decompensated heart failure who have dyspnea at rest. It should not be used to replace diuretics and should not be used repetitively or to improve renal function.
10. Increased urinary output and decreased dyspnea and fatigue are therapeutic effects of digoxin. The constipation needs to be assessed. Mr. F. should not be allowed to consume large amounts of bran or other foods high in fiber because the bran will bind to the digitalis and make less of the drug available for absorption.
11. a. Inamrinone increases the force of contraction (inotropic effect) and relaxes the blood vessels, causing a reduction in afterload, or the force against which the heart must pump to eject its volume.
    b. Phosphodiesterase inhibitors do not stimulate receptors to cause an increase in the force of contraction as other inotropic drugs do; therefore, the drug maintains its effectiveness for a longer period of time. As a result, increased dosages are not needed to maintain positive results, and unwanted cardiac side effects do not occur.
    c. Thrombocytopenia

Case Study

1. Positive inotropic effect: increases myocardial contractility
   Negative chronotropic effect: decreases heart rate
   Negative dromotropic effect: slows the conduction of electrical impulses in the heart
2. Effects on:
   - Stroke volume: increased

- Venous blood pressure and vein engorgement: decreased
- Coronary circulation: increased
- Diuresis: increased due to improved circulation

3. First, you should complete your assessment by checking her apical pulse, heart and lung sounds, and blood pressure. In addition, check her potassium level, because low levels of potassium may lead to digoxin toxicity. If you have not yet given the digoxin dose, hold it and call the physician immediately. Monitor her for signs of digoxin toxicity, especially dangerous dysrhythmias. The digoxin level of 3.5 ng/mL is above the therapeutic range.

CHAPTER 23 Antidysrhythmic Drugs

Chapter Review and NCLEX® Examination Preparation/Critical Thinking and Application

1. d
2. c
3. a
4. d
5. a
6. b
7. 150 mg
8. a, (3); b, (1); c, (2)
9. a. Class II antidysrhythmics, or beta-blockers, are indicated because they have been shown to significantly reduce the incidence of sudden cardiac death after myocardial infarction.
   b. If Mr. K. had asthma, use of most of the class II drugs would be contraindicated. Noncardioselective beta-blockers block not only the $beta_1$-adrenergic receptors in the heart but also the $beta_2$-adrenergic receptors in the lungs. As a result, preexisting asthma could be worsened.
10. Amiodarone is considered a drug to use when other therapies fail. Although it is very effective, amiodarone can penetrate and concentrate in the adipose tissue of any organ in the body, where it may have unwanted effects. It may cause either hypothyroidism or hyperthyroidism, corneal microdeposits, pulmonary toxicity (which is fatal in about 10% of patients), and even dysrhythmias. Amiodarone has a very long half-life and the side effects may take months to subside.
11. a. Lidocaine must be injected intramuscularly or intravenously; when lidocaine is taken orally, the liver converts most of it to inactive metabolites.
    b. Lidocaine is extensively metabolized in the liver. For patients in liver failure or with a history of cirrhosis, a dosage reduction of 50% is recommended.
12. Alicia should not double up on her medication. The physician should be contacted about the missed dose and about Alicia's symptoms of chest pain and dizziness, which are adverse effects of the quinidine.

Case Study

1. As their name implies, they work by inhibiting the slow-channel pathways, or the calcium-dependent channels. As a result, they depress phase 4 depolarization, slow sinoatrial and atrioventricular nodal conduction rates, and thus reduce the incidence of paroxysmal supraventricular tachycardia (PSVT).
2. Prevention or reduction of supraventricular rhythms.
3. Taking phenytoin, an anticonvulsant, along with diltiazem may result in reduced effectiveness of the calcium channel blocker.
4. The physician may prescribe adenosine, which is useful for the treatment of PSVT that has failed to respond to verapamil.

CHAPTER 24 Antianginal Drugs

Chapter Review and NCLEX® Examination Preparation/Critical Thinking and Application

1. c
2. c
3. a, c, d, e
4. d
5. a
6. b
7. DO NOT cut the patch in half! The nurse needs to call the pharmacy to obtain the correct dosage of the transdermal patch, one that delivers 0.2 mg/hr.
8. The nurse will call 911 and assist the patient until the ambulance arrives. He will check the "ABCs" and administer CPR if necessary. At this time the nurse does not know the man's condition, and certainly cannot administer someone else's medication to him. Isordil is available in a sublingual form, but the nurse cannot administer one person's medication to another person, especially to someone with an undetermined condition.
9. Ms. V. might be taking a beta-blocker. Fatigue and lethargy are the most common patient complaints with the use of beta-blockers, and mental depression can be exacerbated, particularly in older adults. Also, one of the central nervous system adverse effects of beta-blockers is the occurrence of unusual dreams.
10. Theresa should always include in her journal a description of the activity she was performing at the time her angina occurred and the number of tablets she had to take before the pain subsided. Also, she must keep the tablets in an airtight, dark glass bottle away from sunlight, because the active ingredient in nitroglycerin is easily destroyed.

Case Study

1. Chronic stable angina, also known as *classic* or *effort angina*, can be triggered by either exertion or stress (cold temperature or emotions).
2. When experiencing an acute anginal attack, he should take 1 sublingual tablet as soon as possible after the pain begins, lie down immediately, remain calm, and rest.
3. If he obtains no relief after taking 1 sublingual tablet, his handball partner should call 911 immediately and have emergency response personnel take him to the hospital. The emergency response team would be better equipped to help him should further complications occur. The patient can take 1 more tablet, while awaiting emergency care, and a third tablet 5 minutes later, but no more than three tablets total.
4. The beta-blockers are most effective in the treatment of typical exertional angina.

CHAPTER 25
Antihypertensive Drugs

Critical Thinking Crossword

Across

1. Secondary
5. Idiopathic
7. Orthostatic
8. Vasodilators

Down

2. Essential
3. Primary
4. Diuretics
6. ACE

Chapter Review and NCLEX® Examination Preparation/Critical Thinking and Application

1. c
2. b, d, e
3. b
4. a
5. d
6. 2 tablets per dose (See Overview of Dosage Calculations, Section II.)
7. Because nitroprusside has a very short half-life (10 minutes), the nurse should first discontinue the infusion. Placing the patient in the Trendelenburg position will also be helpful. Treatment for the hypotension is supportive; pressor drugs can be given to raise the blood pressure quickly if necessary.
8. a. Captopril is probably best for Irene. In critically ill patients, a drug with a short half-life, such as captopril, is better, because if problems arise, they will be short-lived. Also, Irene has liver dysfunction, so captopril has an advantage because it is not a prodrug (a prodrug is inactive in its initial form and must be biotransformed in the liver to its active form to be effective).
   b. Because of his history of poor compliance, Kory would benefit from a drug with a long half-life and long duration of action, which he would need to take only once a day. Therefore, one of the newer ACE inhibitors—benazepril, fosinopril, lisinopril, quinapril, or ramipril—would be best.
9. There is a first-dose effect with prazosin. This means that the patient will experience a considerable drop in blood pressure after taking the first dose, so he should take it while lying down or before bedtime and arise slowly. This effect decreases with time or with a reduction in the dosage, as ordered by the physician.
10. a. Beta-blockers and ACE inhibitors
    b. Calcium channel blockers and diuretics

Case Study

1. Initial drug therapy would include thiazide-type diuretics. Other drugs that may also be started include ACE inhibitors, angiotensin II receptor blockers, beta-blockers, calcium channel blockers, or a combination. Because John is African American, calcium channel blockers and diuretics would be chosen over beta-blockers and ACE inhibitors.
2. He should be taught about the possibility of orthostatic hypotension and instructed to change positions slowly—especially after stooping or bending over or when rising from supine or sitting to standing.
3. Exercise is an important part of a healthy lifestyle. However, the importance of safety and the need to avoid excessive exercise, hot climates, saunas, hot tubs, and hot environments should be emphasized. Heat may precipitate vasodilation and lead to worsening of hypotension with the risk of fainting and injury to self.

CHAPTER 26
Diuretic Drugs

Chapter Review and NCLEX® Examination Preparation/Critical Thinking and Application

1. c
2. f
3. e
4. i
5. g
6. j
7. h
8. a
9. d
10. b
11. a, c, d, e

12. c
13. a
14. d
15. b
16. 150 mL (hint: 20% indicates 20 g per 100 mL)

$$\frac{20g}{100mL} = \frac{30g}{x\ mL}$$

(20 g)(x mL) = (100 mL)(30 g); $20x = 3000$;
$x = 150$ mL
(See Overview of Dosage Calculations, Section III.)

17. a. Ms. A. was probably prescribed a carbonic anhydrase inhibitor (CAI).
    b. An undesirable effect of the CAIs is that they elevate the blood glucose level, causing glycosuria in diabetic patients. They may also interact with some oral antidiabetic drugs.
18. a. For mannitol to be effective in treating acute renal failure, enough renal blood flow and glomerular filtration must exist to enable the drug to reach the tubules.
    b. Mannitol is always administered intravenously through a filter, because it can crystallize when exposed to low temperatures (which is more likely to occur when concentrations exceed 15%). In addition, the fluid container should be visually inspected for precipitants.
    c. Arthur's headache and chills are probably side effects of the mannitol therapy. At this time the therapy should be continued, but Arthur should be monitored for the development of more serious adverse effects.
19. a. Mr. F. will be prescribed spironolactone in high doses; this drug is used often for the treatment of ascites associated with cirrhosis of the liver.
    b. His serum potassium level will need to be monitored frequently because he has impaired renal function. The spironolactone may cause hyperkalemia.
20. a. Impotence and decreased libido are among the side effects of thiazide. Brendan is possibly experiencing these effects.
    b. He should stop eating licorice, because its consumption can lead to an additive hypokalemia in patients taking thiazide. Brendan's fatigue may be the result of severe hypokalemia and should be evaluated.
21. It is likely that Mrs. H.'s neighbor was prescribed one of the potassium-sparing diuretics and thus was not instructed to eat additional potassium-rich foods. Mrs. H. should follow the dietary recommendations provided for her, not for her neighbor.

Case Study

1. These symptoms suggest hypokalemia. Furosemide causes potassium to be excreted along with sodium and water.
2. Foods high in potassium include bananas, oranges, apricots, dates, raisins, broccoli, green beans, potatoes, tomatoes, meats, fish, wheat bread, and legumes.
3. Spironolactone is a potassium-sparing diuretic; it causes sodium and water to be excreted, but potassium is retained.
4. The use of ACE inhibitors or potassium supplements in combination with potassium-sparing diuretics can result in hyperkalemia. When taken together, lithium and potassium-sparing diuretics can result in lithium toxicity. The use of nonsteroidal antiinflammatory drugs with potassium-sparing diuretics can reduce the effectiveness of the diuretics.

CHAPTER 27
Fluids and Electrolytes

Chapter Review and NCLEX® Examination Preparation/Critical Thinking and Application

1. a, b, d, e
2. c
3. d
4. c
5. b
6. b
7. Rate: 42 mL/hour; 11 gtt/min (rounded up from 10.5) (See the Overview of Dosage Calculations, Section V.)
8. **Advantages:** Crystalloids are less expensive than colloids and blood products for replacing fluids and better for emergency short-term plasma volume expansion. They also promote urinary flow. They do not carry the risk of transmission of viral diseases or anaphylaxis and do not promote bleeding. **Disadvantages:** The fluids can leak out of the plasma into the tissues and cells, which results in edema (such as peripheral edema or pulmonary edema). They may dilute plasma proteins, resulting in lower colloid oncotic pressure (COP), and dilute erythrocyte concentration, resulting in decreased oxygen tension. Large volumes are needed to be effective, but prolonged infusions and administration of large volumes may worsen acidosis or alkalosis. Lastly, their effects are relatively short-lived compared with those of colloids.
9. a. Blood products
   b. They are the only fluids that contain hemoglobin.
   c. They are natural products that require human donors, which means that they can be incompatible with a recipient's immune system. These products can also transmit pathogens from the donor to the recipient.
10. a. Tanya is exhibiting early symptoms of hypokalemia.

b. She should eat foods high in potassium, such as bananas, oranges, apricots, dates, raisins, broccoli, green beans, potatoes, tomatoes, meats, fish, wheat bread, and legumes. She may be placed on oral potassium supplements for a short time.

11. a. Hyponatremia
 b. Mr. S. can take in sodium by eating foods high in salt, such as catsup, mustard, cured meats, and potato chips.
 c. Vomiting a possible adverse effect of oral administration of sodium chloride; if vomiting occurs, he needs to be careful about monitoring for further fluid and electrolyte loss.
12. a. Signs of transfusion reaction include apprehension, restlessness, flushed skin, increased pulse and respiration rate, dyspnea, rash, joint or lower back pain, swelling, fever and chills, nausea, weakness, and jaundice.
 b. Although it is possible for pathogens such as that causing acquired immunodeficiency syndrome (AIDS) to be transmitted via blood products, Victor's wife should be reassured that techniques are now used that have drastically reduced the incidence of such problems.
 c. Every 15 minutes or more often if needed
 d. Victor's restlessness and increased pulse need to be reported to the physician immediately, because these are signs of a reaction to the blood product. The nurse will have another nurse notify the physician; she should stop the transfusion immediately and change the infusion to normal saline at a slow rate. The nurse will check the patient's vital signs, and follow the facility's protocol for transfusion reactions.

Case Study

1. The normal total protein level is 7.4 g/dL. If the level drops below 5.3 g/dL, the colloid oncotic pressure becomes less than the hydrostatic pressure, and fluid shifts into the tissues, which results in edema.
2. The albumin will increase the COP and move fluid from outside the blood vessels to inside the blood vessels, thus reducing the edema.
3. Colloids are the choice for this patient. Crystalloids can leak out of the plasma into the tissues and cells, resulting in edema anywhere in the body. Crystalloids also dilute the proteins that are in the plasma, further reducing the COP. Finally, crystalloids are more likely to cause edema because of the larger volumes needed to achieve the desired clinical effect. Colloids reduce edema and expand plasma volume by pulling fluid from the extravascular space into the blood vessels.
4. Colloids can alter the coagulation system, which results in impaired coagulation and possibly bleeding. They have no oxygen-carrying ability and contain no clotting factors, and they may also dilute the plasma protein concentration, which may impair the function of platelets.

CHAPTER 28
Coagulation Modifier Drugs

Chapter Review and NCLEX® Examination Preparation/Critical Thinking and Application

1. k
2. n
3. j
4. l
5. m
6. b
7. a, c
8. c
9. i
10. h
11. e
12. g
13. a, c, d
14. b
15. a
16. c
17. b, c, d, e
18. d
19. 0.8 mL
20. The nurse will assess the site and ask her not to rub it. The injection site should not be massaged or rubbed before or after the injection because this may cause hematoma formation.
21. a. The anticoagulant effects of heparin can be reversed with protamine sulfate.
 b. In general, 1 mg of protamine sulfate can reverse the effects of 100 units of heparin.
 c. The activated partial thromboplastin time is the test most commonly used.
22. a. Vitamin K
 b. Current recommendations are to use the lowest amount of vitamin K possible, based on the clinical situation.
 c. After the use of vitamin K for warfarin toxicity, warfarin resistance will occur for up to 7 days; thus the patient cannot be anticoagulated by warfarin during this period. In such cases, either heparin or an LMWH may need to be added to provide adequate anticoagulation if necessary.
23. The physician will probably prescribe one of the antifibrinolytic drugs, which are used to stop excessive oozing from surgical sites, such as chest tubes.
24. Desmopressin is used in patients with type I von Willebrand's disease; it increases the levels of clotting factor VIII.

25. a. No. Alteplase is present in the body in a natural state, so it does not induce an antigen-antibody reaction.
    b. The alteplase can be readministered because it has a very short half-life of 5 minutes. Because of its short half-life, it is given along with heparin to prevent reocclusion of the infarcted blood vessel.
26. a. They are possible indications of bleeding problems related to the anticoagulation therapy.
    b. Ursula might also be exhibiting a change in pulse rate or rhythm, blood pressure, or level of consciousness.
    c. The nurse will notify the physician immediately. She must not administer any other anticoagulants; if Ursula is receiving a continuous infusion of an anticoagulant, she must stop the infusion. The nurse will take her vital signs and stay with her. She will prepare to administer the appropriate antidote.
27. Heparin is commonly used for DVT prophylaxis in a dose of 5000 units two or three times a day given subcutaneously, and does not need to be monitored when used for prophylaxis.

Case Study

1. Use of aspirin is contraindicated in the presence of peptic ulcer disease. Doug has been started on the clopidogrel therapy to reduce the risk of stroke.
2. He should be taught to watch for signs of abnormal bleeding and should immediately report any of the following signs and symptoms to the health care provider: respiratory difficulty, back pain, skin rash, evidence of gastrointestinal bleeding, any other bleeding abnormality, diarrhea, acute severe headache, and change in vision (blurred vision or loss of vision).
3. He needs to take measures to prevent bleeding, such as using a soft toothbrush and an electric razor, and should take great care when trimming his nails, gardening, and participating in rough or contact sports. He needs to take precautions to protect himself from injury and subsequent bleeding or bruising, which can be extremely dangerous while he is taking antiplatelet drugs.
4. Herbal products that contain garlic, ginger, ginseng, and ginkgo should be avoided because they have anticoagulant properties.

CHAPTER 29
Antilipemic Drugs

Chapter Review and NCLEX® Examination Preparation/Critical Thinking and Application

1. d
2. a, c, d, e
3. a
4. b
5. d
6. c
7. 1.5 tablets
8. a. Fibric acid derivative—it is believed that these drugs work by activating the lipoprotein lipase, an enzyme responsible for the breakdown of cholesterol.
   b. Lipid-lowering drug and vitamin—exact mechanism unknown; beneficial effects are believed to be related to its ability to inhibit lipolysis in adipose tissue, decrease esterification of triglycerides in the liver, and increase the activity of lipase.
   c. HMG-CoA reductase inhibitor—reduces blood cholesterol by decreasing the rate of cholesterol production.
   d. Bile acid sequestrant—binds bile, preventing the resorption of the bile acids from the small intestine. The insoluble bile acid and resin (drug) complex that is formed is excreted in the feces.
9. Unless Mr. H. has additional risk factors, his high level of low-density lipoprotein (LDL) cholesterol alone does not warrant drug therapy at this time. He will be recommended for dietary therapy with an LDL goal of less than 160 mg/dL. All reasonable nonpharmaceutical means of controlling Mr. H.'s LDL level need to be tried and found to fail before he is given drug therapy. Mr. H. needs to find time in his busy schedule to exercise and eat more wisely.
10. Mr. J.'s age and smoking are risk factors, as is the fact that his father died suddenly of heart disease before 55 years of age. Mr. J.'s asthma and arthritis are not risk factors, nor is his blood pressure. Mr. J.'s level of high-density lipoprotein (HDL) cholesterol is above 60 mg/dL, so it is considered a negative risk factor and can be subtracted from the total number of positive risk factors.
11. Mrs. K. is experiencing constipation and belching associated with cholestyramine use (she may also be experiencing heartburn, nausea, and bloating). Mrs. K. requires extra patient teaching and support to help her maintain compliance with the drug therapy; she should be assured that these adverse effects will probably diminish over time.
12. No. Justus is not a candidate for niacin therapy because niacin use is contraindicated in patients with peptic ulcer. Also, when niacin is taken with an HMG–CoA reductase inhibitor, the likelihood of myopathy development is greatly increased, although it is not uncommon to see these drugs used together.
13. Mrs. N. must take her antihypertensive and cholestyramine (Questran) at different times of the day because the bile acid sequestrant may interfere sig-

nificantly with the absorption of other drugs taken at the same time. All other drugs should be taken at least 1 hour before or 4 to 6 hours after the administration of antilipemics.

Case Study

1. No, he is not right. Dietary measures are a part of antilipemic therapy. Nonpharmacologic measures include consumption of a low-fat, low-cholesterol diet; supervised, moderate exercise; weight loss; cessation of smoking or drinking; and relaxation therapy.
2. This drug is used primarily to lower total and LDL cholesterol levels as well as triglyceride levels; it has been shown to raise the HDL level as well.
3. Elevations in liver enzyme levels may also occur, and the patient should be monitored for excessive elevations, which may indicate the need for alternative drug therapy. In addition, total cholesterol level, LDL/HDL ratio, and triglyceride levels need to be monitored to evaluate therapeutic effect.
4. Myopathy (muscle pain) is an uncommon but clinically important side effect that may occur in some patients taking statins. It may progress to a serious condition known as *rhabdomyolysis* in which the breakdown of muscle protein occurs, leading to myoglobinuria and possible renal damage. Patients receiving statin therapy should be taught to report unexplained muscle pain to their health care providers immediately.

CHAPTER 30
Pituitary Drugs

Chapter Review and NCLEX® Examination Preparation/Critical Thinking and Application

1. a. Glucocorticoids, mineralocorticoids, androgens
   b. Corticotropin
   c. Regulates anabolic processes related to growth and adaptation to stressors; promotes skeletal and muscle growth; increases protein synthesis; increases liver glycogenolysis; increases fat mobilization
   d. Somatropin and somatrem
   e. Antidiuretic hormone
   f. Vasopressin and desmopressin
   g. Promotes uterine contractions
   h. Oxytocin
2. d
3. d
4. b
5. d
6. c
7. a
8. a. Dose per week for this child (44 lb = 20 kg) is 6 mg
   b. Dose per injection (6 daily injections) = 1 mg per dose per day for 6 days
9. In addition to information about proper subcutaneous injection techniques, the teaching plan should include a reminder of the dosage form and amount and the importance of compliance with therapy. The nurse will show the parents how to keep a journal of Patricia's growth measurements.

Case Study

1. Mr. Collins will probably be found to have diabetes insipidus; if so, he will benefit from treatment with vasopressin or desmopressin.
2. Assessment strategies should include evaluating pulse, vital signs, intake and output, daily weight, and edema. Desmopressin should be given cautiously in patients with migraine headaches, seizures, and asthma.
3. Treatment will be via nasal spray, 1 to 2 sprays administered into each nostril three times daily. This should increase water resorption in the distal tubules and collecting ducts of the nephron, performing all the physiologic functions of antidiuretic hormone.
4. It should eliminate his severe thirst and decrease his urinary output.

CHAPTER 31
Thyroid and Antithyroid Drugs

Critical Thinking Crossword

Across

3. Secondary
6. Thyroxine
7. Primary

Down

1. Levothyroxine
2. Hyperthyroidism
4. Propylthiouracil
5. Tertiary
6. Thyrotropin

Chapter Review and NCLEX® Examination Preparation/Critical Thinking and Application

1. c
2. d
3. a
4. a, c, d
5. c
6. 0.088 mg
7. Mrs. W. probably has hypothyroidism, which may result in the formation of a goiter, an enlargement of the thyroid gland resulting from its overstimulation by elevated levels of thyroid-stimulating hormone. She may benefit from one of the thyroid drugs, including thyroid, levothyroxine, liothyronine, or

liotrix. Levothyroxine is generally preferred because, as a chemically pure formulation of 100% thyroxine, its hormonal content is standardized; therefore, its effect is predictable.

8. Even if it can be determined that the last several symptoms are due to menopause, the combination of the rest of the symptoms, plus her history, indicates the strong possibility that Ms. H. has hyperthyroidism. This is especially worth investigating because it is often caused by Graves' disease.
9. Surgery to remove all or part of the thyroid gland is an effective way to treat hyperthyroidism, but as a result, lifelong hormone replacement is normally required.
10. Levothyroxine is dosed in micrograms. A common medication error is the write the intended dose in milligrams instead of micrograms. If not caught, this error would result in a thousandfold overdose. Doses higher than 200 **mcg** should be questioned in case this error occurred.

Case Study

1. Her symptoms suggest hypothyroidism, and a thyroid replacement hormone, such as levothyroxine, would be indicated for this condition.
2. The thyroid preparations are given to replace what the thyroid gland cannot itself produce to achieve normal thyroid levels, known as a "euthyroid" condition.
3. Thyroid preparations should be taken at the same time every day to maintain constant blood levels. Taking the medication in the morning will help reduce problems with insomnia, which may result when the medication is taken later in the day or in the evening.

CHAPTER 32 Antidiabetic Drugs

Chapter Review and NCLEX® Examination Preparation/Critical Thinking and Application

1. b
2. d
3. a
4. c
5. a
6. b
7. d
8. Four units (238 – 150 = 88 ÷ 20 = 4.4. (Answer is 4, because 20 divides into 88 four whole times. The "left-over" 8 does not add up to 20, so it does not count toward the insulin dose.)
9. a. Pramlintide, given by subcutaneous injection, works by mimicking the action of the natural pancreatic hormone amylin. Amylin is secreted along with insulin in response to food intake and influences postmeal glucose levels by slowing gastric emptying, suppressing glucagon secretion (which reduces the liver's glucose output), and centrally modulating the senses of appetite and satiety. As a result, blood glucose levels are reduced.
   b. Exenatide is also an injectable medication, which comes in a prefilled pen-type device. It mimics the incretins, a class of hormones that normally enhance glucose-driven insulin secretion from the pancreatic beta cells. The incretins also suppress excessive glucagon secretion and delay gastric emptying. As a result, fasting and postmeal blood glucose levels should be reduced in patients with type 2 diabetes.
   c. Metformin works primarily by inhibiting hepatic glucose production and increasing the sensitivity of peripheral tissue to insulin, thus lowering blood glucose levels.
10. a. Confusion, irritability, tremor, and sweating
    b. The brain needs a constant amount of glucose to function; thus the central nervous system manifestations of hypoglycemia (such as irritability) are often the first to appear.
    c. In the conscious person, oral forms of glucose are used, such as rapidly dissolving buccal tablets or semisolid gel forms designed for rapid mucosal absorption. She could also try corn syrup, honey, fruit juice, a nondiet soft drink, or a small snack such as crackers or half a sandwich.
11. a. The nurse's co-worker should check the order at least three times and have another registered nurse check the prepared injection to be sure it is in accordance with the physician's order.
    b. The nurse, of course. Novolin-R is regular insulin, and regular insulin is clear.
    c. If left at room temperature, the insulin in the vial should have been used within 1 month; otherwise, it should have been refrigerated.
12. a. Mrs. F. needs to make some significant lifestyle changes. She must stop smoking, lose weight, and exercise regularly, which will help with both the high blood glucose level and the hypertension.
    b. Mrs. F. should continue with her exercise and weight loss program; however, because her blood glucose level is still elevated, she also requires an oral antidiabetic drug.
13. a. Hypoglycemia
    b. Dennis may have been drinking alcohol. Sulfonylureas may interact with alcohol in a way that is similar to the interaction with disulfiram, which is used to deter alcohol ingestion in persons with chronic alcoholism. This

disulfiram-type reaction includes vomiting and hypertension.

14. a. Twenty units of NPH insulin plus 4 units regular insulin
    b. No coverage needed
    c. Six units of regular insulin
15. If the patient receiving metformin is to undergo diagnostic studies with contrast dye, the prescriber will need to discontinue the drug prior to the procedure and restart it after the tests, but only after reevaluation of the patient's renal status.

Case Study

1. Glipizide has a rapid onset of action; its effect is thus much like the body's normal response to meals, when greater levels of insulin are rapidly required to deal with the increased glucose in the blood.
2. Glipizide works best if given 30 minutes before meals. This allows the timing of the insulin secretion induced by the glipizide to correspond with the elevation in blood glucose level induced by the meal in much the same way as endogenous insulin levels are raised in a person without diabetes.
3. Mr. D. should contact his physician immediately. He may require a change in his diabetic treatment while he is sick, because vomiting and inability to eat can cause a change in his blood glucose levels.

CHAPTER 33 Adrenal Drugs

Chapter Review and NCLEX® Examination Preparation/Critical Thinking and Application

1. a
2. c
3. a, b, c
4. b
5. d
6. c
7. 2 tablets
8. Ms. R.'s glucocorticoid can interact with aspirin and other nonsteroidal antiinflammatory drugs (NSAIDs), producing additive effects. Also, she should avoid people with infections, because her own immune system is suppressed. The children in the hospital may have infections. In addition, she should report any fever, increased weakness and lethargy, or sore throat.
9. a. The use of systemic glucocorticoids with antidiabetic drugs may reduce the hypoglycemic effect of those drugs. A baseline blood glucose level should be determined, and Peter should be monitored for any problems.
   b. Oral dosage forms should be taken with milk, food, or nonsystemic antacids (such as aluminum-, calcium-, or magnesium-containing antacids), unless contraindicated, to minimize gastrointestinal upset. Another option is for the physician to order a histamine-2 receptor antagonist or proton pump inhibitors to prevent ulcer formation (glucocorticoids may cause gastric ulcers). Patients should be encouraged not to take the drug with alcohol, aspirin, or other NSAIDs to minimize gastric irritation and gastric bleeding.
10. The nurse should intervene. The student nurse should, while wearing gloves, apply the medication with a sterile tongue depressor or cotton-tipped applicator if the skin is intact. If the skin is not intact, a sterile technique should be used.
11. In addition to routine teaching about inhaler administration technique, Nina should be instructed to rinse out her mouth with lukewarm water after using the inhaler to prevent the development of an oral fungal infection.

Case Study

1. One very important point about long-term use of steroids is that they must not be stopped abruptly. These drugs require a tapering of the daily dose, because the administration of these drugs causes the endogenous (body's own) production of the hormones to stop. This is referred to as *HPA* or *adrenal suppression*. This suppression places the patient at risk of developing hypoadrenal crisis (shock, circulatory collapse) in times of increased stress (i.e., surgery, trauma). Tapering of daily doses allows the HPA axis the time to recover and to start stimulating the normal production of the endogenous hormones.
2. Short- or long-term therapy may cause steroid psychosis. In addition, long-term effects cause cushingoid symptoms, including moon face, weight gain, muscle wasting, and increased deposition of fat in the trunk area, leading to truncal obesity (See Table 33-4).
3. Glucocorticoid. Biologic functions of glucocorticoids include antiinflammatory actions, maintenance of normal blood pressure, carbohydrate and protein metabolism, fat metabolism, and stress effects. Biologic functions of mineralocorticoids include sodium and water resorption, blood pressure control, and regulation of potassium levels in and pH of blood.
4. The best time is early in the morning (6:00 AM to 9:00 AM) because this results in the least amount of adrenal suppression.

CHAPTER 34
Women's Health Drugs

Chapter Review and NCLEX® Examination Preparation/Critical Thinking and Application

1. b, c, e
2. a
3. a
4. b
5. b
6. c, e, f
7. 1.25, or 1.3 mL
8. a. The nurse will ask Isabelle if she is taking medication for her depression. Estrogen therapy is indicated for the symptoms of menopause, but the use of estrogen with a tricyclic antidepressant may result in toxicity of the latter drug.
   b. The smallest dose of estrogen that alleviates the symptoms is used for the shortest possible time.
9. a. The physician will probably prescribe medroxyprogesterone, which is indicated for treatment of secondary amenorrhea.
   b. Ms. K.'s dose of antidiabetic drug may need to be adjusted because of a possible decrease in glucose tolerance when progestins and antidiabetic drugs are taken together.
10. a. Perhaps Jacklyn's prescription could be switched to a 28-day form of Ortho-Novum, which is taken for all 28 days of the menstrual cycle rather than for 3 weeks with 1 week off.
    b. One of the benefits of oral contraceptive use is decreased blood loss during menstruation.
11. Choriogonadotropin alfa is often given in a carefully timed fashion after follicle-stimulating hormone–active therapy with a drug such as menotropin or clomiphene, when patient monitoring indicates sufficient maturation of ovarian follicles. Once the ovaries have been sufficiently stimulated, then a single dose of choriogonadotropin alfa is given the next day.
12. Mrs. I. needs to know that smoking can diminish the therapeutic effects of the estrogen she is taking and add to the risk of thrombosis. Also, she should be cautioned to wear sunscreen while in Aruba, because estrogen makes the skin more susceptible to sunburn.
13. a. Mrs. S. is assuming that the medication is estrogen therapy. Alendronate (Fosamax) is indicated to prevent osteoporosis in postmenopausal women. The nurse will need to explain to her that it is a nonestrogen, nonhormonal medication used for prevention of bone loss in the early postmenopausal period. For women who experience early menopause, a dose of 5 mg daily is recommended.
    b. The nurse knows that she experienced early menopause; other risk factors associated with the development of postmenopausal osteoporosis include thin body build, white or Asian race, family history of osteoporosis, and moderately low bone mass. She would need to be assessed for these other risk factors.
14. Megestrol is used in the management of anorexia, cachexia, or unexplained substantial weight loss in patients with acquired immunodeficiency syndrome (AIDS). In addition, it may be used to stimulate appetite and promote weight gain in patients (male or female) with cancer.

Case Study

1. The physician will probably prescribe terbutaline or ritodrine. These drugs work by stimulating the beta-adrenergic receptors located on the uterine smooth muscle. The muscle then relaxes and stops contracting.
2. Ms. O. should be placed in the left lateral recumbent position to minimize hypotension and increase renal blood flow and blood flow to the fetus.
3. Hyperglycemia and hypokalemia are metabolic adverse effects of tocolytic therapy.
4. No, because tocolytic therapy is indicated for premature labor between the 20th and 37th weeks of gestation. At this time, her labor would not be considered premature.

CHAPTER 35
Men's Health Drugs

Chapter Review and NCLEX® Examination Preparation/Critical Thinking and Application

1. b
2. b, d, f
3. a
4. d
5. c
6. a
7. The nurse should administer 1.5 mL, using the 200 mg/mL strength. Using the 100 mg/mL strength would require 3 mL, which may require two separate injections.
8. a. Testosterone's poor performance in the oral dosage form is due to the fact that most of a dose is metabolized and destroyed by the liver before it can reach the circulation.
   b. Methyltestosterone and fluoxymesterone are both testosterone derivatives that are effective when given buccally or orally.
   c. With either drug, contraindications that could apply to Mr. M. include significant cardiac,

hepatic, or renal dysfunction; breast cancer; or known or suspected prostate cancer.

9. a. No. The manufacturer's guidelines suggest that the patient not swallow, chew, or eat the buccal tablet but that it be completely absorbed in the mouth. The part of the drug that is swallowed will not reach the intended site of action because of heavy first-pass metabolism.
   b. Patients taking any hormone-related drug should never abruptly stop the drug. The physician may consider whether a transdermal form is suitable for Mr. M.
10. With finasteride, education about the drug's therapeutic effects as well as adverse effects should be provided at the patient's educational level. Female family members, significant others, and caregivers who are pregnant or of childbearing age should be educated about the need to avoid exposure during handling of this drug, including *not* touching any broken or crushed tablets, which could result in exposure to the drug and the risk of teratogenic effects. Wearing gloves is recommended. Finasteride may be given orally without regard to meals. It should be protected from exposure to light and heat.
11. The Testoderm patch is applied only to the scrotal skin. The skin should be clean, dry scrotal skin that has been shaved for optimal skin contact. These patches are replaced every 22 to 24 hours. Androderm patches should be applied to clean, dry skin on the back, abdomen, upper arms, or thighs; the scrotum and bony areas (shoulder, hip) should be avoided. These patches are often ordered to be changed every 7 days. AndroGel is applied to the shoulders, arms, or abdominal skin daily.

Case Study

1. Sildenafil (Viagra) should be used cautiously in patients with renal disorders, hypertension, diabetes, and cardiovascular disease, and is contraindicated if the patient is taking nitrates because of the potential for severe hypotensive effects.
2. Headache, flushing, and dyspepsia are the most common adverse effects reported. In addition, sildenafil is highly protein bound and may interact with many drugs. Mr. E. should check with the doctor before taking any other medication. In addition, he should report any visual changes immediately.
3. Older individuals experience declining liver function, so drugs may not be metabolized as effectively as when they were younger. In addition, there have been reports of vision loss in men who have been taking this class of drugs.
4. Sildenafil should be taken 1 hour before intercourse and no more than once a day.

CHAPTER 36 Antihistamines, Decongestants, Antitussives, and Expectorants

Chapter Review and NCLEX® Examination Preparation/Critical Thinking and Application

1. a, b, c, e
2. a
3. b, e
4. c
5. b
6. d
7. 15 mL (See Overview of Dosage Calculations, Section II.)
8. The antihistamines cannot push off histamine that is already bound to its receptor. Because they compete with histamine for unoccupied receptors, they work best when given early in a histamine-mediated reaction, before all of the histamine binds to receptors.
9. Yes. The traditional antihistamines have anticholinergic effects, which may make them more effective in some cases. Patients respond to and tolerate these drugs quite well. Also, because many traditional antihistamines are generically available at this time, they are often much less expensive.
10. No. Mrs. L. is likely experiencing rebound congestion caused by sustained use of the naphazoline for several days.
11. Keith is exhibiting symptoms of the cardiovascular effects that can occur when a topically applied adrenergic nasal decongestant is absorbed into the bloodstream. Usually the amount absorbed is too small to cause systemic effects at normal dosages. Excessive dosages of these medications, however, are more likely to cause systemic effects elsewhere in the body. These may include cardiovascular effects such as hypertension and palpitations and CNS effects such as headache, nervousness, and dizziness. These systemic effects are the result of alpha-adrenergic stimulation of the heart, blood vessels, and CNS.
12. Benzonatate's mechanism of action is entirely different from that of the other drugs. It suppresses the cough reflex by numbing the stretch receptors, which keeps the cough reflex from being stimulated in the medulla. It is associated with fewer drug interactions than the opioid antitussives and dextromethorphan.
13. The nurse will ask Irene whether she is taking any thyroid medication. A drug interaction (an additive hypothyroid effect) can occur if she takes an expectorant with an antithyroid drug. Irene should call her physician before she goes to the drugstore.
14. First, Lisa's brother received Robitussin A-C, an opioid antitussive containing codeine, for his cough. Lisa has been prescribed Robitussin, an expectorant, for her nonproductive cough associated with

bronchitis. Second, even if the two children were prescribed the same drug, Lisa is only 5 years old and requires a smaller dosage than her brother. Prescription medications should not be shared among family members.

15. Antihistamines should generally be used with caution lactating mothers. The decision will be made by weighing the drug's potential effect on the baby versus the need for her to take the medication.

Case Study

1. James's diabetes should not affect his treatment.
2. The topical diphenhydramine might come in combination with a drug such as calamine, camphor, or zinc oxide.
3. He should be informed that taking any of the sedating antihistamines may precipitate drowsiness, and so he should be instructed to avoid driving or operating heavy machinery should these side effects occur or until he knows how he responds to the medication.
4. James should also be informed not to consume alcohol or take other central nervous system depressants because they may interact with the diphenhydramine to exacerbate drowsiness and sedation.

CHAPTER 37
Bronchodilators and Other Respiratory Drugs

Chapter Review and NCLEX® Examination Preparation/Critical Thinking and Application

1. b, d, e, f
2. d
3. d
4. b
5. c
6. a
7. After 25 days (8 puffs per day, divided into 200 doses)
8. The cause of idiopathic (or intrinsic) asthma is unknown; allergic asthma is caused by hypersensitivity to an allergen in the environment. Idiopathic asthma is not mediated by immunoglobulin E, whereas allergic asthma is.
9. Tom is exhibiting some side effects of theophylline therapy, and the level in his blood is probably too high (the common therapeutic range for theophylline is a blood level of 10 to 20 mcg/dL). Tom may require a reduction in dosage.
10. Sylvia is exhibiting dose-related adverse effects of the albuterol, probably because she used it too frequently. Sylvia needs to be reminded to use her medication exactly as prescribed.
11. a. Anticholinergics, corticosteroids, and beta-agonists
    b. Of concern is Mrs. V.'s glaucoma. Use of anticholinergics is contraindicated in patients with glaucoma.
12. a. The disadvantage of administering the corticosteroids orally is that they can then lead to systemic effects, such as adrenocortical insufficiency, increased susceptibility to infection, fluid and electrolyte disturbances, endocrine effects, dermatologic effects, and nervous system effects. They can also interact with other systemically administered drugs. The advantage to administering corticosteroids by inhalation is that their action is limited to the topical site of action—the lungs. Thus they have no systemic effects and cannot interact with other systemically administered drugs.
    b. Yes. The use of an inhaled corticosteroid frequently allows for a reduction in the daily dose of the systemic corticosteroid. This reduction should be gradual.
13. It depends. Theophylline tablets come in regular and extended-release forms. The extended-release form, of course, cannot be crushed.
14. The albuterol is a beta-agonist that can be used to treat acute bronchospasms. The fluticasone is a corticosteroid and is not effective for acute bronchospasm. Fluticasone is useful for long-term management of asthma and works to reduce inflammation.
15. He needs to be reminded about foods and beverages that contain caffeine (e.g., chocolate, coffee, cola, cocoa, tea), because their consumption can exacerbate CNS stimulation.

Case Study

1. These drugs are not direct bronchodilators; they work to reduce the inflammatory response in the lungs.
2. They are primarily used for oral prophylaxis and chronic treatment of asthma and are not recommended for treatment of acute asthma attacks.
3. There are no interactions between ibuprofen and montelukast; however, Jennie should continue to check with her physician before taking other over-the-counter medications.
4. These drugs should be taken every night on a continuous schedule, even if symptoms improve.

CHAPTER 38
Antibiotics Part 1

Critical Thinking Crossword

Across

3. Prophylactic

6. Tetracycline
7. Penicillin
8. Bactericidal
9. Cephalosporin

Down

1. Macrolide
2. Sulfonamide
4. Bacteriostatic
5. Superinfection

Chapter Review and NCLEX® Examination Preparation/Critical Thinking and Application

1. b, d, e
2. a
3. b
4. c
5. d
6. d
7. b, c, d
8. 25 mL per dose. Each dose will contain 500,000 units (every 6 hours will be 4 doses per day; divide 2 million units per day by 4 to get 500,000 units per dose). (See Overview of Dosage Calculations, Section III.)
9. Cefoxitin (Mefoxin) is frequently used in patients undergoing abdominal or colorectal surgeries because it can effectively kill intestinal bacteria such as gram-positive, gram-negative, and anaerobic bacteria.
10. a. Sean should not take the doxycycline with milk because that can result in a significant reduction in the oral absorption of the drug. Sean should also be aware that tetracyclines can cause photosensitivity; he should stay out of the sun.
    b. The diarrhea is probably the result of alteration of the intestinal flora caused by the drug therapy.
11. She is experiencing a superinfection because the antibiotics she has been taking for her bronchitis have reduced the normal vaginal bacterial flora, and the yeast that is usually kept in balance by this normal flora has an opportunity to grow and cause an infection.

Case Study

1. He should be assessed for renal problems and blood dyscrasias. Also, the use of co-trimoxazole is contraindicated in cases of known drug allergy to sulfonamides or chemically related drugs such as sulfonylureas (used for diabetes), thiazide and loop diuretics, and carbonic anhydrase inhibitors.
2. If he is taking a sulfonylurea for his type 2 diabetes, close monitoring is needed, because sulfonamides can potentiate the hypoglycemic effects of sulfonylureas in patients with diabetes. In addition, although he is currently receiving intravenous heparin and not warfarin, he may be switched to oral anticoagulants soon, so you should keep in mind that sulfonamides can potentiate the anticoagulant effects of warfarin and lead to hemorrhage.
3. These antibiotics achieve very high concentrations in the kidneys, through which they are eliminated. Therefore, they are primarily used in the treatment of urinary tract infections.
4. Sulfonamides do not actually destroy bacteria but inhibit their growth. For this reason they are considered bacteriostatic antibiotics. Bactericidal antibiotics kill bacteria.

CHAPTER 39
Antibiotics Part 2

Chapter Review and NCLEX® Examination Preparation/Critical Thinking and Application

1. c
2. b
3. a
4. a, b, c, d
5. a, b, e
6. 40 mL (See Overview of Dosage Calculations, Section II.)
7. The current practice is once-a-day aminoglycoside dosing. The nurse can tell her that studies have shown that once-daily dosing provides a sufficient plasma drug concentration to kill bacteria and also has either an equal or lower risk of toxicity compared with multiple daily dosing. Hopefully this type of dosing will be safer and more effective for her.
8. A blood sample for measurement of "trough" level is drawn at least 18 hours after a dose is given (24 hours if the patient has renal impairment). The therapeutic goal is a trough level at or below 1 mcg/mL. If the trough level is above 2 mcg/mL, then the patient is at greater risk for ototoxicity and nephrotoxicity. Trough levels are normally monitored initially then once every 5 to 7 days until the drug therapy is discontinued. The patient's serum creatinine level should also be measured at least every 3 days as an index of renal function, and drug dosages should be adjusted as needed for any changes in renal function.
9. Yes. In patients who receive amiodarone therapy, dangerous cardiac dysrhythmias are more likely to occur when quinolones are taken. Hopefully another drug besides levofloxacin has shown effectiveness against the bacteria that is causing his infection.
10. Nitrofurantoin is used primarily to treat urinary tract infections because it is renally excreted and concentrates in the urine. It can cause significant renal impairment.

Case Study

1. Ototoxicity and nephrotoxicity. Symptoms of ototoxicity include dizziness, tinnitus, and hearing loss.

Symptoms of nephrotoxicity include urinary casts, proteinuria, and increased blood urea nitrogen and serum creatinine levels. Keeping the drug blood levels (peak and trough) within a specific therapeutic range can help prevent those toxicities.

2. The aminoglycosides and penicillins are often used together because they have a synergistic effect; that is, the combined effect of the two drugs is greater than that of either drug alone.
3. Yes, there is a concern! The desired trough level is 1 mcg/mL, so a level of 3 mcg/mL could mean that he is receiving a dose that is too high. The increased serum creatinine level is also a concern because it could be an indication of impaired renal function. The physician should be notified immediately and doses of the aminoglycoside withheld until the physician responds.

CHAPTER 40
Antiviral Drugs

Chapter Review and NCLEX® Examination Preparation/Critical Thinking and Application

1. d
2. d
3. a
4. c
5. a, b
6. 5 mL
7. Any drug that kills a virus can also kill healthy cells. Viruses must enter cells to replicate. Therefore, antiviral drugs must also enter the host cells. Few drugs can kill only the virus and leave the body's cells unharmed. Viruses are also difficult to kill because often by the time they are discovered, they have finished replicating. At that point, it is too late for antiviral drugs, which interfere with viral replication, to work.
8. Yes. Zidovudine, one of the few anti–human immunodeficiency virus (HIV) drugs known to prolong patient survival, can be used for maternal and fetal treatment. During the pregnancy, Amy can receive the oral form of the drug. During labor she can receive the drug intravenously. Drug therapy for the infant can begin within 12 hours of delivery and continue for 6 weeks.
9. a. Acyclovir (Zovirax) is indicated for the herpes zoster (shingles).
   b. Bailey's daily fluid intake should be at least 2400 mL while she is taking the acyclovir. Also, acyclovir capsules may be taken with food.
   c. Bailey will be treated with acyclovir again; it is the drug of choice for treatment of both initial and recurrent episodes of shingles.
10. a. Ribavirin is used to treat infections caused by respiratory syncytial virus.
    b. Yes. Brenda's treatment will last at least 3 days but not longer than 7 days.
11. The patient may be experiencing zidovudine's major dose-limiting adverse effect, which is bone marrow suppression.
12. No. The nurse's co-worker is doing fine. Acyclovir administered by intravenous infusion is first diluted in the solution recommended by the manufacturer and is administered slowly over at least 1 hour to prevent renal damage.
13. No. Therapy with oseltamivir (Tamiflu) should begin within 2 days of the onset of influenza. It is probably too late for this medication to be effective for Stacy.
14. Ganciclovir may be administered to *prevent* CMV disease (generalized infection) in high-risk patients, such as those receiving organ transplants.

Case Study

1. Mr. C. should use a glove when applying topical acyclovir (Zovirax) to the affected area, which should be kept clean and dry. Also, he should not use any other creams or ointments on the area.
2. Mr. C.'s herpes infection cannot be "cured," although the acyclovir will help to manage the symptoms.
3. Stress the importance of treatment for Mr. C. and his sexual partner, and discuss with him how to prevent transmission of the virus.
4. There are several viruses in the *Herpesviridae* family, including herpes simplex type 1 (HSV-1), which causes mucocutaneous herpes—usually blisters around the mouth; varicella-zoster virus (herpes simplex type 3, or HSV-3), which causes both chickenpox and shingles; herpesvirus type 4 (also called Epstein-Barr virus or EBV); and herpesvirus type 8, which is believed by some to cause Kaposi's sarcoma, a cancer associated with acquired immunodeficiency syndrome (AIDS).

CHAPTER 41
Antitubercular Drugs

Chapter Review and NCLEX® Examination Preparation/Critical Thinking and Application

1. a
2. b
3. a, b, c
4. c
5. a
6. 3 tablets (See Overview of Dosage Calculations, Sections I & II.)
7. a. Liver function studies should be performed because isoniazid can cause hepatic impairment.

A complete blood count, including hemoglobin level and hematocrit value, should be checked because of the hematologic disorders isoniazid can cause. In addition, an eye examination is important because the drug may cause visual disturbances.

b. Diane may be a slow acetylator. Acetylation, the process by which isoniazid is metabolized in the liver, requires certain enzymes to break down the isoniazid. In slow acetylators, who have a genetic deficiency of these enzymes, the isoniazid accumulates. The dosage of isoniazid may need to be adjusted downward in these patients.

8. a. Streptomycin is administered intramuscularly, deep into a large muscle mass, and the sites are rotated.
   b. The side effects and adverse effects of streptomycin are ototoxicity, nephrotoxicity, and blood dyscrasias.
   c. Although it may not be a concern in terms of Ms. I.'s streptomycin therapy, oral contraceptives become ineffective when given with rifampin. If rifampin is part of her therapy, Ms. I. should switch to another form of birth control.
9. A thorough eye examination may be called for before therapy is initiated, because ethambutol can cause a decrease in visual acuity resulting from optic neuritis, which is also a contraindication to the use of ethambutol. In addition, isoniazid may cause optic neuritis and visual disturbances.
10. a. Mr. F. needs to know that his compliance with therapy is essential for achieving a cure. Although he is keeping his follow-up appointments, Mr. F. also needs to take his medication as ordered. He should be warned not to consume alcohol, and he should be encouraged to take care of himself by ensuring adequate nutrition, rest, and relaxation.
    b. The therapeutic response can be confirmed by results of laboratory studies (sputum culture and sensitivity tests) and chest radiographic findings.
11. a. Frannie, like all patients taking antitubercular drugs, needs to be compliant with the therapy regimen and keep her follow-up appointments. She should be reminded that she can spread the disease (during the initial period of the illness); she should wash her hands frequently and cover her mouth when coughing or sneezing. Frannie also needs adequate nutrition and rest.
    b. It is likely that Frannie is on rifampin therapy. She should be told that her urine, stool, saliva, sputum, sweat, and tears may become red-orange-brown in color and that this is an effect of rifampin therapy.

Case Study

1. George's gout is a consideration; pyrazinamide can cause hyperuricemia, so gout or flare-ups of gout can occur in susceptible patients. His diabetes is a concern too; ethambutol should be used cautiously in patients with diabetes. A baseline hearing test should be performed if streptomycin is considered, because this drug may cause ototoxicity.
2. An individual with a genetic deficiency of the liver enzymes that metabolize drugs can be classified as a "slow acetylator." When isoniazid is taken by slow acetylators, the drug accumulates because there are not enough of the enzymes to break down the isoniazid. As a result, the dosage of isoniazid may need to be reduced.
3. Results of liver function studies should be assessed carefully before therapy is initiated, because some drugs (isoniazid, pyrazinamide) are hepatotoxic. Liver function test results should be monitored closely during therapy as well.
4. Patients should take pyridoxine (vitamin B_6) as prescribed by the physician to prevent some of the neurologic side effects of isoniazid, such as numbness and tingling of the extremities (peripheral neuritis).

CHAPTER 42
Antifungal Drugs

Chapter Review and NCLEX® Examination Preparation/Critical Thinking and Application

1. j
2. e
3. f
4. g
5. a
6. c
7. h
8. i
9. d
10. b
11. c
12. b, c, e
13. d
14. b
15. a
16. 50 mL/hour (See Overview of Dosage Calculations, Section V.)
17. Mycotic infections are very difficult to treat and research into new drugs has occurred at a slow pace, in part because the necessary chemical concentrations of the experimental drugs cannot be tolerated by humans.
18. a. Fluconazole (Diflucan), unlike itraconazole and other azoles, can pass into the cerebrospinal fluid, which makes it useful in the treatment of cryptococcal meningitis.

b. Unfortunately, Mr. K. will need to remain on the medication (at a reduced dosage) for 10 to 12 weeks after the negative results on his cerebrospinal fluid culture.

19. a. The amphotericin B should be diluted according to the manufacturer's guidelines and administered using an infusion pump. The nurse must not use solutions that are cloudy or that have visible precipitates.
    b. Fever, chills, hypotension, tachycardia, malaise, anorexia, nausea and vomiting, and headache are possible adverse effects.
    c. No. Almost all patients experience these effects. To decrease their severity, the patient may be pretreated with antipyretic (e.g., acetaminophen), antihistamines, and antiemetics.
20. Lewis should be aware that he will be taking the medication for 2 to 6 weeks, until the infection clears. During that time, he should avoid alcohol because of the increased risk for hepatoxicity, and he should take the medication with food to avoid gastrointestinal upset. Some antifungal medications also causes photophobia, so Lewis should avoid the sun or use sunscreen and sunglasses with ultraviolet protection.
21. Nystatin oral troches or lozenges should be dissolved slowly and completely in the mouth for the best effects and should not be chewed or swallowed. Chrissie needs a review of how to use this medication.
22. Lipid formulations of amphotericin B have been developed in an attempt to decrease the incidence of its adverse effects and increase its efficacy. The disadvantage is that they are more expensive than conventional amphotericin B.

Case Study

1. Voriconazole is used to treat major fungal infections in patients who do not tolerate or respond to other antifungal drugs.
2. Use of voriconazole is contraindicated in patients taking other drugs that are metabolized by cytochrome P-450 enzyme 3A4 (e.g., quinidine) because of the risk of inducing serious cardiac dysrhythmias.
3. Careful cardiac monitoring should be performed if Sally is also taking quinidine while taking this antifungal drug.

CHAPTER 43 Antimalarial, Antiprotozoal, and Anthelmintic Drugs

Chapter Review and NCLEX® Examination Preparation/Critical Thinking and Application

1. a
2. b
3. c
4. b, e
5. d
6. c
7. The dose is 280 mg (4 mg/kg × 70 kg); the nurse will draw up 4.6 mL of the diluted solution for the infusion. (See Overview of Dosage Calculations, Section III.)
8. Malaria is caused by Plasmodium organisms. During the asexual stage of the Plasmodium life cycle, which occurs in the human host, the parasite resides for a while outside the erythrocyte; this is called the *exoerythrocytic phase*. The most effective drug for eradicating the parasite during this phase is primaquine.
9. Before primaquine is administered, Professor H. should be given a pregnancy test. This is a pregnancy category C drug, so you will need to know if certain precautions are needed in Professor H.'s case. She should also be assessed for hypersensitivity, anemia, lupus erythematosus, methemoglobinemia, porphyria, rheumatoid arthritis, methemoglobin reductase deficiency, and glucose-6-phosphate dehydrogenase (G6PD) deficiency.
10. Mefloquine is indicated for the treatment of chloroquine-resistant malaria. Quinine, an older drug, may also be used. Quinine can be used alone but is more commonly given in combination with pyrimethamine, a sulfonamide, or a tetracycline (such as doxycycline).
11. Each of these three patients has a protozoal infection. The patient with the intestinal disorder has giardiasis. The patient with acquired immunodeficiency syndrome (AIDS) has pneumocystosis. The patient with the sexually transmitted disease has trichomoniasis. See Table 43-3 for specific drugs used to treat these diseases.

Case Study

1. Intestinal roundworms are diagnosed based on symptoms and examination of stool specimens.
2. Contraindications include allergy to the medication and pregnancy. Even though she is only 15 years of age, she should be assessed for possible pregnancy before this medication is given. In addition, her liver function test results should be assessed, because use of pyrantel is contraindicated in patients with liver disease.
3. Based on her weight of 57 kg, the dose for her would be 627 mg (11 mg × 57 kg).
4. Adverse effects of pyrantel therapy include headache, dizziness, insomnia, and skin rashes, as well as anorexia, cramps, diarrhea, nausea, and vomiting.

CHAPTER 44
Antiinflammatory and Antigout Drugs

Chapter Review and NCLEX® Examination Preparation/Critical Thinking and Application

1. b
2. b
3. a, b, d, e
4. c
5. d
6. a
7. a. Yes. The safe range of acetaminophen dosage for this infant is 27 to 40.5 mg (based on 2.7 kg weight); 30 mg falls within this range.
   b. 0.3 mL per dose of 30 mg (See Overview of Dosage Calculations, Section IV.)
8. Symptoms of both salicylism (chronic salicylate intoxication) and acute salicylate overdose are similar except that the effects are often more pronounced and occur more quickly in the acute form. Acute salicylate overdose results from the ingestion of a single toxic dose. Chronic salicylate intoxication occurs as a result of either high dosages or prolonged therapy with high dosages.
9. Treatment of acute salicylate overdose consists of removing the salicylate from the gastrointestinal tract and preventing its absorption; correcting fluid, electrolyte, and acid-base disturbances; and implementing measures to enhance salicylate elimination, including hemodialysis.
10. Mr. C. has an acute overdose of a nonsalicylate nonsteroidal antiinflammatory drug (NSAID). If the condition progresses, symptoms can include intense headache, dizziness, cerebral edema, cardiac arrest, and even death.
11. His treatment will consist of removing the NSAID from the gastrointestinal tract, followed by administration of activated charcoal. Supportive and symptomatic treatment will be implemented. Hemodialysis, however, is not helpful with this type of overdose.
12. Mr. H. needs to know that compliance with the entire medical regimen is important for the success of his treatment for gout. Allopurinol should be taken with meals to help prevent the occurrence of gastrointestinal symptoms such as nausea, vomiting, and anorexia. Fluids should be increased to 3 liters per day, and hazardous activities should be avoided if dizziness or drowsiness occurs with the medication. Also, alcohol and caffeine should be avoided, because these drugs will increase uric acid levels and decrease the levels of allopurinol.
13. Ketorolac (Toradol) is indicated for the short-term management (up to 5 days) of moderate to severe acute pain that requires analgesia at the opioid level. It is not indicated for treatment of minor or chronic painful conditions.
14. The main adverse effects of ketorolac (Toradol) include renal impairment, gastrointestinal pain, dyspepsia, and nausea. These problems limit the length of time that the medication can be used.
15. The vinegary odor means that the aspirin has experienced some chemical breakdown, and she should not use it! She should discard it safely and purchase a new bottle.

Case Study

1. The specific COX-2 selectivity of these drugs allows them to control the inflammation and pain without producing some of the toxicity associated with NSAID therapy.
2. The most common adverse effects include fatigue, dizziness, lower extremity edema, hypertension, dyspepsia, nausea, heartburn, and epigastric discomfort. Any stomach pain, unusual bleeding, or blood in vomit or stool should be reported to the physician immediately. Chest pain, palpitations, and any gastrointestinal problems should be reported as well.
3. Celecoxib should not be used in patients with known sulfa allergy.
4. She should avoid alcohol and aspirin while taking this medication and should check with her physician before taking any over-the-counter medications.

CHAPTER 45
Immunosuppressant Drugs

Chapter Review and NCLEX® Examination Preparation/Critical Thinking and Application

1. b
2. c
3. c
4. a
5. a, c, d, e
6. a
7. a. 750 mg for this dose
   b. 15 mL (See Overview of Dosage Calculations, Section II.)
8. a. Daclizumab can help prevent organ rejection. If her immune system cannot recognize the new kidney as foreign, it will not mount an immune response against it.
   b. Laboratory tests should include hemoglobin level, hematocrit, white blood cell count, and platelet count. These studies should be done before, during, and after therapy. If the leukocyte count should drop below 3000/mm^3, the drug should be discontinued after the physician is notified.

c. The antifungal drug is added several days before surgery as prophylaxis for Candida infections.
9. Encourage the patient to take the drug with meals or mixed with chocolate milk, milk, or orange juice to prevent stomach upset.
10. Styrofoam containers or cups should be avoided, because the drug has been found to adhere to the inside wall of such containers. The nurse needs to find a glass or cup that is not made of Styrofoam.
11. Tess is experiencing symptoms consistent with adverse effects of muromonab-CD3. The nurse will need to monitor her closely for signs of fluid retention and pulmonary edema.
12. Glatiramer acetate is the only immunosuppressant drug that is currently indicated for the treatment of relapsing-remitting multiple sclerosis. Hopefully it will help to reduce the frequency of his relapses.

Case Study

1. Yes, immunosuppressant therapy will be lifelong.
2. White patches on the tongue, mucous membranes, and oral pharynx would be indicative of candidiasis.
3. Mr. K. needs to be seen by a physician immediately. These symptoms could indicate that he has a severe infection.
4. If the leukocyte count drops below 3000/mm^3, then the drug should be discontinued, because he is experiencing a severely immunosuppressed state.

CHAPTER 46
Immunizing Drugs and Biochemical Terrorism

Chapter Review and NCLEX® Examination Preparation/Critical Thinking and Application

1. a. Zoster vaccine (Zostavax)
   b. Active
   c. Active
   d. *Haemophilus influenzae* type b prophylaxis
   e. Hepatitis B virus vaccine (inactivated)
   f. Rh_0(D) immune globulin
   g. Passive
   h. Active
   i. Tuberculosis prophylaxis
   j. Active
   k. Diphtheria, tetanus, and pertussis prophylaxis, pediatric
   l. Passive
   m. Postexposure passive tetanus prophylaxis
   n. Active
   o. Diphtheria and tetanus prophylaxis (pediatric and adult)
2. b
3. d
4. a
5. a
6. c
7. a, c
8. 0.005 mg (See Overview of Dosage Calculations, Section I.)
9. Sometimes, after vaccination, the levels of antibodies against a particular pathogen decline over time and a second dose of the vaccine is given to restore the antibody titers to a level that can protect the person against the infection. This second dose is referred to as a *booster shot*.
10. Each year a new influenza vaccine is developed that contains three influenza virus strains that represent the strains most likely to circulate in the United States in the upcoming winter. The vaccination from the previous year may not be effective for the influenza virus strains occurring in the current year.
11. Carl may experience localized swelling, redness, discomfort, and warmth at the injection site. Acetaminophen and rest are recommended for the relief of these side effects, and application of warm compresses to the injection site may also help ease some of the discomfort.
12. There are three routes of inoculation (what the neighbor calls "types") of anthrax: cutaneous, inhalational, and gastrointestinal. Of the three, anthrax contracted by inhalation of the bacterial spores is the most deadly and has a mortality rate of more than 80%.
13. Paul is experiencing more than the expected adverse effects of his vaccinations. He is probably experiencing "serum sickness," which may occur after repeated injections of equine-derived immunizing drugs. Because his symptoms may indicate respiratory impairment, he needs to be taken to the hospital for evaluation and monitoring. He may receive analgesics, antihistamines, epinephrine, and/or corticosteroids to treat this reaction.

Case Study

1. Rabies is a very potent virus.
2. Those at high risk for rabies exposure, such as veterinarians, will receive the rabies virus vaccine (Imovax, RabAvert) as preexposure prophylaxis, followed by booster shots every 2 to 5 years based on blood titers. This is a type of active immunization.
3. You will receive drugs that give both active and passive immunization. Postexposure prophylaxis consists of injections of the rabies virus vaccine (see answer 2) and also rabies immune globulin (Imogam Rabies-HT). Because rabies can progress so rapidly, the body does not have time to mount an adequate immune defense—death occurs before it can do so. The passive immunization confers a temporary protection that is usually sufficient to keep the invading organism from causing death, even though it does

not stimulate an antibody response. The active immunization you receive will stimulate an antibody response.

4. The rabies virus vaccine will be given intramuscularly on the day of exposure (day 0) and on days 3, 7, and 14, with 1 dose of rabies immune globulin given within 8 days of the first vaccine dose. The rabies immune globulin is given as a single dose (20 international unit/kg); as much of the dose as possible is infiltrated into the bite wound area, and the remainder is given intramuscularly—but not in the same injection site as the rabies vaccine.

CHAPTER 47
Antineoplastic Drugs Part 1: Cancer Overview and Cell Cycle–Specific Drugs

Critical Thinking Crossword

Across

3. Spread
4. Folic
7. Extravasation
8. Nadir
9. Limiting
10. Leukemia

Down

1. Malignant
2. Leucovorin
5. Nonspecific
6. Benign
7. Emetic

Chapter Review and NCLEX® Examination Preparation/Critical Thinking and Application

1. a, b, c, e, f
2. d
3. a
4. b
5. c
6. d
7. a. 8.2 mg
   b. 8.2 mL

Case Study

1. Methotrexate is an antimetabolite—specifically, a folic acid antagonist. It inhibits the action of an enzyme that is responsible for converting folic acid to a substance used by the cell to synthesize DNA for cell reproduction. As a result, the cell dies.
2. Laboratory test results should be checked for white blood cell and red blood cell counts, hemoglobin level and hematocrit, platelet counts, and renal and liver function studies.
3. The concurrent administration of nonsteroidal antiinflammatory drugs (NSAIDs) and methotrexate may lead to severe bleeding tendencies. Allen should be instructed to avoid all NSAIDs, including aspirin, while taking methotrexate.
4. Antiemetic therapy and antacids are often needed to decrease nausea, vomiting, and gastrointestinal upset. Because methotrexate may cause hyperuricemia (increased uric acid levels) associated with tumor lysis syndrome, allopurinol (Zyloprim) may be given. Leucovorin may be used to protect the patient from potentially fatal bone marrow suppression, a toxic effect of methotrexate.

CHAPTER 48
Antineoplastic Drugs Part 2: Cell Cycle–Nonspecific and Miscellaneous Drugs

Chapter Review and NCLEX® Examination Preparation/Critical Thinking and Application

1. c
2. a
3. b
4. a, c, e, f
5. a
6. d
7. 46 mL/hr (rounded up from 45.5) (See Overview of Dosage Calculations, Section V.)
8. Cytoprotective drugs help to reduce the toxicity of various antineoplastics. As a result, the adverse effects may be reduced or increased dosages of the antineoplastic medication may be tolerated, which allows greater cancer cell kill. Examples include:
   - Amifostine (Ethyol) used during therapy with cisplatin
   - Dexrazoxane (Zinecard), used during therapy with doxorubicin
   - Leucovorin (Wellcovorin) and allopurinol (Zyloprim), used during therapy with methotrexate (Chapter 47)
9. Patients receiving bleomycin must be monitored closely for the development of pulmonary fibrosis and pneumonitis. Mrs. S. needs to be assessed carefully for these possible problems.
10. No! In most facilities, institutional guidelines direct that the pharmacy department mix these drugs. Special requirements must be met for the safety of those working with these drugs, including the use of a laminar airflow hood and appropriate personal protection equipment (such as gown, mask, and gloves). It would not be safe for the nurse or for those around her to mix the chemotherapy drug on the nursing unit.
11. The nurse will stop the infusion immediately but won't pull out the intravenous catheter quite yet. The physician should be notified immediately, and the nurse should expect to receive orders to treat this extravasation of mechlorethamine by injecting a

solution of 10% sodium thiosulfate and sterile water (see Table 48-2) through the existing line into the extravasated site (then remove the line) as well as multiple subcutaneous injections into the site. Over the next few hours, the patient will receive repeated subcutaneous injections into the area, and cold compresses should be applied to the site.

Case Study

1. Nephrotoxicity (possible damage to the kidneys), peripheral neuropathy (possible damage to peripheral nerves), and ototoxicity (possible damage to hearing).
2. Baseline renal studies should be performed, because this drug is highly nephrotoxic. If Dottie is receiving any other drugs that are potentially nephrotoxic (such as aminoglycoside therapy), dosage changes will need to be considered. If she has gout, concurrent use of cisplatin may result in hyperuricemia or worsening of the gout. Baseline auditory studies should be performed, as well as baseline liver function studies and measurement of white blood cell count, hemoglobin level, hematocrit, and platelet level, because of the anticipated bone marrow suppression.
3. Because peripheral neuropathies may occur, numbness, tingling, or pain in the extremities should be reported to the physician immediately to prevent complications and enhance comfort.
4. Yes, this is a concern, because dehydration while taking cisplatin may lead to renal damage. Patients who are at home after treatment with this drug should be reminded of the importance of hydration and should be told to contact the physician if they experience dry mucous membranes, very dark amber urine, or little or no urinary output, or vomiting of large amounts over a period of 8 hours or less. It may be a challenge, but she needs to try to take in 3000 mL of fluid per day to prevent dehydration.

CHAPTER 49
Biologic Response–Modifying and Antirheumatoid Drugs

Chapter Review and NCLEX® Examination Preparation/Critical Thinking and Application

1. e
2. a
3. g
4. b
5. h
6. d
7. c
8. d
9. b
10. a, b, c, d, e
11. c
12. 1.3 mL (See Overview of Dosage Calculations, Section III.)
13. The major dose-limiting side effect of interferons is fatigue. Patients taking high dosages become so exhausted that they are often confined to bed. Sonja needs to know this before she starts the therapy.
14. Colony-stimulating factors (CSFs) such as filgrastim (Neupogen), pegfilgrastim (Neulasta), and sargramostim (Leukine) can be given for chemotherapy-induced leukopenia. These drugs should be administered 24 hours after the chemotherapy drugs have been given, because the myelosuppressive effects of the chemotherapy drugs tend to cancel out the therapeutic benefits of the CSFs.
15. She will receive oprelvekin (Neumega), which is given via subcutaneous injections daily for up to 21 days. Because she has severe thrombocytopenia, however, the nurse must be careful to prevent excessive bleeding and bruising at the injection sites and to teach Brittany measures to reduce bleeding risks.
16. Methotrexate is given *weekly*, not daily! The nurse needs to clarify and correct this mistranscribed order. It is very important to note that the drug is given once per week, not once per day. Serious medication errors, including deaths, have occurred when the drug is given daily instead of once a week.

Case Study

1. Epoetin alfa is a synthetic derivative of the human hormone erythropoietin, which is produced primarily by the kidneys. It promotes the synthesis of erythrocytes (red blood cells) by stimulating the production of red blood cell precursors.
2. Hemoglobin level and hematocrit should be monitored carefully. If therapy is not halted when the target hemoglobin level of 12 g/dL is reached or if the hemoglobin level and hematocrit rise too quickly, hypertension and seizures can result.
3. The drug is synthetically manufactured in mass quantities by means of recombinant DNA technology. This technology allows the drug to be essentially identical to its endogenously produced counterpart in the body.
4. Epoetin can be given either intravenously or subcutaneously; for administration at home, she will need to be taught subcutaneous administration.
5. Darbepoetin alfa (Aranesp) can be given weekly, so that the number of injections is reduced.

CHAPTER 50
Acid-Controlling Drugs

Chapter Review and NCLEX® Examination Preparation/Critical Thinking and Application

1. h
2. e
3. i
4. k
5. c
6. a, b
7. f
8. d
9. b
10. g
11. b
12. c
13. d
14. b, d, e
15. b
16. 200 mL/hr (See Overview of Dosage Calculations, Section V.)
17. You need to let him know that long-term self-medication with antacids may mask symptoms of serious underlying diseases. He needs to be evaluated for possible bleeding ulcer or even a malignancy, but you may not want to scare him with those possibilities! If his current self-treatment is no longer working, he needs a medical evaluation.
18. Omeprazole should be taken before meals, and the capsule should be taken whole, not crushed, opened, or chewed. Omeprazole may also be given with antacids, if ordered.
19. Patients with heart failure or hypertension should use antacids that are low in sodium. He should also be told to take the antacid alone, not at the same time as other medications (unless specifically instructed to do so), because the antacid will interfere with the absorption of the other medications. Antacids should be taken 1 hour before or 1 to 2 hours after other medications. If symptoms continue or worsen, he should consult his health care provider.
20. Antacids may promote premature dissolving of the enteric coating; if the coating is destroyed early in the stomach, gastrointestinal upset may occur. He should take the aspirin tablets with food, not with antacids.
21. Regimen 1 therapy is one of eight FDA-approved regimens for eradication of *Helicobacter pylori*. It consists of therapy with both the proton pump inhibitor omeprazole and the antibiotic clarithromycin in specific dosages for each.

Case Study

1. Although histamine-2 (H_2) antagonists are available over the counter, the dose of the over-the-counter preparation will not be the same strength as the usual dose of the prescription formulation.
2. The drug effects of the H_2 blockers are limited to specific blocking actions on the parietal cells of the gastric glands in the stomach. As a result, hydrogen ion production is decreased, which leads to an increase in the pH of the stomach (i.e., decreased stomach acid).
3. Use of H_2 receptor antagonists is contraindicated in patients with known drug allergy or impaired renal function or liver disease. Cautious use is recommended in patients who are confused, disoriented, or older. Interactions may occur with drugs that have a narrow therapeutic range. Caution should be used if she is taking theophylline for her asthma. Patients requiring these medications should avoid aspirin and other nonsteroidal antiinflammatory drugs, alcohol, and caffeine because of their ulcerogenic or gastrointestinal tract–irritating effects.
4. Smoking has been shown to decrease the effectiveness of H_2 blockers because the absorption of H_2 antagonists is impaired in individuals who smoke. Hopefully if she herself is not smoking, this will not be a problem for her, but spending several hours in a smoke-filled room may have an effect. Also, the beer and possibly spicy pizza may aggravate the underlying condition.

CHAPTER 51
Bowel Disorder Drugs

Critical Thinking Crossword

Across

6. Emollient
7. Probiotic
8. Saline
9. Bulk-forming

Down

1. Adsorbent
2. Opiates
3. Hyperosmotic
4. Stimulant
5. Anticholinergic

Chapter Review and NCLEX® Examination Preparation/Critical Thinking and Application

1. d
2. a
3. d
4. c
5. a, d
6. 7.5 mL (See Overview of Dosage Calculations, Section II.)
7. Darkening of the tongue or stool is a temporary and harmless side effect associated with the use of bismuth subsalicylate (Pepto-Bismol).

8. Use of the belladonna alkaloid preparations, such as Donnatal, are contraindicated in patients with narrow-angle glaucoma. She should not use this drug.
9. Several factors may be causing Hillary's constipation: lack of proper exercise, poor diet (which might involve inadequate roughage and an excess of dairy products), use of aluminum-containing antacids, and stress.
10. a. The bulk-forming laxatives tend to produce normal stools, have few systemic effects, and are among the safest available.
    b. Ira should mix the medication with at least 6 to 8 oz of fluid and drink it immediately. He should never take it dry.
11. a. Because glycerin is very mild, it is often used in children.
    b. Abdominal bloating and rectal irritation
12. a. It will probably be determined based on Kyle's weight.
    b. She should not give Kyle any more medication, and she should contact the physician immediately.

Case Study

1. Antibiotic therapy destroys the balance of normal flora in the intestines, and diarrhea-causing bacteria proliferate.
2. *Lactobacillus acidophilus* is indicated for diarrhea caused by antibiotic treatment that has destroyed the normal intestinal flora.
3. Exogenously supplying these bacteria helps restore the balance of normal flora and suppress the growth of diarrhea-causing bacteria.
4. It is considered a dietary supplement. It is often used to treat uncomplicated diarrhea, although this is an off-label use (not approved by the Food and Drug Administration).

CHAPTER 52
Antiemetic and Antinausea Drugs

Chapter Review and NCLEX® Examination Preparation/Critical Thinking and Application

1. a
2. c, e
3. d
4. c
5. b
6. d
7. 30 mL (See Overview of Dosage Calculations, Section II.)
8. a. Petra should take the metoclopramide 30 minutes before meals and at bedtime.
   b. Petra should be cautioned about taking her medication with alcohol because of the possible toxicity and central nervous system depression that can occur.
9. This drug comes in oral, intramuscular, intravenous, and rectal forms, but because she on "nothing-by-mouth" status and has no intravenous access, the intramuscular route was ordered. The nurse can call her physician to get an order for an alternate route but cannot change the route without an order, because the dosage may also be different.
10. Dronabinol is a synthetic derivative of the major active substance in marijuana. The nurse explains to him that it is used to stimulate appetite and weight gain in patients with acquired immunodeficiency syndrome (AIDS).

Case Study

1. There are no significant drug interactions associated with the serotonin blockers such as ondansetron.
2. Antiemetics are often administered before a chemotherapy drug is given, frequently 1/2 to 3 hours before treatment.
3. The headache is caused by the ondansetron and can be relieved with acetaminophen.

CHAPTER 53
Vitamins and Minerals

Chapter Review and NCLEX® Examination Preparation/Critical Thinking and Application

1. c
2. g
3. b
4. h
5. e
6. k
7. i
8. d
9. j
10. a
11. l
12. f
13. a, d, e
14. b
15. d
16. d
17. 1 mL (See Overview of Dosage Calculations, Section III.)
18. By "endogenous," the physician meant the form of vitamin D synthesized in the skin through exposure to ultraviolet radiation. Dietary sources of vitamin D include fish oils, salmon, sardines, and herring; fortified milk, bread, and cereals; and animal livers, tuna fish, eggs, and butter.
19. a. Pernicious anemia

   b. The oral absorption of cyanocobalamin (vitamin B_{12}, or extrinsic factor) requires the presence of intrinsic factor, which is a glycoprotein secreted by gastric parietal cells. Damage to the gastrointestinal tract may reduce the amount of intrinsic factor available.
   c. The patient education card for Ms. E. should focus on foods containing cyanocobalamin; these include foods of animal origin such as liver, kidney, fish, shellfish, meat, and dairy products.
20. To avoid venous irritation, calcium should be properly diluted and given via an infusion pump when given intravenously. It should be infused slowly (less than 1 mL/min for adults) to avoid cardiac dysrhythmias and cardiac arrest. The physician is correct in ordering infusion with 1% procaine. This will reduce vasospasm and dilute the effects of calcium on surrounding tissues. In either case, monitor for extravasation; if it occurs, you should discontinue administration immediately.

Case Study

1. Broad-spectrum antibiotics can inhibit the intestinal flora, which provide the body with vitamin K_2. As a result, a deficiency may occur. Vitamin K can be given either orally or by injection in adults.
2. Vitamin K is essential for the synthesis of blood coagulation factors, which takes place in the liver.
3. Deficiency states can also be seen in newborns because of malabsorption attributable to inadequate amounts of bile. The deficiency may also be seen in patients receiving specific anticoagulants (i.e., warfarin) that inhibit hepatic vitamin K activity.
4. Dietary sources of vitamin K are green leafy vegetables (cabbage, spinach, etc.), meats, and milk.

CHAPTER 54
Nutritional Supplements

Critical Thinking Crossword

Across

1. Erythromycin
4. Anabolism
5. Gastrostomy
8. Absorptive
10. Fatty acid
11. Essential
12. Nitrogen

Down

2. Catabolism
3. Enteral
6. Semiessential
7. Metabolism
8. Arginine
9. Phlebitis

Chapter Review and NCLEX® Examination Preparation/Critical Thinking and Application

1. a
2. c
3. a, c, d, e
4. c
5. a
6. d
7. 1680 mL over 24 hours
8. a. Advantages of the newer tubes are that they are thinner, have a smaller diameter, and are more pliable for better patient tolerance. However, they also make checking for gastric aspiration more difficult.
   b. Patients who suffer from this condition experience cramping, diarrhea, abdominal bloating, and flatulence with the ingestion of lactose. In this case, lactose-free solutions should be used.
   c. The residual should not be more than 2 hours' worth of feeding—in this case, no more than 100 mL. You should return the aspirate, withhold the feeding, elevate the head of the bed, and notify the physician.
9. Mr. R. shows signs of fluid overload. The first thing you should do is slow his infusion rate, then remain with him and contact the physician immediately. Continually assess his vital signs. Next time you can prevent this by maintaining intravenous rates, assessing the intravenous infusion every hour, and monitoring the patient's fluid status.

Case Study

1. If total parenteral nutrition is discontinued abruptly, rebound hypoglycemia may occur because the pancreas has not had time to adjust to the reduced blood glucose levels. Hypoglycemia is manifested by cold, clammy skin; dizziness; tachycardia; and tingling of the extremities.
2. To prevent hypoglycemia, hang a solution of 5% to 10% glucose to infuse until bag No. 4 is ready. You should also call to make sure the pharmacy is preparing the infusion bag.
3. During this infusion, her blood glucose levels should be monitored on a regular basis. You should assess for signs of both hyperglycemia and hypoglycemia, signs of infection, and signs of fluid overload.

CHAPTER 55
Anemia Drugs

Chapter Review and NCLEX® Examination Preparation/Critical Thinking and Application

1. d
2. b
3. c

4. a, b, c
5. b, c, d
6. a
7. 26 mg (rounded up from 25.95) (See Overview of Dosage Calculations, Section III.)
8. Anyone who is about to receive his first dose of iron dextran is at risk for fatal anaphylaxis. Because of this, a test dose of 25 mg of iron dextran should be administered by the chosen route and appropriate method. An anaphylactic reaction should occur within a few moments, although waiting at least 1 hour before giving the rest of the initial dose is recommended. Intramuscular iron should be administered deep in a large muscle mass using a Z-track method and a 23-gauge 1 1/2-inch needle.
9. Eggs, corn, beans, and many cereal products containing chemicals known as phytates may impair absorption of iron from other iron-containing foods or iron supplements. However, it should also be noted that both beans and eggs are themselves common dietary sources of iron. Antacids and milk products decrease the absorption of iron.
10. The orange juice contains ascorbic acid (vitamin C), which enhances the absorption of iron.
11. Treatment should include suction and maintenance of the airway, correction of acidosis, and control of shock and dehydration with intravenous fluids or blood, oxygen, and a vasopressor. Abdominal radiographs can allow visualization of the tablet. A serum concentration of more than 300 mcg/dL will place David at serious risk for toxicity. His stomach should be emptied immediately. Because many of the iron products are extended-release formulations that liberate their contents in the intestines rather than in the stomach, whole-gut lavage is generally believed to be superior to and more effective than gastric lavage. This is followed by a saline cathartic or possible surgical removal of ingested iron tablets.
12. The risk of anaphylaxis for both drugs is much less than with iron dextran and a test dose is not required.

Case Study

1. Oral forms should be given with juice (but not antacids or milk) between meals for maximal absorption. Should gastrointestinal distress occur, however, the iron can be taken with meals.
2. She should be reminded that use of any iron product will cause the stools to turn tarry and black.
3. She should be told that one iron product cannot be substituted for another because each product contains different forms of the iron salt in different amounts.
4. Liquid oral forms of iron should be diluted per the manufacturer's instructions and taken through a plastic straw to avoid discoloration of tooth enamel.

CHAPTER 56
Dermatologic Drugs

Chapter Review and NCLEX® Examination Preparation/Critical Thinking and Application

1. a
2. b
3. a
4. b
5. a, b, d
6. d
7. a
8. 167 mL/hour (See Overview of Dosage Calculations, Section V.)
9. The nurse may first ask Mr. M. about any allergies to other forms of drugs. If he has an allergy to a particular antibacterial drug, that drug should not be used topically either. If culture and sensitivity testing is to be carried out, the nurse must be sure to collect the specimen before the first application of the antibacterial drug. In this case, the nurse can simply apply a thin film of clindamycin and monitor for signs of allergy to clindamycin.
10. Gloves are used not only to prevent contamination from secretions but also to prevent absorption of the medication through the skin of the person applying the medication.
11. Mr. L. and his children are being treated for head lice. Tell him the following: "Leave the shampoo on for 4 minutes, then rinse and dry the hair. Then use a nit comb to remove nits (eggs) from the hair shafts." Other measures he should take include decontaminating the clothing and personal articles of the infested people. All clothing, linens, stuffed toys, and so on should be washed in hot, soapy water or dry-cleaned.
12. A patient taking any anti-acne drug should avoid ultraviolet light, weather extremes, sunlight, abrasive cleansers, and other keratolytic products. Sunscreen should be worn during therapy. Tretinoin is available in many topical formulations, including creams, gels, and a liquid. Because of its potential to cause severe irritation and peeling, it may initially be applied once every 2 or 3 days, often starting with a lower-strength product. Benzoyl peroxide generally produces signs of improvement in 4 to 6 weeks, and side effects are infrequent and rarely a problem. Most are confined to the skin and involve peeling of the skin, redness, or a sensation of warmth. Benzoyl peroxide is applied sparingly one to four times daily and is available as a cleansing bar, liquid, lotion, mask, cream, gel, and cleanser.
13. The patient should be assessed for allergy to iodine. Cadexomer iodine (Iodosorb) is used to chemically débride the wound by absorbing exudates. It is not harmful to viable cells, but it does stain tissue.

14. It is possible that the patient is not a candidate for surgery at this time or is taking anticoagulants, which could cause the area to bleed excessively if surgical débridement is performed. The prescribed medication selectively removes necrotic tissue without harming normal tissue and can be used on infected wounds.

Case Study

1. Judy's allergies, especially any allergies to sulfonamide drugs, should be assessed. This cream should be applied only to areas that have been cleansed and débrided. The wound bed may need to be débrided before the cream can be applied.
2. The dressing helps keep the medication at the intended site and provides protection to the wound. In addition, it keeps the cream from soiling the clothing.
3. No! He should prevent contamination of the medication and avoid exposure to Judy's wound secretions. He should apply the cream with a sterile, gloved hand.
4. The side effects of silver sulfadiazine are similar to those of other topical drugs and include pain, burning, and itching.

CHAPTER 57
Ophthalmic Drugs

Chapter Review and NCLEX® Examination Preparation/Critical Thinking and Application

1. c
2. h
3. j
4. k
5. a
6. d
7. b
8. f
9. g
10. e
11. c
12. b
13. b
14. d
15. b, c, d, e
16. c
17. 19 gtt/min (See Overview of Dosage Calculations, Section V.)
18. The effect is less pronounced in individuals with dark eyes (brown or hazel), because pigment absorbs the drugs and dark eyes have more pigment than light eyes (blue).
19. a. Dipivefrin (Propine), a prodrug of epinephrine, has better lipophilicity than epinephrine and can penetrate into the anterior chamber of the eye. It is 4 to 11 times more potent than epinephrine in reducing intraocular pressure.
    b. Mrs. N. should report any stinging, burning, itching, lacrimation, or puffiness of the eye.
    c. No. Systemic effects are rare; they include cardiovascular effects and possibly headaches and faintness.
20. Ned may have had an allergic reaction to a preservative, such as benzalkonium chloride, in the first drug that was tried. Timolol is available in a preservative-free product.
21. a. Purulent drainage or exudate would inhibit the product's effectiveness.
    b. The solution must have been cloudy; in that case, it should be discarded—only clear solutions should be administered.
22. The nonsteroidal antiinflammatory drugs are considered less toxic, and they are preferred over the corticosteroids as initial topical therapy for injuries.
23. Stinging is normal after instillation of the drops. Ms. L. should not wear her contact lenses while taking this medication.

Case Study

1. The ointment should be applied to the conjunctival sac, not directly onto the cornea or eyeball, moving from the inner canthus to the outer edge of the eye. Excess medication can be removed with a tissue, but he should not rub his eyes. See Chapter 10 for specific instructions.
2. Ointments may cause a temporary blurriness to the vision because of the film that bathes over the eye. This film will decrease once absorbed, and vision should become clearer. He will need to be careful and prevent falling if his vision is blurry. In addition, he should not touch the tip of the medication container to his eye or to his fingers in order to prevent contamination of the medication.
3. Burning and stinging are common but transient effects of ophthalmic antimicrobial drugs, and they should subside shortly.
4. He should *not* take this medication! It is most likely contaminated, and is not ordered for his current problem. In addition, if the drops were a corticosteroid, there could be immunosuppressive effects, which may interfere with the antimicrobial's action.

CHAPTER 58
Otic Drugs

Chapter Review and NCLEX® Examination Preparation/Critical Thinking and Application

1. a, b, d, e
2. d

3. b
4. a
5. c
6. a. 375 mg
   b. Low range (20 mg/kg): 220 mg; high range (40 mg/kg): 440 mg
   c. Yes, 375 mg is in the range of 220 and 440 mg. (See Overview of Dosage Calculations, Section III.)
7. The patient needs medical care immediately. His symptoms may be indicative of head trauma.
8. To take advantage of the steroidal antiinflammatory, antipruritic, and antiallergic drug effects.
9. a. Clean the ear, remove all cerumen by irrigation, and ensure that the dropper is clean. The drops also need to be at room temperature.
   b. He might become dizzy, so he should be supine when the drops are instilled.
10. a. The hydrocortisone will help reduce the inflammation and itching associated with the infection.
    b. A drug hypersensitivity or a perforated eardrum
11. Many ear disorders involve pain and inflammation; the anesthetic effect of the local anesthetic drugs makes them beneficial in treating these conditions.
12. a. The instructions are different for each boy. The pinna should be held up and back during instillation of eardrops in children older than 3 years of age, like Drew. For children 3 years of age or younger, like Ben, the pinna should be gently pulled down and back.
    b. Reduced pain, redness, and swelling are therapeutic effects of the medication.
13. a. Esther's husband should warm the eardrops to body temperature by holding the bottle under warm running water, not by soaking it in hot water—especially because he should be careful not to let water get into the bottle or damage the label.
    b. Esther should not sit up right away. She should lie down on the side opposite the side of the affected ear for about 5 minutes after the drug is instilled. As an alternative, she can gently insert a small cotton ball into the ear canal to keep the drug in place, but the cotton ball should not be forced into the ear canal.

Case Study

1. Mark probably has an impaction of earwax in his ear canal. Such a buildup can cause pain and temporary deafness.
2. He should be taught that he should not insert anything into his ear canal. He will need to know how to clean his ears properly and how to use cerumen removal drugs. You may need to irrigate his ear canals before medication therapy is started.
3. This medication is given as otic (ear) drops. He will need to follow the manufacturer's recommendations for administration. He should lie on the side opposite of the affected ear for about 5 minutes after instillation of the drug. A small cotton ball may be inserted gently into the ear canal to keep the drug there, but it should not be forced or jammed down into the ear canal. When administering the drops, he should pull the pinna of his ear up and back.
4. The carbamide peroxide will slowly release hydrogen peroxide and oxygen, and this effervescent effect will mechanically act to loosen the cerumen. In addition, the glycerin will soften the cerumen, making it easier to remove.

OVERVIEW OF DOSAGE CALCULATIONS

Introduction

Interpreting Medication Labels

1.	Generic name:	simvastatin
	Trade name:	Zocor
	Unit dose:	40-mg tablets
	Total in container:	60 tablets
	Route:	oral (It is assumed that tablets are oral route.)
2.	Generic name:	amoxicillin
	Trade name:	Amoxil
	Unit dose:	200 mg per 5 mL
	Total in container:	50 mL (when reconstituted)
	Route:	oral
3.	Generic name:	medroxyprogesterone acetate suspension
	Trade name:	Depo-Provera
	Unit dose:	400 mg per mL
	Total in container:	10 mL
	Route:	intramuscular use only
4.	Generic name:	hydrocortisone sodium succinate
	Trade name:	Solu-Cortef
	Unit dose:	250 mg
	Total in container:	250 mg per 2 mL (when mixed)
	Route:	intravenous or intramuscular

Section I

Basic Conversions Using Ratio and Proportion

1. 600,000 mcg
2. 1,500,000 mcg
3. 5 mg

4. 5000 mg
5. 2500 mg
6. 0.9 g *(Don't forget the leading zero.)*
7. 8000 g
8. 0.75 L *(Don't forget the leading zero.)*
9. 975,000 mL
10. 0.5 L *(Don't forget the leading zero.)*
11. 960 mg
12. 1.5 gr
13. 20 mL
14. 12 tsp
15. 6 tbsp
16. 90 mL
17. 0.2 oz *(Don't forget the leading zero.)*
18. 198 lb
19. 68.2 kg *(rounded to tenths)*
20. 24.2 lb

Section II

Calculating Oral Doses

1. 1 tablet
   0.5 g = 500 mg; each tablet is 500 mg; therefore 1 tablet is needed
2. 2 tablets
   0.5 mg = 500 mcg;
   250 mcg : 1 tablet :: 500 mcg : *x* tablet
   Proof: 250 × 2 = 500; 1 × 500 = 500
3. 0.5 tablet
   0.25 g = 250 mg;
   500 mg : 1 tablet :: 250 mg : *x* tablet
   Proof: 500 × 0.5 = 250; 1 × 250 = 250
4. 20 mL
   12.5 mg : 5 mL :: 50 mg : *x* mL
   Proof: 12.5 × 20 = 250; 5 × 50 = 250
5. 2 tablets
   600 mg = gr x; gr v : 1 tablet :: gr x : *x* tablet
   Proof: gr v × 2 = gr x; 1 × gr x = gr x
   NOTE: With this problem, since most are more familiar with metric doses, you may convert the dose on hand, gr v, to 300 mg. Then set up your problem:
   300 mg : 1 tab :: 600 mg : *x*
6. 4 mL
   0.1 g = 100 mg; 125 mg : 5 mL :: 100 mg : *x* mL
   Proof: 125 × 4 = 500; 5 × 100 = 500
7. 3 tablets
   0.3 g = 300 mg;
   100 mg : 1 tablet :: 300 mg : *x*
   Proof: 100 × 3 = 300; 1 × 300 = 300
8. 22.5 mL
   20 mEq : 15 mL :: 30 mEq : *x*
   Proof: 20 × 22.5 = 450; 15 × 30 = 450
9. 3 capsules
   0.15 g = 150 mg;
   50 mg : 1 capsule :: 150 mg : *x*
   Proof: 50 × 3 = 150; 1 × 150 = 150
10. 4 tablets
   2 g = 2000 mg;
   500 mg : 1 tablet :: 2000 mg : *x*
   Proof: 500 × 4 = 2000; 1 × 2000 = 2000

Section III

Reconstituting Medications

1. 2 mL
   100 mg : 1 mL :: 200 mg : *x*
   Proof: 100 × 2 = 200; 1 × 200 = 200
2. 1.5 mL
   40 mg : 1 mL :: 60 mg : *x*
   Proof: 40 × 1.5 = 60; 1 × 60 = 60
3. 0.8 mL
   10,000 units : 1 mL :: 8000 units : *x*
   Proof: 10,000 × 0.8 = 8000; 1 × 8000 = 8000
4. 1.5 mL
   500 mg : 1 mL :: 750 mg : *x*
   Proof: 500 × 1.5 = 750; 1 × 750 = 750
5. 20 mL
   125 mg : 5 mL :: 500 mg : *x*
   Proof: 125 × 20 = 2500; 5 × 500 = 2500
6. Choose the concentration using 4.6-mL diluent. Using the 9.6-mL diluent would necessitate giving 3 mL intramuscularly versus 1.5 mL using the 4.6-mL diluent.
   1.5 mL
   200,000 units : 1 mL :: 300,000 units : *x* mL
   Proof: 200,000 × 1.5 = 300,000; 1 × 300,000 = 300,000
7. 0.75 mL
   First: Convert mcg to mg : 750 mcg = 0.75 mg
   1:1000 indicates 1 g in 1000 mL, or 1000 mg in 1000 mL, or 1 mg/mL.
   1 mg : 1 mL :: 0.75 mg : *x*
   Proof: 1 × 0.75 = 0.75; 1 × 0.75 = 0.75
8. 1 mL
   NOTE: 1:5000 indicates 1 g in 5000 mL, or 1000 mg in 5000 mL, or 0.2 mg/mL.
   0.2 mg : 1 mL :: 0.2 mg : *x*
   Proof: 0.2 × 1 = 0.2; 1 × 0.2 = 0.2
9. 9 mL
   NOTE: 10% indicates 10 g per 100 mL, or 0.1 g/mL.
   Need to ensure units that are alike: 900 mg = 0.9 g
   0.1 g : 1 mL :: 0.9 g : *x*
   Proof: 0.1 × 9 = 0.9; 1 × 0.9 = 0.9
10. 8 mL
   NOTE: 50% indicates 50 g per 100 mL, or 0.5 g/mL.
   0.5 g = 1 mL :: 4 g : *x*
   Proof: 0.5 × 8 = 4; 1 × 4 = 4

Section IV

Pediatric Calculations

1. a. 0.46 to 47.3 mg/hr
   40 lb = 18.2 kg
   Low dose: 0.025 mg/kg/hr × 18.2 kg = 0.455, rounded to 0.46 mg/hr
   High dose: 2.6 mg/kg/hr × 18.2 kg = 47.32, rounded to 47.3 mg/hr
   b. Yes, the ordered dose of 1 mg/hr falls within the safe range for this child.
2. a. 75 to 150 mg/dose
   33 lb = 15 kg
   Low dose: 5 mg/kg/dose × 15 kg = 75 mg/dose
   High dose: 10 mg/kg/dose × 15 kg = 150 mg/dose
   b. 600 mg (40 mg × 15 kg = 600 mg/kg/24 hr)
   c. Yes, the ordered dose of 120 mg falls within the safe and therapeutic range for this child.
3. a. 3180 to 4770 mg/24 hr
   70 lb = 31.8 kg
   Low dose: 100 mg/kg/24 hr × 31.8 kg = 3180 mg/24 hr
   High dose: 150 mg/kg/24 hr × 31.8 kg = 4770 mg/24 hr
   b. 1060 to 1590 mg/dose
   Three doses in 24 hours; 3180 ÷ 3 = 1060 mg/dose; 4770 ÷ 3 = 1590 mg/dose
   c. No. 1.7 g = 1700 mg, which exceeds the safe dosage range for this drug for this child. (Did you remember to convert g to mg?)
4. a. 0.14 to 0.34 mg/day
   15 lb = 6.8 kg
   Low dose: 0.02 mg/kg/day × 6.8 kg = 0.136 rounded to 0.14 mg/day
   High dose: 0.05 mg/kg/day × 6.8 kg = 0.34 mg/day
   b. 0.07 to 0.17 mg/dose
   "bid" doses are given twice in 24 hours. 0.14 ÷ 2 = 0.07 mg/dose; 0.36 ÷ 2 = 0.17 mg/dose
   c. Yes, 150 mcg = 0.15 mg, which falls within the safe and therapeutic dosage range for this child. (Did you remember to convert mcg to mg?)
5. a. 15.5 to 34.1 mg/kg/dose
   34 lb = 15.5 kg
   Low dose: 1 mg/kg/dose × 15.5 kg = 15.5 mg/dose
   High dose: 2.2 mg/kg/dose × 15.5 kg = 34.1 mg/dose
   b. Yes, the ordered dose of 30 mg is within the safe and therapeutic dose range for this child.
6. a. 90.8 to 113.5 mcg/kg/day
   50 lb = 22.7 kg
   Low dose: 4 mcg/kg/day × 22.7 kg = 90.8 mcg/day
   High dose: 5 mcg/kg/day × 22.7 kg = 113.5 mcg/day
   b. No. The ordered dose, 0.2 mg = 200 mcg, which exceeds the safe and therapeutic dosage range for this child. (Did you remember to convert mcg to mg?)

Section V

Basic Intravenous Calculations

1. Start at STEP 1. You need to calculate the hourly rate.
   a. 167 mL/hr
   1000 mL :: 6 hr :: x : 1 hr
   (1000 × 1) = (6 × x); 1000 = 6x;
   x = 1000/6 = 166.66 (Round to nearest whole number.)
   Proof: 1000 × 1 = 1000; 6 × 167 = 1002 (slight difference due to previous rounding)
   (Alternate method: 1000 mL ÷ 6 hr = 166.67 or 167 mL/hr)
   b. 42 gtt/min (Round to nearest whole number.)
   STEP 2:
   $\frac{\text{drop factor}}{\text{time (min)}}$ × hourly rate = 15/60 × 167 = 1/4 × 200 = 41.75 (rounded to nearest whole number)
2. Start at STEP 1. You need to calculate the hourly rate.
   a. 200 mL/hr
   600 mL : 3 hr :: x : 1 hr
   (600 × 1) = (3 × x); 600 = 3x;
   x = 600/3 = 200
   Proof: 600 × 1 = 600; 3 × 200 = 600
   (Alternate method: 600 mL ÷ 3 hr = 200 mL/hr)
   b. 33 gtt/min (Round to nearest whole number.)
   STEP 2:
   $\frac{\text{drop factor}}{\text{time (min)}}$ × hourly rate = 10/60 × 200 = 1/6 × 200 = 33.33 (rounded to nearest whole number)
3. Start at STEP 1. You need to calculate the hourly rate.
   a. 83 mL/hr
   1000 mL : 12 hr :: x : 1 hr
   (1000 × 1) = (12 × x); 1000 = 12x; x = 1000/12 = 83.33 (Round to nearest whole number.)
   Proof: 1000 × 1 = 1000; 12 × 83 = 996 (slight difference due to previous rounding)
   (Alternate method: 1000 mL ÷ 12 hr = 83.33 or 83 mL/hr)
   b. 21 gtt/min (Round to nearest whole number.)

STEP 2:

$\frac{\text{drop factor}}{\text{time (min)}}$ × hourly rate = 15/60 × 83 = 1/4 × 83 = 20.75 (rounded to nearest whole number)

4. Start at STEP 1. You need to calculate the hourly rate.
   a. 100 mL/hr
      200 mL : 2 hr :: x : 1 hr
      (200 × 1) = (2 × x); 200 = 2x;
      x = 200/2 = 100
      Proof: 200 × 1 = 200; 2 × 100 = 200
      (Alternate method: 200 mL ÷ 2 hr = 100 mL/hr)
   b. 100 gtt/min
      STEP 2:
      $\frac{\text{drop factor}}{\text{time (min)}}$ × hourly rate = 60/60 × 100 = 1 × 100 = 100
   c. The drop factor for microdrip tubing is 60 gtt/mL.
5. Start at STEP 2. The hourly rate has been provided (75 mL/hr).
   13 gtt/min (Round to nearest whole number.)
   STEP 2:
   $\frac{\text{drop factor}}{\text{time (min)}}$ × hourly rate = 10/60 × 75 = 1/4 × 75 = 12.75 (rounded to nearest whole number)
6. Start at STEP 2. The hourly rate has been provided (75 mL/hr).
   19 gtt/min (Round to nearest whole number.)
   STEP 2:
   $\frac{\text{drop factor}}{\text{time (min)}}$ × hourly rate = 15/60 × 75 = 1/4 × 75 = 18.75 (rounded to nearest whole number)
7. Start at STEP 2. The hourly rate has been provided (75 mL/hr).
   25 gtt/min
   STEP 2:
   $\frac{\text{drop factor}}{\text{time (min)}}$ × hourly rate = 20/60 × 75 = 1/3 × 75 = 25 (rounded to nearest whole number)
8. As the drop factor increases, the gtt/min also increases.
9. a. 100 mL/hr
   b. and c. Since the infusion pump delivers in mL/hr, it is unnecessary to calculate gtt/min.
      Start at STEP 1. You need to calculate the hourly rate. Remember, 30 min = 0.5 hr.
      50 mL : 0.5 hr :: x mL : 1 hr
      (50 × 1) = (0.5 × x); 50 = 0.5x;
      x = 50/0.5 = 100
      Proof: 50 × 1 = 50; 0.5 × 100 = 50
      (Alternate method: 50 mL ÷ 0.5 hr = 100 mL/hr)
10. Start at STEP 1. You need to calculate the hourly rate.
   a. 125 mL/hr
      500 mL : 4 hr :: x : 1 hr
      (500 × 1) = (4 × x); 500 = 4x;
      x = 500/4 = 125
      Proof: 500 × 1 = 500; 4 × 125 = 500
      (Alternate method: 500 mL ÷ 4 hr = 125 mL/hr)
   b. 125 gtt/min
      STEP 2:
      $\frac{\text{drop factor}}{\text{time (min)}}$ × hourly rate = 60/60 × 125 = 1 × 125 = 125 (rounded to nearest whole number)

Practice Quiz

1. 0.75 mg
   1000 mcg : 1 mg :: 750 mcg : x mg
   Proof: 1000 × 0.75 = 750; 1 × 750 = 750
2. 8000 mg
   1 g : 1000 mg :: 8 g : x mg
   Proof: 1 × 8000 = 8000; 1000 × 8 = 8000
3. 113.6 kg
   1 kg : 2.2 lb :: x kg : 250 lb
   Proof: 1 × 250 = 250; 2.2 × 113.6 = 249.92 (rounds to 250)
4. 165 lb
   1 kg : 2.2 lb :: 75 kg : x lb
   Proof: 1 × 165 = 165; 2.2 × 75 = 165
5. 15 mL
   1 tsp : 5 mL :: 3 tsp : x mL
   Proof: 1 × 15 = 15; 5 × 3 = 15
6. 600 mg
   gr i (1) : 60 mg :: gr x (10) : x mg
   Proof: 1 (gr i) × 600 = 600; 60 × 10 (gr x) = 600
7. 10 mL
   25 mg : 5 mL :: 50 mg : x mL
   Proof: 25 × 10 = 250; 5 × 50 = 250
8. 1 tablet
   STEP 1: Convert g to mg : 0.5 g = 500 mg
   500 mg : 1 tablet :: 500 mg : x tablet
   Proof: 500 × 1 = 500; 1 × 500 = 500
9. 2 mL
   50 mg : 1 mL :: 100 mg : x mL
   Proof: 50 × 2 = 100; 1 × 100 = 100
10. 5 mL
   1% indicates 1 g in 100 mL, which equals 1000 mg/100 mL, or 10 mg/1 mL.
   10 mg : 1 mL :: 50 mg : x mL
   Proof: 10 × 5 = 50; 1 × 50 = 50
11. 0.25 mL
   1:1000 indicates 1 g in 1000 mL, which equals 1000 mg/1000 mL, or 1 mg/mL.
   1 mg : 1 mL :: 0.25 mg : x mL
   Proof: 1 × 0.25 = 0.25; 1 × 0.25 = 0.25

12. 1.5 mL
    10,000 units: 1 mL :: 15,000 units: x mL
    Proof: 10,000 × 1.5 = 15,000; 1 × 15,000 = 15,000
13. a. 0.2 to 0.8 mg/dose
    b. No, the dose of 1 mg exceeds the safe and therapeutic dosage range for this child.
       22 lb = 10 kg
       Low range: 0.02 mg/kg/dose × 10 kg = 0.2 mg/dose
       High range: 0.08 mg/kg/dose × 10 kg = 0.8 mg/dose
14. a. 63 mL/hr
       500 mL ÷ 8 hr = 62.5 (rounded to 63 mL/hr)
    b. 16 gtt/min
       $\frac{\text{drop factor}}{\text{time (min)}}$ × hourly rate = 15/60 × 63 = 1/4 × 63 = 15.75 (rounded to nearest whole number)
15. a. Infusion pumps deliver mL/hr.
    b. 50 mL/hr (as stated in the question)
16. a. 42 mL/hr
       1000 mL ÷ 24 hr = 41.67 (rounded to 42 mL/hr)
    b. 42 gtt/min (Remember that if the drop factor is 60, the rate is the same as the gtt/min.)
       $\frac{\text{drop factor}}{\text{time (min)}}$ × hourly rate = 60/60 × 42 = 1 × 42 gtt/min
17. a. 1 g
    b. 2.5 mL
       200 mg : 1 mL :: 500 mg : x mL
       Proof: 200 × 2.5 = 500; 1 × 500 = 500
18. a. 200,000 units/mL
    b. 23 mL
    c. 1 mL (concentration is 200,000 units per 1 mL)
    d. Label the multidose vial with the date, time, amount of diluent used, and user's initials.
19. a. 6 mL
       100 mg : 1 mL :: 600 mg : x mL
       Proof: 100 × 6 = 600; 1 × 600 = 600
    b. Up to 1410 mg/24 hr
       31 lb = 14.1 kg; 14.1 kg × 100 mg/kg/day = 1410 mg/24 hr (safe dose)
    c. 705 mg/dose
       There are two doses per day; 1410 mg ÷ 2 = 705 mg/dose
    d. Yes
       The ordered dose of 600 mg does not exceed the 705 maximum dose.
20. 2.5 mL
    125 mcg = 0.125 mg
    0.05 mg : 1 mL :: 0.125 mg : x mg
    Proof: 0.05 × 2.5 = 0.125 × 0.125 = 0.125